The Horse Dictionary

The Horse Dictionary

*English-Language Terms Used
in Equine Care, Feeding, Training,
Treatment, Racing and Show*

by
VIVIENNE M. EBY

McFarland & Company, Inc., Publishers
Jefferson, North Carolina, and London

The present work is a reprint of the library bound edition of The Horse Dictionary: English-Language Terms Used in Equine Care, Feeding, Training, Treatment, Racing and Show, *first published in 1995.*

Illustrations not drawn by the author are reprinted with the kind permission of the following companies from their catalogs: Chick's, Jeffers, Kennel Vaccine Vet Supply Co., and Omaha Vaccine Co., Inc.

Library of Congress Cataloguing-in-Publication Data

Eby, Vivienne M.
    The horse dictionary : English-language terms used in equine care, feeding, training, treatment, racing and show / by Vivienne M. Eby.
       p.   cm.

    ISBN-13: 978-0-7864-1145-0
    (softcover : 50# alkaline paper) ∞

    1. Horses—Dictionaries.   2. Horsemanship—Dictionaries.
I. Title.
SF278.E28   2001
636.1'003—dc20   95-10730

British Library cataloguing data are available

Manufactured in the United States of America

McFarland & Company, Inc., Publishers
  Box 611, Jefferson, North Carolina 28640
    www.mcfarlandpub.com

To my parents, who introduced me
to my first horse at the age of three
and taught me how to ride from the
excellence of their own experience

PREFACE

The horse has been a part of human life for some 10,000 years, from the time when horses in the Americas were hunted as a source of food and hides. Once efforts at domestication proved successful, horses became an essential part of a great range of activities: among other services, they carried soldiers into battle, provided a means of rapid transportation, made advances in agriculture and industry possible, and contributed to sports and leisure activities. It is difficult to imagine how differently human history might have developed had not these versatile animals been present.

For centuries the horse has been among the most frequent subjects of paintings and books, and it is hardly surprising that there now exists within the English language an enormous vocabulary of exclusively equine words, as well as a great number of words in general usage that possess specifically equine meanings. Despite the abundance of horse books in print, this body of horse-related language has not heretofore been comprehensively collected and defined. It was with the intention of filling this void that this dictionary was written. It serves as a quick, concise, up-to-date reference to words that relate to any aspect of the horse or equestrian culture — physiological and medical terms, words associated with sports and recreational activities, words relating to feed and tack, the various breeds and prehistoric ancestors of the horse, and many others.

The definitions, including those of technical terms, are constructed so as to be easily understood by the nonspecialist reader, and are often accompanied by illustrations for clarity. Cross-references are provided when the defined word is closely related to one or more other terms. As in a traditional dictionary, parts of speech are identified (except for multiple-word phrases) and all forms of a term are listed. As a practical matter, however, certain other features common to general dictionaries had to be omitted, principally syllabification, phonetic spellings, and etymologies. Nonetheless, in occasional instances when the pronunciation of a word differs dramatically from what one might expect, a phonetic spelling is provided. If a word has two or more accepted spellings, it is found under the most common form with alternate spellings immediately following the first.

Although many words describing diseases, injuries and the like are defined in terms of their symptoms and causes, curative instructions have been deliberately omitted. This information is best left to veterinary books and to veterinarians themselves.

More than seven years of research went into the compilation of this dictionary. From equine books purchased or borrowed, supply catalogs, encyclopedias and countless horse magazines I have extracted the approximately 6,600 terms that appear here. To ensure accuracy I cross-checked information in multiple sources. It is my hope that the resulting volume will be of use to anyone seeking a compact yet comprehensive guide to equine vocabulary.

THE DICTIONARY

− A −

abasia *n*. lack of muscular coordination in walking

abdomen *n*. the part of the body between the chest and pelvis — **abdominal** *adj*.

abdominal cavity the part of the body containing all of the abdominal organs

abdominocentesis *n*. the suction of fluid through a needle from the abdominal cavity

abduct *vt*. in relation to muscles, to pull (a part of the body) away from the midline (opposite of adduct) — **abductive** *adj*. — **abductor** *n*.

aberrant *adj*. deviating from the normal — **aberration** *n*.

abirritant *n*. a medicinal agent that relieves irritation

ablactation *n*. the end of a period when breast milk is produced — *see also* **weaning**

ablation *n*. the surgical removal of a body part, such as a limb; a horse is usually destroyed when an injured leg cannot be saved, but modern surgical methods have made it possible to amputate a leg and fit the horse with a prosthesis — **ablate** *vt*.

ablatio placentae premature separation of the placenta from the uterine wall

abocclusion *n*. *see* **malocclusion**

abort *vi*. to give birth prematurely to a dead fetus — *vt*. to remove (a dead fetus) as a veterinary procedure — **abortion** *n*.

abortifacient *n*. a drug that causes abortion — *adj*. causing abortion

above the bit a position in which a horse's head is raised with the muzzle pushed outward, evading bit pressure

abrade *vt., vi*. to rub off, as the skin — **abrasion** *n*. a scrape or rubbed break in the skin or cornea of the eye

abscess *n*. a pus-filled area in body tissue — *vi*. to form an abscess — **abscessed** *adj*.

abscission *n*. the surgical removal of a body part — **abscise** *vi., vt*.

absolute dry matter in analyzing feed, the result of subtracting the percentage of water from 100 percent

acalcerosis *n*. an unsound condition of the body caused by lack of calcium

acampsia *n*. inability to bend or extend a joint

acanthocyte *n*. a deformed red blood cell

acanthocytosis *n*. a condition in which the blood contains an abnormal number of acanthocytes

acariasis *n*. a skin disease caused by mites called acarids; causes constant

1

itching of the skin, mane and or tail
—*see also* **mange**

acataposis *n.* difficulty in swallowing
brought on by a pathology or choking

accelerometer *n.* a device that measures a hoof's potential for absorbing
shock

accessory carpal bone the bone that
forms the sharp ridge at the back of
the knee

acclimate, acclimatize *vi.* to become
accustomed to a different environment
or climate — *vt.* **acclimation, acclimatization** *n.*

account for in hunting, to kill (a fox)

accumulator *n.* in racing, a collective
bet on two or more horses to win

accumulator competition in jumping, competition over a course comprising 6–10 jumps successively increasing in difficulty

acellular *adj.* not made up of cells;
e.g., hair

acephalia *n.* a rare condition of the
fetus in which the skull does not
develop normally, usually resulting in
the fetus being aborted or born dead

Acepromazine *n.* trade name for acetylpromazine, a tranquilizer

acetabulum *n.* the hip socket into
which the head of the femur fits

acetylcholine *n.* a chemical released
by nerves which activates the muscles

acetone *n.* a chemical substance found
in rare cases in the body — **acetonemia**
n. the condition in which acetone is
present in the body.

acetylpromazine *n.* generic name for
a tranquilizer

acetylsalicylic acid aspirin

acey deucey in racing, a term which
refers to a jockey's stirrups when they
are unequal in length

achievement signals chemical reactions between the horse and parasites
which allow the parasites to grow and
live within their host

Achilles tendon the tendon which
joins muscles of the gaskin to the point
of hock

achromatism *n.* lack of color;
achromia —**achromatize** *vt.* to cause
lack of color —**achromatous, achromic**
adj. —*see also* **leucoderma**

achromia *see* **achromatism**

Achromycin *n.* trade name for tetracycline

acid *n.* 1. something that is sour to the
taste 2. a chemical that can react with
a base to form a salt

acidemia *n.* the lowering of blook pH
to an abnormally low, or acidic, level

acid firing a method of firing in which
sulfuric acid is applied on a shaved
area to be treated, as for sprained tendons, etc. —*see also* **cauterize; firing**

acidosis *n.* a condition of the body in
which acid content is unbalanced due
to faulty metabolism and elimination
of acid chemicals

acne *n.* a pus formation of pimples or
boils that form at the seat of inflamed
hair follicles; chiefly caused by friction
with harness or other tack but also by
injury from a clipping machine or flies
—*see also* **contagious acne**

aconite, aconitum *n.* a drug formerly
used as a respiratory sedative and administered unprofessionally with drastic and fatal results

acorn *n.* the fruit of the oak tree that
contains tannic acid and small quantitites of volatile oil; horses love to eat
acorns but they can cause colic, particularly when green

acridine *n.* a compound derived from
coal tar and used in medicinal preparations

acriflavin *n.* a brownish powder derived from acridine and used as an antiseptic

acromastitis *n.* inflammation of either
of the mare's nipples

acrylic resin a thermoplastic used to fill hoof cracks

ACTH adrenocorticotropic hormone, a hormone secreted by the pituitary gland to stimulate corticosteroid secretion and growth of the adrenal glands

actin *n.* a protein in muscles — *see also* **actomyosin**

acting master a stand-in for a permanent master who makes arrangements for a hunt

Actinobacillus equuli a type of bacteria that causes foal abortion or death shortly after birth and occasionally attacks adult horses — *see also* *Bacterium viscosum equi*

actinomycosis *n.* a rare pus-filled swelling that may affect the tongue, the spermatic cord following castration, or the submaxillary lymphatic glands, the latter being the most common site; wooden tongue

action *n.* the amount of flexion of the knees and hocks; a style of moving; a horse is said to have high action when it lifts its legs high — *see also* **daisy cutting**

active hyperemia a condition brought on by a sudden oversupply of blood to the brain caused by any of a number of stimulants such as overexertion, excitement, embolism, etc.; the horse becomes over-excited, plunging about and perhaps out of control; the eyes stare with dilated pupils, pulse increases and head feels hot

actomyosin *n.* a combination of two proteins (actin and myosin) in muscles which, with ATP, are responsible for muscular contractions

acupressure *n.* the application of pressure to a precise point on the body for the purpose of reducing pain

acute *adj.* in relation to disease, severe but rapid, not chronic — **acuteness** *n.* — **acutely** *adv.*

Adayer *n.* one of two subdivisions of the Kazakh breed

added money in rodeos and racing, the money given by the rodeo or racing committee and added to the entry fees paid by the contestants or racehorse owners, the total of which makes up the stakes

Addison's disease a degenerative disease caused by deficiency or failure of the adrenal glands

additive *n.* something added to a substance, as a vitamin to grain

adduct *vt.* to move (a part of the body, such as a leg) toward the midline, as by a muscle; to draw inward — **adduction** *n.* — **adductive** *adj.* — **adductor** *n.*

adductor muscles a group of thigh muscles that adduct the thigh

adenitis *n.* inflmmation of a gland

adenocarcinoma *n.* a cancerous tumor that originates in a gland

adenoma *n.* a benign tumor that arises from glandular tissue — **adomatous** *adj.*

adenosarcoma *n.* a sarcoma, or malignant tumor, with glandular elements

adenosine deaminase an enzyme that activates energy transfer

adenosine triphosphate *see* ATP

adenovirus *n.* any of a group of viruses that cause respiratory and gastrointestinal diseases; can be dormant in the body

adequan *n.* a polysulfated glycosamenoglycan (PSGAG) drug, synthesized from the traceal cartilages of cattle, and used for treatment of arthritis by intraarticular (into joint) or intramuscular (into muscle) injection; its effect is to protect cartilage by enhancing many of the natural biochemical processes of the joint

adhesion *n.* the abnormal sticking together, by fibrous tissue, of body structures that are normally separate;

usually results from inflammation —
adhesive *adj.*

adipose *n.* fat in connective body tissues —*adj.*

adiposity *n.* the condition of being fat

adjuvant *n.* something that helps, as an agent added to a drug to help its action

adrenal *adj.* relating to the adrenal glands —*n.* an adrenal gland

adrenal cortex the outer layer of the adrenal gland

adrenal gland either of two small, flat organs, located in front of the kidneys, which produce hormones

adrenaline *n.* a hormone secreted by the adrenal gland; acts chiefly as a stimulant; synthetic adrenaline is produced and used to increase heart rate; can also be locally applied to stop hemorrhage; epinephrine

adrenal medulla the inner part of the adrenal gland that stores and releases hormones

adrenergic *adj.* 1. of sympathetic nerve fibers that release epinephrine or a similar substance   2. chemically similar to epinephrine, as an adrenergic drug

adrenocortical *adj.* pertaining to the cortex of the adrenal glands

adrenocorticotrophic, -tropic *adj.* able to stimulate the cortex of the adrenal glands

adrenocorticotrophic (*or* -tropic) hormone *see* ACTH

adrenocorticotrophin *n. see* **corticotrophin**

adult *n.* a horse fully grown; i.e., over five years old —*adj.*

adynamia *n.* pathological weakness and debilitation —**adynamic** *adj.*

adynamic fever a low fever that causes debilitation and depression; asthenic fever

aedes *n.* a genus of mosquitoes that can transmit equine encephalomyelitis

A-Equi-1, A-Equi-2 two strains of the equine influenza virus

aerobe *n.* a microorganism that is dependent on oxygen to live and grow

aerobic *adj.* 1. dependent on oxygen to live and grow   2. pertaining to exercise that lies within the horse's current capacity to supply oxygen to the cells

aerobic exercise exercise which is performed within the limits of the body's ability to supply adequate amounts of oxygen to the cells; this is maintained during exercise at relatively slow, steady rates, which develops endurance

aerobic glycolysis a steady energy system that depends on a continuous supply of oxygen to the cells for burning of carbohydrates and triglycerides

aerobics *n.* a method of physical training using gradually increasing exercise to condition the body to use more oxygen

aerophagia *n. see* **wind-sucking**

afebrile *adj.* without fever

affection *n.* 1. a fondness for or attachment to another horse (*see* **bond**) or to a person. A horse that has no equine pasture mates is usually likely to demonstrate more affection for its human caretaker than one kept with other horses. —**affectionate** *adj.*   2. an ailment or disease

afferent nerve the nerve which conducts impulses from the body's surface inward to the brain and spinal cord

aflatoxin *n.* a type of toxin produced by the fungus fusarium, which grows on grain, especially corn, and poisons horses who ingest the affected feed; the first signs of poisoning are depression, general lethargy and aimless walking about; by the time these signs are detected or become apparent, the horse stands only a 50-50 chance of survival; then cirrhosis of the liver develops, with the appearance of constipation, abnormal sweating, abdominal discomfort, dark urine and jaundiced gums and nostrils; finally, in the last stage, leucoencephalomalacia sets in with resultant blind staggering, pressing of the head against a solid surface, convulsions, coma and death

African horse-sickness a fatal disease transmitted by insects and having symptoms of pneumonia and enteritis, fever, labored breathing, patchy sweating and dry cough

afterbirth *n. see* **placenta**

Against the Clock in show-jumping, describes a timed competition in which the competitor with the least number of faults in the fastest time wins

agalactia *n.* a failure of lactation — **agalactic** *adj.*

agalorrhea *n.* the stoppage of lactation or milk flow

agar *n.* a gelatin-like substance made from seaweed and used as a medium for bacterial cultures

agar gel immuno-diffusion test a test to detect specific antibodies in the blood using agar gel as a medium; Coggins test

aged *adj.* past the age of 9 as of January 1 of a given year; fully mature, as opposed to old (often loosely used, however, to describe an old horse)

agent *n.* a substance that causes a physical or chemical reaction

agglutinate *vi., vt.* to clump together by agglutination — *adj.* clumped together

agglutination *n.* the clumping together of separate or suspended particles, such as blood cells, microorganisms, etc. — **agglutinative** *adj.*

agglutination titer the highest dilution of a serum that causes agglutination

agglutinin *n.* a substance or antibody that causes agglutination

agglutinogen *n.* any antigen that stimulates the production of agglutinins — **agglutinogenic** *adj.*

agonist *n.* a muscle whose action is counteracted by the opposite action of another muscle, the antagonist

AHR Arabian Horse Registry

AHSA American Horse Show Association

AI artificial insemination

aid *n.* the signals given by a rider to the horse through the use of his legs, hands (reins), weight (seat), and voice; artificial aids include a crop, spurs, martinagale, etc.

air *n.* the horse's correct posture and rhythm of movement when in action; **artificial airs** are those which, as opposed to natural gaits, are learned from special training by the rider

air above the ground any of several haute école performances with the forelegs or with the fore and hind legs off the ground; they include the **levade, courbette, capriole, ballotade,** and **croupade**

air cast a bag which is wrapped around an injured limb and inflated to reduce movement, stop bleeding, and protect against further injury

airer *n.* a saddle stand which may be made of wood or metal; some, made of fiberglass, have heating elements for quickly drying the panel; also called saddle airer

akaryocyte *n.* a red blood cell

Akhal-Teke *n.* a Russian breed noted for great endurance and adaptability to desert conditions; 14.2–15.2 h.h.

a la brida a style of horsemanship wherein the rider sits straight-legged, feet somewhat forward in a saddle having a high pommel and cantle; a severe curb bit is used, having a high port and shanks as long as 15 inches

aladdin's slipper effect the turned-up shape of a foundered toe

a la gineta a Moorish style of horsemanship using a ring bit called la gineta

alanine *n.* an amino acid found in many proteins

alar cartilage a band of firm-edged but flexible cartilage that surrounds the opening of the nostril

alazan *adj.* (Spanish) a chestnut color with red or dark flaxen points

Albino *n.* a horse having totally white hair and pink skin due to genetically caused lack of pigment; a true albino has pink iris of the eye but some have blue eyes; **albinism** may occur in any breed but the Albino is deliberately bred in the U.S.A. as what the breeders consider a distinct breed, starting with the foundation sire called Old King (1906), allegedly of Arab-Morgan stock; Albinos may have a predisposition to such weaknesses as poor vision and poor resistance to skin infections — **albinic** *adj.*

albumin *n.* a protein contained in most animal and vegetable tissues

albuminuria *n.* the presence of albumin in urine, characterized by inflamed kidneys or infection of the urinary tract

aldosterone *n.* a steroid secreted by the adrenal cortex

alert *adj.* watchful and ready to act — **alertness** *n.* — **alertly** *adv.*

alfalfa *n.* a legume used as fodder; an excellent source of vitamins; **lucerne**

algae *n.pl.* various small plants that grow in ponds or in water containers that are not kept scrubbed out

aliment *n.* food — *vt.* to nourish

alimentary colic *see* **colic**

alimentary tract the food canal beginning at the mouth and extending to the anus; gastrointestinal tract

alkali 1. any soluble hydroxide base that gives a high concentration of hydroxyl ions in solution 2. a soluble mineral salt found in soils

alkali disease a disease caused by an excessive amount of selenium in the diet, which results in hair loss in the mane and tail and deterioration and deformity of the hooves; bobtail disease

alkaline *adj.* the opposite of acid; having the properties of an alkali — **alkalinity** *n.* — **alkalize, alkalinize** *vt.*

alkaloid *n.* a bitter organic alkaline substance found in some plants; can be toxic to horses — **alkaloidal** *adj.*

alkalosis *n.* the opposite of acidosis; a condition in which there is an insufficiency of acid or an excess of bicarbonate in the blood

allantochorion *n.* in pregnancy, that part of the placenta that is connected to the uterus, handles waste disposal and protects the fetus

allantoic fluid a brown or yellowish-brown fluid formed jointly by placenta and fetal urine and surrounds the fetus although separated from it by amnion

allantoic sac the fluid-filled part of the placenta

allantois *n.* a membrane that contributes to the formation of the placenta **allantoic** *adj.*

allele *n.* one of a pair of genes occupying the same position on a pair of chromosomes; they are responsible for traits that are inherited alternatively because each allele has a corresponding allele on the chromosome's paired counter part; for example: one allele responsible for white hair color will have one corresponding allele representing white, brown or chestnut hair color — **allelic** *adj.*

allelomimetic behavior in herds, the aping by one horse of another horse's actions

allelomorph *n.* allele — **allelomorphic** *adj.*

allergen *n.* any substance that causes an allergic reaction — **allergenic** *adj.*

allergic bronchiolitis an inflammation of the smallest bronchioles of the bronchial tubes in the lungs; induced by an allergy to some environmental substance

allergy *n.* a hypersensitivity or abnormal sensitivity to an allergen or specific substance, as pollen, dust, drug, or feed, etc.

all on in hunting, a term used by the whipper-in to advise the huntsman that all hounds are together

allopathy *n.* medical treatment of a disease using agents that produce effects opposite to those produced by the disease; opposite of homeopathy — **allopathic** *adj.* — **allopathically** *adv.*

all-round cow horse a horse trained to perform expertly in response to a cowboy's requirements

aloe *n.* a plant whose leaves have an anti-bacterial gel useful for healing wounds, burns, or infections; there are many species, the most widely used of which is aloe vera

alopecia *n.* loss of hair where it is normally present

alpha blocker a drug that blocks specific undesirable nerve signals

alpha horse the dominant horse in a herd

alsike *n.* a species of clover that is toxic to horses

also ran in racing, a competing horse that did not place

Altan *n.* trade name for danthron

alter *vt.* to castrate or geld (a horse)

alternaria *n.* a species of fungus the growth of which in the lungs causes irritation, inflammation and allergic reaction

Alter Real a Portuguese breed that resembles the Andalusian, its foundation breed; popularly used for dressage; 15–15.3 h.h.

alum *n.* a substance which produces constriction and is used medicinally for diarrhea as well as in medicinal lotions

alveolar emphysema damaging enlargement of the alveoli in the lungs

alveolar periostitis a condition which usually occurs in the cheek teeth and causes pain and sometimes loose teeth; if the upper teeth are involved, the sinuses can be affected, causing an odorous nasal discharge; pyorrhea

alveolus *n., pl.* -li a minute air cavity, as an air sac in the lung, tooth socket, etc. — **alveolar** *adj.*

amateur *n.* a non-professional

amateur class a class in which every riding contestant who has reached 18 years of age enjoys amateur status

amateur rodeo a rodeo not sanctioned by the PRCA (Professional Rodeo Cowboys Association)

amaurosis *n.* partial or total blindness caused by a diseased optic nerve but unapparent in the external eye — **amaurotic** *adj.*

amble *vi.* a very slow gait that is just faster than a walk; the legs move in lateral pairs: near-fore, near-hind almost together — **ambler** *n.* — **ambling** *adj.*

American *n.* a type of light wagon driven one- or two-in-hand

American Albino Horse Club a group organized in Nebraska in 1937 to preserve the breeding of Albino horses

American Bashkir Curley *see* **Bashkir**

American Horse Council a national organization that represents American horsemen and advises on government legislation on equestrian affairs

American Horse Show Association (AHSA) an organization which controls all recognized shows, lists judges and publishes a yearly book of rules regarding horse shows; also keeps a list of all breed organizations

American Indian Horse a breed whose lineage goes back to Columbus and the Spanish conquistadores of the 15th and 16th centuries who brought them to North America; at that time they were crosses of Barb, Arabian, and Andalusian breeds. Through the years the Indians acquired them, hence their name; although herds were killed by the U.S. Cavalry in their efforts to conquer the Indians, these tough horses managed to survive and contributed to the foundation of various breeds, such as the Morgan, Saddlebred, and Tennessee Walker. A registry was established in 1961 in an effort to rekindle the survival of the breed that was almost extinct, and as of 1992 about 1,600 existed worldwide, of which 1,200 were in the United States. 13–15 h.h. Also called Spanish Horse.

American Saddle Horse *see* **Saddlebred**

American Shetland a more refined, taller version of the Scottish Shetland imported and crossed with American Hackneys; used as a child's mount and in trotting races, and often shown in halter and harness classes, for which the tail is sometimes nicked for an artificially high carriage; 11.2 h.h.

American skin disease *see* **contagious acne**

amikacin sulfate an antibiotic effective against bacterial infections of the mare's uterus and clitoris and of foals

amine *n.* a compound derived from ammonia — **aminic** *adj.* — **amino** *adj.* of amine

amino acids organic compounds which are the basic structural units of proteins

amino glycosides a class of powerful antibiotics

ammonia *n.* a gas composed of nitrogen compounds which is used for medicinal purposes both externally and internally

ammonia vapor a gas given off by decomposing dung; injurious to a horse in poorly ventilated quarters

amnion *n.* the fetal membrane; a bluish-white bag lining the placenta and enveloping the fetus; filled with watery fluid (amniotic fluid) — **amniotic** *adj.*

amnionitis *n.* a fungal or bacterial infection of the amnion which causes inflammation and a thicker than normal membrane

amniotic fluid the clear fluid that surrounds a fetus in a mare's womb

amoxicillin trihydrate an antibiotic that can be used to treat foals for diarrhea or septicemia; trade name Clamoxyl

amphetamine *n.* a drug used to overcome fatigue by stimulating the central nervous system, to reduce appetite, or to reduce nasal congestion; examples are Benzedrine, Dexedrine, Methedrine

amphiarthrosis *n.* a type of jointing in which cartilage connecting bones allows very limited movement — **amphiarthrodial** *adj.*

amphoric respiration respiratory sound heard on auscultation of the lungs

amphotericin B an antibiotic used to counteract fungus infections

ampicillin *n.* a generic name for a semisynthetic form of penicillin

ampule *n.* a sealed glass container used for a sterile preparation for hypodermic injections

ampulla *n., pl.* -**pullae** an enlarged part of a body canal, such as of a milk duct — **ampullar** *adj.*

amsinckia *n.* a poisonous weed which affects the intestines; fiddleneck

amylase *n.* an enzyme that contributes to the digestion of sugar; found in saliva, pancreatic juice, etc.

amyloid *n.* a waxy deposit from tissue degeneration

amyloid liver rare liver disease; usually results from pneumonia or pleurisy

amylolysis *n.* the conversion of starch into a soluble substance by enzyme action or by action with dilute acids — **amylolytic** *adj.*

anabolic *adj.* relating to the process by which food is converted into living tissue — **anabolism** *n.* — **anabolic steroid** a steroid that stimulates the growth of living tissue

anaerobic *adj.* 1. able to live without oxygen, as some bacteria 2. pertaining to exercise that lies beyond the horse's current capacity to supply oxygen to the cells

anaerobic exercise a level of exertion performed at such a strenuous rate as to demand muscle function without oxygen, a level which cannot be kept up for more than three minutes; respiration and heart rate escalate dangerously

anaerobic glycolysis a breakdown of carbohydrates and glucose in the muscles which occurs in the absence of enough oxygen, resulting in the production of lactic acid

anaerobic threshold the work rate beyond which a horse will begin to produce lactic acid in the muscles

anaesthesia *n. see* **anesthesia**

anal *adj.* pertaining to the anus

analeptic 1. *adj.* stimulating 2. *n.* a stimulating drug

analgesia *n.* a lack of feeling pain although fully conscious

analgesic *n.* a drug that relieves pain — *adj.* causing analgesia

analysis *n.* 1. an examination of a substance, such as urine, blood, etc. 2. the report of the results of this examination — **analyze** *vt.*

anamnesis *n.* the case history of a patient — **anamnestic** *adj.*

anaphylaxis *n.* an extreme allergic reaction, often fatal, to a substance to which the horse has been previously exposed and sensitized; results in shock — **anaphylactic** *adj.*

anasarca *n.* an edema (dropsy) of the legs, chest and abdomen — **anasarcous** *adj.*

anasarcous fever *see* **purpura**

anastomosis *n.* interconnection between blood vessels or internal organs — **anastomotic** *adj.* — **anastomose** vt., vi.

anatomization *n.* 1. the dissection of an animal's body for analysis 2. detailed analysis — **anatomize** *vt., vi.*

anatomy *n.* 1. the science of the structure of the body 2. the structure of the body

ancestor *n.* 1. a horse early in the family line from which one is descended, one farther back than a grandparent 2. an early type of horse from which later types have evolved

ancestry *n.* a horse's parentage back through a number of generations

anchylosis *n. see* **ankylosis**

anconeus muscle muscle which extends the elbow joint

Andalusian *n.* a Spanish breed that has an ancient heritage dating back to the Moorish invasion of Spain when North African Barbs were crossed with native Spanish horses. Andalusians have formed the foundation of many breeds in Europe, as well as North and South America when Spanish colonists took them there; the Paso Fino, Peruvian Paso, Criollo, Mustang, and Appaloosa all came originally from Andalusians. They excel in dressage. Spirited but gentle, the Andalusian is a very fine looking horse with heavy mane and tail and is usually gray or bay; 15.1–15.3 h.h.

androgen *n.* a male sex hormone —**androgenic** *adj.*

androgenous *adj.* tending to produce male offspring

androsterone *n.* a steroid in the urine of both male and female horses which carries male characteristics

anemia *n.* a low count of red blood cells; usually caused by inordinate bleeding, a poor diet, parasites, or infection; characterized by a lack of energy —*see also* **equine infectious anemia; swamp fever**

anesthesia *n.* 1. partial or total loss of physical feeling produced by a disease 2. a loss of feeling due to the administration of an anesthetic either limited to a specific area (local anesthesia) or encompassing unconsciousness (general anesthesia)

anesthetic *adj.* relating to anesthesia —*n.* a drug used to produce anesthesia

anesthetize *vt.* to administer an aesthetic to

anestrus *n.* the period of sexual inactivity during a mare's sexual cycle during which she will refuse a stallion

aneurysm, -ism *n.* a localized dilation of the wall of an artery, restricting the blood flow; caused by disease or injury; the most common form in horses is parasitic aneurysm —**aneurysmal, aneurismal** *adj.*

angioma *n.* a tumor mainly of blood and lymphatic vessels; rare in horses

angleberry *n. see* **sarcoid**

angle pelham a pelham bit with a straight bar having right-angle bends at the ends

Anglo-Arab *n.* a cross between the Thoroughbred and the Arabian or their subsequent recrossing (originally known in France as the Tarbenian). Valued worldwide for its intelligence, physical excellence, and versatility that make it ideal for a variety of competitions such as jumping, dressage, hunting, 3-day events, etc. About 16 h.h.

anhidrosis *n.* failure of the sweat glands; may affect horses brought from a temperate to a tropical climate; if exercised without care the horse staggers and dies; characterized by increased respiration and temperature; drycoat, puff disease

anhydrase *n.* an enzyme which stimulates the removal of water from a compound —**anhydrous** *adj.*

animation *n.* a lively, brisk quality demonstrated by a high neck and tail carriage and high stepping action —**animated** *adj.*

anisocytosis *n.* having red blood cells of irregular size

ankylosis, anchylosis *n.* stiffening of a joint due to fusion of bones or fibrous parts incurred by disease, injury, or surgery —**ankylose, anchylose** *vt., vi.* —**ankylotic, anchylotic** *adj.*

annular *adj.* relating to a ring or encircling shape in the body, as an **annular ligament,** which encircles tendons where they pass over a joint

anodynes *n.* any of various medicines given to relieve pain, as from colic

anomaly *n.* an abnormality, particularly as resulting from a congenital defect

anophthalmia *n.* a very rare congenital deformity in which both eyes are absent —*see also* **microphthalmia**

anorchid *n.* a male having no testicles in the scrotum —**anorchidism** *n.* the condition thereof

anorexia *n.* loss of appetite; causes may include fever, pain or digestive disorders

anovulation *n.* failure to ovulate or produce and release an ovum (egg) — **anovular** *adj.*

anoxia *n.* lack of oxygen

antacid *n.* a substance that relieves excessive acidity of the gut

antagonist *n.* a muscle, drug, etc. that resists or counteracts another

antalkaline *adj.* counteracting alkalinity — **antalkali** *n.*

antepost bet a bet placed on a racehorse before race day

anterior *adj.* relating to the front of the body or part thereof; opposite of posterior

anteroposterior *adj.* from front to back

anteroposterior deviation abnormal vertical formation or crookedness of a limb involving the flexor/extensor apparatus of tendons and or ligaments; this may be exemplified by a shortening of the back of the foreleg resulting in a pastern that is too upright or a knee that is, in extreme cases, buckled forward

anthelmintic *n.* a drug that kills intestinal worms; vermicide; vermifuge — *adj.*

anthrax *n.* an infectious disease caused by *Bacillus anthracis* and characterized by black pustules; very rare in horses now; usually fatal

anthropomorphism *n.* the explanation of equine behavior in human terms

anthropozoonosis *n.* a disease that can be contagious between man and animal; examples in relation to horses are: glanders, encephalomylitis

antiabortifacient *n.* a drug used to prevent abortion

antiandrogen *n.* a hormone that reduces the effect of an androgen, i.e., decreases masculinity

antibacterial *adj.* able to check or kill bacteria

antibiotic *adj.* destructive of bacteria and other organisms — *n.* a drug composed of a chemical substance produced by a microorganism used to counteract bacterial infection

antibody *n.* a substance produced in the body to counteract or produce an immunity to an attacking antigen; immune body

antibody titer a measurement of the amount of an antibody in blood serum or other fluid — *see also* **titer**

anticoagulant *n.* a substance that prevents blood clotting

anticonvulsant *n.* a drug that counteracts convulsions; used for newborn foals with this problem

antidiuretic hormone a pituitary hormone that influences the kidney to conserve water

antidote *n.* 1. a remedial substance given to counteract a poison 2. anything that is effective in correcting an undesirable condition

antiendotoxin *n.* an antibody that counteracts the poison of certain intestinal bacteria

antifungal *n.* a substance used to counteract fungal infections — *adj.*

antigen *n.* a substance which, when it invades the body, causes a defense reaction by the body's immune system which in turn then combats it with an antibody; an antigen may be an animal or vegetable product, a toxin, a bacterium, an enzyme, etc. — **antigenic** *adj.*

anti-grazing reins sidecheck reins that can be attached to a Western or English saddle and installed on any browband bridle to prevent a horse from dropping its head to graze, which can be a very annoying habit

antihemorrhagic *n.* a drug that stops hemorrhage — *adj.*

antihistamine *n.* a medication to relieve effects of histamine

anti-lug bit a jointed snaffle bit with one side shorter than the other; used on racehorses who tend to turn to one side, the long side of the bit being used on the side to which the horse hangs

antimonytrichloride *n.* a strong chemical sometimes used under a vet's supervision on the frog and hoof in a case of thrush

anti–over–reach shoe a shoe that is used to counteract overreaching of the hind feet; the back edge of the shoe's toe is rounded and the shoe set back on the foot with the toe rasped down

antiprostaglandin *n.* a non-hormonal anti-inflammatory drug that counteracts the action of prostaglandins, cell-produced substances that cause inflammation in response to injury

antipruritic *n.* a substance that relieves itching — *adj.*

antipyretic *n.* any medication that reduces fever — *adj.*

antiseptic *n.* an agent used to inhibit infection by microorganisms — *adj.* sterile; free from infectious organisms

antisepticize *vt.* to make antiseptic or apply antiseptics to

antiserum *n.* a serum having antibodies taken from an animal that has been immunized against a particular antigen

antispasmodic *n.* a drug that prevents spasms of the gut — *adj.*

antitoxin *n.* 1. an antibody formed by the body which acts against a toxin 2. a serum containing an antitoxin — **antitoxic** *adj.*

antiviral *n.* a substance that destroys viruses — *adj.*

antrum *n.* a cavity, as the bony cavity that forms the sinus in the cheek

anuria *n.* a condition that arrests the excretion of urine

anus *n.* the outlet of the alimentary canal or end of the rectum

anvil *n.* an iron block having a smooth flat top on which a farrier hammers and shapes horses' shoes

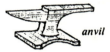

anvil

aorta *n.* the main artery that carries blood from the heart to branching arteries of the body — **aortic, aortal** *adj.*

apathy *n.* inert disinterest in surroundings, symptom of illness — **apathetic** *adj.*

apex *n., pl.* **apexes, apices** the highest point or the tip of a body part

aphonia *n.* loss of voice as due to an operation to relieve roaring — **aphonic** *adj.*

aphtha *n.* a small, fungal pustule; **apthous** *adj.* — *see also* **stomatitis**

aplasia *n.* a birth deformity

aplastic anemia a condition wherein there are insufficient numbers of red blood cells due to the body's inability to make new ones; usually unresponsive to therapy

apnea, apnoea *n.* temporary stoppage of respiration — **apneic, apnoeic** *adj.*

Apocalypse, Four Horsemen of the famous creatures described in the last book of the Bible's New Testament; God holds a scroll sealed with 7 seals; 4 of these are opened to reveal 4 mounted horsemen and their horses are white (rider carries a bow representing conquest), red (rider carries a sword representing slaughter), black (rider carries a pair of scales representing famine), and pale-colored (death); these horsemen are well known in art and literature

apocrine *adj.* (of a glandular secretion) carrying away part of the secreting cell

apocrine glands sweat glands; mammary glands (which secrete milk through a mare's nipples) are a type of apocrine gland

apomorphine *n.* derivative of morphine

apoplexy *n.* brain hemorrhage

Appaloosa *n.* an American breed that was introduced to America by the Spaniards around 1600; derives its name from the Palouse river in Idaho where it was bred by the Nez Percé Indians and was known to the white settlers as Palouseys. The outstanding characteristic of this breed is its spotted coloring which may comprise a variety of patterns including dark spots all over a white background (leopard), light spots on dark background (snowflake), a dark forehand with a blanket that has no spots or very few (white blanket), spots on quarters and loins only (spotted blanket), dark base color when born, which fades to nearly white, except for some darker marks on face and legs (marble), or dark base color with either frost or white spots on loins and hips (frosted tip). A fine all-purpose saddle horse, sometimes called "raindrop" horse; about 15 h.h.

appetite *n.* desire for food; a depraved appetite is a desire for something other than food, such as tree bark (wood chewing), dung (coprophagy), etc. *—see also* **thirst**

apple ducking race a mounted game in which each participant races to a bucket containing a floating apple, dismounts, grabs the apple by mouth, remounts and races back to the starting point with the apple

apple picker *see* **manure fork**

appointment card in hunting, a card sent out by the hunt secretary to prospective participants in hunts giving them details of planned meets

appointments *n.pl.* equipment and clothing required for a specific class, event or style of riding

apricot dun *see* **dun**

apron *n.* a covering made of strong horse-hide worn by farriers to protect the front of the body while shoeing

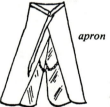

apron

apron face a face with a white marking which narrows between the eyes and the widens to cover the whole muzzle

aprosopia *n.* facelessness; a rare deformity in which eyes, nostrils, and mouth have not developed in a fetus. The foal usually dies right after birth.

AQHA American Quarter Horse Association

aqueous humor the fluid in the anterior part of the eye between the cornea and the lens; regulates pressure within the eye

Arab, Arabian *n.* an Arabian breed of ancient origins, the oldest purebred in the world now bred worldwide and crossed with other breeds to improve them. Intelligent and known for exceptional beauty and presence, it is generally considered to be the most noble of all breeds; also famous for its tremendous endurance and wonderful disposition which is proud and spirited but gentle and affectionate. The head is small with a distinctive face that has a concave ("dished") profile called the jibbah, formed by the bulge between the eyes up to the forehead and down across the first third of the nasal bone; large, expressive and gentle eyes are set low and wide apart; cheeks are large, muzzle small and very soft; nostrils are large and capable of considerable extension; ears are somewhat broad in the middle, tapering and curving to alert points; the strong neck is arched at the crest and joins the head in an angle that is called the mitbah; the back is short, having one fewer vertebra than other breeds (five instead of six), and there is also one fewer pair of ribs; the girth is deep, chest broad and muscular; the croup is level, generous quarters are round and muscular; the tail is set high, carried elegantly, and like the mane, is very fine and silky; the legs are very fine but strong; colors are solid, mostly chestnut and bay, but many are gray; 14.1–15 h.h.

arabella hypoplasia a disease, probably inherited, which affects Arabs as well as several other breeds

arachnid *n.* an arthropod of the class *Arachnida,* as a tick, mite, scorpion, or spider

arcade *n.* a row of teeth

arch 1. *n.* a convex curve 2. *vt.* to bend with an upward curve —**arched** *adj.* as an arched neck or back

Ardennais *n. see* **Ardennes**

Ardennes *n.* a cold-blood draft breed (also called Ardennais) that originated in the Ardennes Mountains between France and Belgium and is thus indigenous to both those countries; they have a very old heritage, perhaps 2,000 years; large-boned with strong, short legs and known for an extremely gentle temperament; there is also a **Swedish Ardennes**; 15.1–16.1 h.h.

areflexia *n.* lack of reflexes

arena *n.* an area, either outdoors or indoors, in which a horse show or show-jumping competition is held

arena director the person appointed to direct a rodeo according to the rules

Ariegeois *n.* a semi-wild French breed indigenous to the mountainous area around the Ariege River; a registry for those that have been domesticated dates back to 1948; usually black; also called Merens; about 14 h.h.

armor *n.* heavy, metal protective cover-ing used on horses (and knights) long ago in battle; in bullfights today horses used in the ring are covered with a type of armor consisting of very thick padding for protection against the bull's horns

arrhythmia *n.* lack of rhythm, especially of the heartbeat —**arrhythmic** *adj.* —**arrhythmically** *adv.*

arsenic *n.* a poisonous chemical, compounds of which are used in medicines, particularly worm medicines

arterialize *vt.* to oxygenate (venous blood) and thereby change (it) into arterial blood —**arterialization** *n.*

arteriole *n.* a small artery

arteriosclerosis *n.* a thickening of the arterial walls, which become brittle and may rupture; a type of this condition may be caused by the larvae of strongyle parasites —**arteriosclerotic** *adj.*

arteriovenous *adj.* relating to both an artery and a vein

arteriovenous (AV) shunt a passageway between an artery and vein that bypasses the capillary bed which that artery normally supplies; anastomosis

arteritis *n.* a contagious disease characterized by discharge from eyes and nose (pink eye), fever (shipping fever), possible pneumonia (stable pneumonia), sometimes edematous swelling on the trunk and legs (epizootic cellulitis), corneal cloudiness depression, lack of appetite; fatality is moderate; also called equine infectious arteritis

artery *n.* a vessel that carries blood from the heart —**arterial** *adj.* —**arterially** *adv.*

arthritis *n.* inflammation of a joint or joints, causing pain and stiffness —**arthritic** *adj.* —*see also* **open arthritis** and **closed arthritis**

arthrocele *n.* a swollen joint

arthrocentesis *n.* the introduction of an instrument into a joint to aspirate fluid

arthrodesis *n.* an orthopedic technique which permanently fuses a joint in a stable position; it can be used in cases of severe sesamoid fracture; the joint is thus pain free but it is immobilized so that the horse can never be ridden but can freely move about on its own

arthropod *n.* an invertebrate animal that has jointed legs and segmented body, such as an insect; may be a parasite to a horse, suck blood and be a vector of disease

arthroscope *n.* an instrument that has lights and mirrors used for examining or operating on a joint by insertion into that joint

arthroscopy *n.* a procedure using an arthroscope for examination or operation on a joint — **arthroscopic** *adj.*

arthrosis *n.* erosion and wearing away of joint cartilage

articular cartilage cartilage covering joints

articulation *n.* a joint; so called because one end of a bone articulates with the end of another bone by means of a joint — **articulate** *vi.* — **articular, articulated** *adj.*

artificial air *see* **air**

artificial insemination the artificial introduction of a stallion's semen into a mare's uterus when she is in estrus

arytenoid cartilage one of two cartilages in the larynx which are attached to the vocal cords

ascariasis *n.* infestation with ascarids

ascarids *n.* a parasitic roundworm

ascitis *n.* an abnormal collection of fluid in the peritoneal cavity of the abdomen — **ascitic** *adj.*

ascorbic acid vitamin C, which is found in most green forage; necessary for capillary strength and formation of collagen

asepsis *n.* a germ-free state — **aseptic** *adj.*

asking the question in competitive events, asking a horse to make a supreme effort when the horse is being pushed to its limit

ask off in jumping, a rider's aids asking a horse to jump

aspartate aminotransferase (AST) an enzyme of the liver and muscles

aspergillosis *n.* infection of body organs by the fungus aspergillus; characterized by irritation, inflammation, and allergic reaction in the lungs

asphyxia *n.* suffocation

asphyxia fetalis suffocation of a fetus

asphyxiant *n.* something that causes asphyxia — *adj.* causing asphyxia

asphyxiate *vt.* 1. to cause asphyxia in 2. to suffocate — *vi.* — **asphyxiation** *n.*

aspirate *vt.* 1. to inhale (something like dust) into the lungs 2. to remove (fluid) from the body by suction — **aspiration** *n.*

aspiration pneumonitis inflammation of the lungs due to inhaled substances

aspirator *n.* the apparatus used for removing fluid from the body

aspirin *n.* a white powder, acetylsalicylic acid, used for relief of pain and reduction of fever

ass *n.* *see* **donkey**

Assateague *n.* an American wild pony breed that lives on the island of Assateague off the coast of Virginia — *see also* **Chincoteague**

assay *n.* 1. an analysis 2. a substance to be analyzed 3. the resulting report of an analysis — *vt.* to analyze or test

Assyrians *n.pl.* the first people to use cavalry horses and chariots in battle

asthenia *n.* weakness of the body —**asthenic** *adj.*

asthenic fever a low fever which causes debilitation and depression; adynamic fever

asthma *n.* a disorder characterized by wheezing and difficulty in breathing; usually an allergic reaction; can be accompanied by bronchitis —*see also* **broken wind**

astride *adv.* on a horse with a leg over each side of the animal

astringent *n.* an externally applied agent that induces contraction or constriction of tissues —*adj.* having the quality of an astringent —**astringency** *n.* —**astringently** *adv.*

astrocyte *n.* a star-shaped cell; found in nervous tissue, as in the brain

asymptomatic *adj.* without symptoms

ataractic/ataraxic *n.* a tranquilizer —*adj.*

atavism *n.* the inheritance of a characteristic from a remote ancestor —**atavistic** *adj.* —**atavistically** *adv.*

ataxia *n.* failure of muscle coordination (as seen in wobbles) —**ataxic** *adj.* —*see also* **coastal ataxia**

at bay in hunting, the position of the hounds when kept off the quarry

atelectasis *n.* a collapsed, or partly collapsed, condition of a lung, or part thereof —**atelectic** *adj.* —*see also* **broken wind, neonatal maladjustment syndrome**

at grass pastured, as opposed to stabled

atheroma *n.* a nodule; a condition wherein small nodules form on the inner walls of arteries —**atheromatous** *adj.*

atherosclerosis *n.* a hardening of the inner lining of arteries; may occur in the horse's aorta with resultant heart murmurs or ruptures of the artery

Atherstone girth a baghide girth used on an English saddle shaped to prevent galling at the elbows; similarly shaped is the **Balding girth**

atlas *n.* the first vertebra in the neck which articulates with the skull

ATP a chemical, adenosine triphosphate, found in muscle tissue, a source of energy as for muscular contractions

atresia *n.* failure of development of a normal opening of an organ, such as the rectum (**atresia ani**) or the colon (**atresia coli**)

atrial fibrillation heart arrhythmia; results in reduced performance and probably eventually an enlarged heart and death

artrial flutter a very fast heartbeat

atrio-ventricular *adj.* of or relating to the auricle and ventricle of the heart

atrium *n., pl.* **atria** a cavity in the body, especially the left and right atria of the heart —**atrial** *adj.*

atrophy *n.* a degeneration, especially of body tissues, organs, etc., or lack of development —*vi.* to degenerate —*vt.* to cause atrophy —**atrophic** *adj.*

atropine, atropin *n.* a chemical obtained from belladonna and similar plants and used to relax muscle spasms and to treat eye diseases, hemorrhages, etc.

attenuate *vt.* to reduce the potency of (often applied to a micro-organism, as in the preparation of a vaccine) — **attenuation** *n.* —**attenuated** *adj.*

atypical *adj.* not typical, especially in relation to symptoms of a disease or to behavioral characteristics

atypical myoglobinuria an inflammation of a muscle or muscles, commonly the croup and loins, characterized by lameness after exercise begins or after a full day of hard work. The muscles feel hard and raised with little tremors; the horse can move only with much difficulty not to be confused with typical or true myoglobinuria (azoturia), although it is partially present. A horse suffering this condition may be said to be set fast, tied up, cording up.

aural *adj.* of or relating to the ear or hearing

aural plaque a small gray or white spot on the inner surface of the external ear

auricle *n.* 1. the external part of the ear 2. an atrium of the heart.

auscultation *n.* the monitoring of sounds within the body, often with a stethoscope — **auscultate** *vt., vi.*

Australian Pony a native of Australia developed from crosses of Welsh, Arab, Thoroughbred, Timor, and Shetland breeds; 12–14 h.h.

Australian Stock Horse *see* **Waler**

Australian stock saddle a type of saddle with a high cantle, high pommel with typically no horn (although some are made Western style with a horn), English type stirrups with leathers about 2½ inches wide, and the unusual feature of knee pads which project outward from just below the pommel

Australian stock saddle

autoclave *n.* an apparatus used for sterilizing instruments by process of steam

autogenous *adj.* self-generated

autogenous vaccine a vaccine manufactured from bacteria taken from the horse's own body

autoimmune response the production of antibodies against the body's own tissues

autoimmunization, autoimmunity *n.* immunity generated by a substance developed within the horse's own body — **autoimmune** *adj.*

automatic timing apparatus an electrical device used for show-jumping competitions; the horse triggers a timer by breaking a concentrated light beam at the start and stops the timer in a similar way at the finish

autonomic nervous system that part of the nervous system that controls involuntary functions, including those of the heart, glands, smooth muscles, etc.

autopsy *n.* a dissection and examination of a dead body to determine the cause of death; post-mortem

autorisation speciale a pink card issued to a rider by his or her national equestrian federation granting permission to enter an international dressage, show-jumping, or combined training event

autosome *n.* a paired chromosome as opposed to an unpaired chromosome, as a sex chromosome — **autosomal** *adj.*

Autumn Double two races (Cesarewitch Stakes and Cambridgeshire Stakes) held every year in England in the autumn

Auxois *n.* a French draft breed; 15.2–16 h.h.

avascular *adj.* lacking in blood

Avelignese *n.* a breed indigenous to Italy, chiefly the hill country where it is used as a light draft horse; very tractable and long living; 13.3–14 h.h.

average *n.* in rodeo, money won by contestants; when there is more than one go-around, contestants win money for each of their go-rounds plus the average which is the aggregate of their go-round scores. Ex: if a competitor wins a score of 5 for each of two go-rounds, his or her average would be 10

avitaminosis *n.* a condition caused by vitamin deficiency

avoidance response behavior to avoid possible punishment

Av shunt *see* **arteriovenous shunt**

avulsion *n.* the tearing away of tissue

axial plexus veins in the digital cushion of the foot

axilla *n.* the area between the shoulder and chest, analogous to the human armpit

axis *n.* 1. the angle of the hoof wall 2. an imaginary line through the center of the body 3. the second cervical vertebra

axon *n.* the extension of a nerve cell through which impulses are transmitted

azoturia *n.* a severe form of muscle cramps characterized by stiffness and staggering, pain, and muscle tremor, usually involving the hindquarters but sometimes also the forequarters; usually caused by irregular work schedules coupled with a high grain diet that has not been reduced during rest periods; appears usually when first exercised, never at rest —*see also* **myoglobinuria**

Azteca *n.* a Mexican breed founded by Antonio Areza Canadilla, a Spaniard who settled in Mexico; by crossing Andalusian stallions with Quarter Horse mares; these horses have the beauty and nobility of the Andalusian, with long, thick manes and tails, and the well muscled hindquarters and chests, power, speed and docile temperament of the Quarter Horse. The Azteca's registry was created in 1982. This is an all-purpose breed suitable for dressage, driving, pleasure riding, and ranch work. 14.3–15 h.h.

azygous *adj.* odd, as not one of a pair; e.g., an azygous muscle

— B —

babbling *n.* in hunting, unnecessary baying by the hounds

Babesia caballi a protozoan transmitted by ticks to the horse's red blood cells; causes equine piroplasmosis; also called *Piroplasma caballi*; *Babesia equi* is a species of the same protozoa which causes the most serious form of piroplasmosis, developing rapidly

babesiosis *n. see* **piroplasmosis**

bachelor herd a herd of male horses

bacillus *n., pl.* **-cilli** bacteria that are rod-shaped and often occur in chains; can cause various diseases

back¹ *n.* that part of the body that extends from the base of the withers to the point where the last rib is attached

back² *vi.* to move rearward; may be used with "-up"; in cueing a horse to back, the rider should sit deep in the saddle, squeeze the legs as for impulsion but simultaneously pull on the reins with an intermittent pressing action (like squeezing a sponge), releasing pressure with each step backward that the horse makes; rein-back

back³ *vt.* to place a bet on (a horse) in competition; **backer** is the person who places the bet

back⁴ *vt.* to train (an unbroken horse) to get used to the saddle and weight of a rider

back band as part of a harness, a strap that runs over or through the pad and supports the traces

back blood an existing hereditary trait which may influence horses bred from the affected parents; also called back breeding

backbone *n.* the column of separate bones (vertebrae) along the center of the back, connected by muscles and tendons; spine

back breeding *see* **back blood**

backgammon board a seat on a coach at the rear and on the roof

back hander in polo, a stroke in which the player traveling forward hits the ball backwards in the opposite direction

back jockey on a Western saddle, the leather skirt at the back and side of the cantle

back-raking *n.* a procedure involving the manual removal of feces from the rectum either as a preparation for treatment or for diagnostic purposes

bacteremia *n.* a condition wherein bacteria exist in the bloodstream

bacteria *n.pl., sing.* **-rium** microscopic plants of the class *Schizomycetes*; some cause diseases, such as pneumonia, etc. — **bacterial** *adj.*

bactericide *n.* an anti-bacterial substance — **bactericidal** *adj.*

bacterin *n.* an immunizing agent prepared from bacteria that have been killed without removing their antigenic properties

bacteriolysis *n.* the destruction of bacteria

bacteriophage *n.* a virus that disintegrates bacteria — **bacteriophagy** *n.*

bacteriostasis *n.* a condition in which bacterial growth is halted

bacteriostatic *n.* an anti-bacterial drug, as an antibiotic — *adj.* causing bacteriostasis

Bacterium viscosum equi a microorganism that can infect the newborn foal; symptoms are excessive sleepiness and long periods of lying down immobile; damages kidneys, liver, and other organs but is not contagious; shigella infection, sleepy foal disease — *see also Actinobacillus equuli*

Baden-Wurttemburg *n.* a German breed developed with Trakehner blood for competition and pleasure riding; 15.3–16.2 h.h.

Badge of Honour the prize awarded by the F.E.I. to riders taking part in Prix des Nations events; points awarded are 5 (Bronze), 25 (Silver) 50 (Gold)

badikins *n.pl. see* **singletree**

bag *n.* the udder of a mare

bag fox in hunting, a fox held in captivity in preparation for a hunt — *see also* **bagman**

bagging up swelling of the udder prior to foaling

baghide *n.* cowhide which has a pattern on it to hide imperfections

bagman *n.* a person who brings a fox to the hunt in a bag due to lack of game in the area

balance *n.* 1. physical stability; the stability of a horse when in motion; a balanced horse is one that carries its own weight and that of the rider almost equally over all four legs 2. equal proportions, as in reference to the feet when they are said to be well balanced when the hoofs match up properly — **balanced** *adj.* — *see also* **balanced hoof**

balanced hoof a hoof in the same angle as that of the pastern

balanced rig a horse trailer with axles properly centered, thereby maintaining the trailer in a balanced position; a minimum of 15 percent of total trailer weight (loaded or unloaded) must be on the tongue

balanced seat a seat wherein a mounted rider sits on his seat bones in the center of the saddle, legs in a natural bent position, ankles flexed, balls of feet resting in the stirrups and held close to the inside, arms bent at elbows and reins held over the horse's withers

balanitis *n.* inflmmation of the balanus — *see also* **balanus**

balanopreputial *adj.* relating to the head and foreskin of the penis

balanus *n.* the head (glans) of the penis — **balanic** *adj.*

bald *n.* a large, uneven white facial marking that includes both eyes; referred to as a "bald face"; the entire face may be white, contrasting with another body color, extending from the top of the face to the muzzle

Balding girth a girth used on an English saddle which is split into three and crossed in such a way as to prevent galling at the elbows; named after William Balding who perfected it

bale *n.* a standardized quantity of hay, compressed and bound up into a rectangular shape called a square bale — *vt.* to bind up (cut grass) into bales

Balearic pony an ancient breed indigenous to Majorca, one of the Balearic Islands; has a short, arched neck with upright mane; lean; gentle; under 14 h.h.

balk *vi.* to refuse to move on command — **balky** *adj.*

ballast *n.* a rider's weight, which can be shifted to help balance the horse and also to act as an aid as when the rider leans slightly into a turn

balling *n.* a hard mass of snow compacted on the sole of the horse's foot within the shoe; may be prevented by generously greasing the sole before a ride

balling gun a device for administering pills

ballotade *n.* in dressage, an air above the ground; the horse half rears, then jumps forward, drawing the hind legs up before landing on all four feet

ballottement *n.* palpation by a veterinarian to detect pregnancy, a tumor, or any of various other conditions

banana relay race a mounted team race in which competitors speed to a given point with a ripe banana and pass it to a team member who continues. The banana should be kept in one piece to avoid penalties; if any sections are broken off, the rider must dismount and collect them. At the finish, each broken piece incurs a 2-second penalty, and a lost piece incurs a 5-second penalty.

band *n.* a group of horses — *vi., vt.* to group together

bandage *n.* a cloth strip used for many purposes such as dressing wounds, leg wraps for support and protection, wrapping the tail to protect it (as in polo) or keep it neat — *vt.*

banding *n. see* **mane banding**

bandy legs *see* **bowlegs** — **bandylegged** *adj.*

banged tail a tail that has been pulled until it is even with the hocks; it is pulled rather than cut for a more natural look

bangs *n. see* **brucellosis**

bank a jump to land on top of a jump before continuing off it

bar *n.* 1. a straight mouthpiece of a bit; bar mouth 2. one of either cheekpieces of a curb bit 3. one of the metal strips to which stirrup leathers are attached on a saddle 4. either of the side portions of a saddle tree 5. one of the four toothless spaces in the mouth that lie between the incisors and molars in mares and between canines and molars in stallions and geldings; bit pressure bears down on these bars 6. any of the dark stripes on the legs in such breeds as buckskins; zebra striping 7. either of the two ridges between the frog and wall of the hoof

Barb *n.* a breed of ancient origins native to Barbary, North Africa, a region which today comprises Morocco, Algeria, and Libya; has influenced many other breeds, including the Andalusian and Thoroughbred, and was a popular import into Europe and England in the 17th century; hardy and an easy keeper but quick-tempered; has a straight, long head with large muzzle, sloping hindquarters and low-set tail; very fast on short distances; 14–15 h.h.

barbed wire strands of fencing wire twisted together and having barbs spaced closely apart; it is sometimes inadvisably used to contain horses, thereby risking injury to them — **barb-wire** *n.*

bard *n.* 1. armor for a warhorse 2. an ornamental covering for a horse

Bardigiano *n.* an Italian breed with an old heritage; 13.2–14.2 h.h.

bareback *adj., adv.* riding without a saddle

bareback bronc riding in rodeo, an event in which contestants ride a bucking horse, the only rigging being a special surcingle around the horse's girth; the rider is allowed to hold onto a rawhide handle on top of the rigging with one hand and should remain on for eight seconds to complete the ride

bareback pad a riding pad with stirrups, girth, and handhold

bareback pad

barefoot *adj., adv.* without shoes; barefooted

bareme *n.* an international term for any of the three tables of rules which govern the judging of show-jumping

barge horse a horse used to tow a boat along a canal

barium *n.* an opaque substance that shows up on an X-ray; administered orally and may be used to diagnose conditions causing dysphagia

barker-foal syndrome *see* **neonatal maladjustment**

barley *n.* 1. a cereal grass 2. the grain of cereal grass used as feed

barn-sour *adj.* describes a horse which is reluctant to be ridden away from its living area and which, when returning, resists the rider's restraining aids in an effort to hurry home, possibly to the point of running away

bar plate a wide metal plate that connects the ends of a horseshoe

barrage *n.* a jumping obstacle

barrel *n.* 1. the trunk of the horse or area between fore- and hindquarters 2. a wooden, cylindrical container with round, flat ends; used in barrel racing

barrel racing a timed contest in which a horse and rider weave around three barrels set in a cloverleaf pattern; a 5-second penalty is added for knocking over a barrel; in playday barrel racing, the barrels may also be set in a straight line

barrel racing special *see* **outside rim shoe**

barren *adj.* 1. not in foal 2. sterile; unable to produce offspring

barrier *n.* 1. in racing, the gate behind which the contestants stand in line ready to start 2. in rodeo calf-roping and steer-wrestling competitions, the line behind which the horse and roper wait for the calf, or steer, to be let out from its stall; when it comes out and crosses the scoreline, the barrier, made of thin rope, is released; it is attached in such a way that if the horse starts too soon and breaks it, he will not be injured but the rider will receive a penalty of 10 seconds; the barrier may also be a light beam 3. a jumping obstacle

barrier boot a protective horse's boot used in cases of injury to the hoof, loss of a shoe while waiting to be shod, etc. *barrier boot*

bar shoe a horseshoe with a bar, a wide metal plate between the heels, thereby having no opening

Barthais *n. see* **Landais**

bascule *vi.* 1. to flex or engage the lumbosacral joint and arch the back, thereby becoming collected; this activates impulsion and results in a smooth ride 2. to achieve bascule 3. to arch the neck and back while jumping — *n.*

baseball race a timed playday event in which a competitor rides up to a barrel set upside down with a baseball set on top in sand; he grabs the ball as he circles around the barrel and races back to an open barrel, near the starting point, into which he tosses the ball

base narrowed a leg conformation fault wherein there is a wider distance between the legs at the top than at the bottom

base widened a leg conformation fault wherein there is a wider distance between the legs at the bottom than at the top

base narrowed   *base widened*

Bashkir *n.* a Russian pony breed of ancient heritage; used for riding, pack and farm work. Young mares produce so much milk (3–6 gallons daily) that they are milked by the Bashkiri people; also found in the U.S.A., particularly Nevada; the Russian ponies have very thick manes and tails, whereas those of American ponies are fine and kinky and shed in summer; the coats are curly; 13.3 h.h.

basophil *n.* a white blood cell

basophilism *n.* abnormal increase in basophils *see* **Cushing's disease**

Basque *n.* a French pony breed of ancient heritage which roams free in the mountainous regions of the Pyrenees between France and Spain. In order to survive in their tough environment, foals mature early (1–2 years). Basques adapt well to domestication and are used as childrens' mounts. This breed's registry began only in the 1970s; 11.2–13 h.h. Also called Pottock.

basse école an exercise preparatory to haute école in which the horse practices regularity of gaits on one and two tracks

bastard strangles a form of strangles that progresses from head to chest and abdomen where it can form abscesses

basterna *n.* a Roman sedan chair carried by two horses, one on each end

Basuto *n.* a breed native to Lesotho (Basutoland), where it is used for polo and general riding; about 14.2 h.h.

bat *n.* a riding crop

Batak *n.* a pony breed of Sumatra in Indonesia; about 12–13 h.h.

Bavarian Warm-blood a German breed, formerly known as the Rottaler, of ancient heritage; a heavyweight riding horse of good temperament; 16 h.h.

bay[1] *n.* a horse of medium brown color with black mane and tail; there are light bays and dark bays and they often have black lower legs — *adj.*

bay[2] *vi.* in hunting, to bark (said of dogs)

baz-diri *n.* a Mongolian mounted game involving a number of contestants riding for several hours, trying to grab a goat's carcass from each other and race off with it to a finishing point

bean *n.* a small ball of waxy secretion which sometimes develops in a depression in the head of a gelding's penis and which may interfere with staling if not cleaned out

bean *vt.* to camouflage unsoundness in (a horse), as by inserting a small, sharp object in a sound hoof to cause tenderness and "equalize" it with the corresponding unsound hoof, making the horse seemingly step soundly on both feet

beanbag fracture a multiple fracture of a joint involving such fragmentation that the area resembles a beanbag

bearing *n.* 1. a support; in relation to the horse, either (a) the upper side of a shoe that contacts the hoof or (b) the bottom of the foot that contacts the ground 2. the horse's way of standing or carrying himself

bearing in (*or out*) going in an inner or (outer) direction

bearing rein 1. a rein applied against the horse's neck in the direction of a turn 2. a fixed rein between the bit and saddle used to hold the head up and arched in an attractive head-set — *see also* **check rein**

beat *vt.* 1. to strike, as with a whip, (a) to make a horse run faster or (b) as a punishment 2. to form a path underfoot by repeated treading 3. to defeat (another contestant or contestants) in competition

Beberbeck *n.* a German breed; about 16 h.h.

bedding *n.* materials used on the floor of a stall, such as straw or wood shavings

bee *n.* an insect whose sting can cause a lump-like swelling on a horse's body, sometimes oozing pus, that can take days to disappear

bee

beet poisoning a condition caused by the oxalic acid of fresh, unwilted beet tops; characterized by paralysis, salivation, inability to swallow, etc.

behind the bit a position in which a horse arches its neck, usually opening its mouth to drop the bit, and tucks its chin close to its chest in an effort to back off the bit pressure; makes control by the rider difficult

Belgian Half-Blood a riding horse whose registry was started in 1920 and developed mainly from imported Arabs, Anglo-Arabs, Thoroughbreds, and Selle Francais; 15.2–16.1 h.h.

belladonna *n.* a poisonous plant with bell-shaped flowers that are purplish or reddish, and black berries; rarely

eaten by horses, except occasionally when mixed, in dried form, with hay, ingestion of which is extremely harmful; atropine is the chief derivative — *see also* **atropine**

bell boots boots that protect the heels from boots over-reaching, faulty gaits, and conformation defects; also called quarter boots

bell boots

bell bottom a style of Western stirrup curved in the shape of a bell

bell bottom
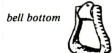

belly *n.* 1. the underside of the horse's body 2. abdomen 3. stomach

belly-ache *n.* see **colic**

belly band girth or cinch

belly brush a stiff brush fastened onto a stallion's belly to discourage masturbation; since it causes the horse to associate pain with sexual expression, it can have a very negative effect on breeding

Belmont Stakes one of America's Classic Races, run in early June at Belmont Park, New York; originally run at Jerome Park in 1867, then at Morris Park from 1890 to 1905 when Belmont Park opened

Belorussian *n.* a small, light Russian cold-blood breed weighing about 1000 lbs.; about 14.3 h.h.

bemegride sodium a medicinal stimulant; trade name Megimide

bench knees the condition wherein the cannon bone deviates laterally from under the knee; conducive to splint formation

bending race a gymkhana game popular in England involving 4–6 participants who race in slalom effect through a line of poles 10–12 feet apart and return the same way to the starting point

benzamine penicillin a white powder used as an antibacterial medication; trade names Dibencil, Penidural

benzimidazole *n.* generic name for a dewormer

benzoin *n.* a resin extracted from balsam fir; used to protect the skin from irritations derived from chemicals or tape burns

benzyl benzoate a treatment for sarcoptic mange; trade name Spasmodin

benzylpenicillin *n.* a type of penicillin used to combat gram-positive bacteria; trade names Crystapen, Falapen, Penavlon, Solupen

Bermuda grass any of several rhizome type perennial grasses grown in the warm temperatures of southern U.S.; used for hay —*see also* **coastal hay**

bet *n.* in racing a wager placed on a horse; "antepost" betting begins before race day; "post" betting is made after the numbers of the competitors are posted —*vi.* to make a wager

beta *n.* the second in a group; a **beta horse** is one which occupies second place, after the alpha horse, in a herd

Betadine *n.* brand name for a type of iodine

beta hemolysis the clear zone around the growth of streptococci on blood agar

betamethasone *n.* an anti-inflammatory agent and very potent steroid; regulates the function of carbohydrates and proteins

betting shop a place away from a racecourse where a licensed bookmaker takes bets on horseraces

bezoar *n.* a ball of hair, plant fibers, or inorganic matter in the large colon

bhoosa *n.* a chaff of barley or wheat straw; tibben

Bhutia, Bhotia *n.* a pony breed native to the Himalayan mountains of India 13.1 h.h.

bib *n.* a rubber or plastic cover for a horse's muzzle to prevent chewing or gnawing of bandages, blankets, etc.; attaches to a halter

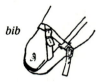

bib

bib martingale a running martingale in which the split is filled in with baghide; web martingale

bicarbonate *n.* a salt of carbonic acid present in the bloodstream which neutralizes acid in the blood

biceps *n.* large muscle in the upper leg — **bicipital** *adj.*

biceps brachii powerful muscle in the front of the foreleg, which aids in controlling the shoulder and elbow joints

biceps femoris powerful muscle in the back of the hind leg; related to the femur (thigh bone), part of which flexes the stifle

bicipital bursa a fluid-filled sac that encloses the biceps brachii muscle where it curves around in the front of the shoulder joint

bicipital bursitis acute inflammation of the bicipital bursa; characterized by severe lameness caused by slipping back of the leg from a retracted position, putting considerable tension on the biceps tendon within the bursa, tearing tissue and causing inflammation and pain —*see also* **bursitis**

bicornuate *adj.* shaped like two horns; e.g., a bicornuate uterus

bicuspid *n.* two cusps or points; used in reference to the valve of the heart or to certain teeth

b.i.d. *bis in die;* twice daily, as in medicinal prescriptions

bifurcate croup a croup that has a distinct dip down the middle

big head disease a condition wherein the head bones get enlarged; caused by excessive phosphorous or insufficient calcium in the diet. Soft, fibrous tissue forms in the bones. First signs are lameness, arching of the back, and creaking joints; eventually broken bones and sprained tendons may develop and finally the face may become enlarged, hence the name; bran disease; miller's disease; osteodystrophia fibrosa; hyperparathyroidism

bight of the reins that part of the reins passing between the thumb and fingers and out of the top of the hand

big knee a swelling of the knee; popped knee; capped knee — *see also* **hygroma**

big leg *see* **lymphangitis**

Bigourdan *n.* *see* **Tarbenian**

big race the chief race of the day at a race meeting

bike *n.* a racing sulky having wheels like those of a bicycle

bile *n.* the yellowish-brown or greenish fluid secreted by the liver; aids digestion, particularly in the absorption of fats

bile duct a tube which carries bile from the liver to the small intestine

biliary *adj.* 1. relating to bile 2. bile-carrying 3. bilious

biliary fever *see* **piroplasmosis**

bilious *adj.* 1. relating to bile 2. having an ailment of the liver — **biliousness** *n.*

bilirubin *n.* bile pigment which is normally changed by the liver into biliverdin but in cases of jaundice may be present in urine and tissues

bilirubinemia *n.* excessive bilirubin in the blood

bilirubinuria *n.* excessive bilirubin in the urine

biliverdin *n.* green pigment formed by liver from bilirubin before passing to intestines

billet strap a strap on an English saddle that attaches saddle to girth; girth strap

bimastic *adj.* having two mammary glands, as does a mare

biniodide of mercury a derivative of mercury used in absorbent ointments

binocular vision vision which uses both eyes to give one image and enables depth perception

bioassay *n.* a method of testing the power of a drug by studying its effects on the growth of an organism

bioelectric impulse an electric current generated by living tissue

biologic *n.* a medical preparation (including a serum, vaccine, antigen, antitoxin) produced from living organisms and their products — **biological** *adj.* — **biologically** *adv.*

biologically inert ineffective against body reaction, such as that involved in a surgical implant

biology *n.* the science of living matter, including animals

biometrics *n.* the branch of biology in which data is expressed mathematically — **biometric, biometrical** *adj.*

biomicroscopy *n.* the microscopic examination of living tissue

biophysics *n.* the study of living processes

biopsy *n.* surgical removal of living tissue for diagnostic examination

biopsy punch surgical instrument used to obtain a sample of tissue for analysis

biorhythms *n.pl.* the cycles governing bodily or mental changes or rhythms; may be daily (circadian cycle), seasonal or annual; they affect a horse's health, disposition and performance

biotin *n.* a water-soluble vitamin first identified as an essential dietary requirement in 1927 and first isolated in 1935. It is needed for the body to synthesize glucose fatty acids and helps in the synthesis of proteins. Some biotin is manufactured in the horse's intestines, but because this takes place at a point beyond the site of protein absorption, it is too late to be effective for this particular function; biotin is, therefore, sometimes given to horses as a supplement, especially to improve the hoof.

Birdsville horse disease a disease caused by the ingestion of large quantities of the indigofera plant and seen to occur mostly in central Australia; characterized by sudden loss of weight and appetite, lethargy and imbalance; indigofera poisoning

birth *n.* the process of producing offspring; parturition — *vi.* to foal; mares usually birth during the night

bishoping *n.* a dishonest dealer's method of altering a horse's teeth to camouflage its age; a drill is used to recreate incisor infundibula (cups) which are then stained dark with a hot iron

bis in die twice a day (used in medicinal prescriptions); b.i.d.

bismuth *n.* a medicinal powder used internally to line the stomach and intestines and externally as a protective ointment, lotion, or powder; trade name Forgastrin

bit *n.* the metal mouthpiece on a bridle; there are numerous kinds including the **snaffle, curb, bridoon** (or **bradoon**), **spade, kimblewicke, pelham, weymouth, Tom Thumb, anti lug**, etc. — *vt.* to put a bit in (a horse's mouth); when a horse takes the bit in its teeth, it clenches it between its teeth, thereby taking control away from the rider

bit burr a round leather piece, fitted around the mouthpiece of a bit, that has bristles pointing inward; used to deter a horse from hanging to one side; brush pricker

bite *vt., vi.* to cut with the teeth or to sting, as an insect does — *n.* 1. the act of biting 2. a wound or bruise incurred by a bite 3. in dentistry, the way the upper and lower teeth meet

bit gnathitis chewing on the bit

bit guards *see* **lozenges**

Bitjug *n.* a Russian breed, probably the oldest; originated by crossing native mares of the Bitjug River area with Dutch cold-blood stallions; about 15.3 h.h.

bitting rig a combination of bridle, harness pad and crupper; used to teach horses to flex at the poll

black *adj.* having a coat color that is the complete opposite of white; applied only to a horse having a true black coat, mane and tail, with no other color or light areas, except perhaps white face or leg markings; not to be confused with what is termed brown

black patch disease the common term for a fungal toxic growth, *Rhizoctonia leguminicola,* on certain legumes, which can affect horses who graze on infected plants or eat hay from infected sources; toxic reaction causes drooling, tearing, diarrhea, frequent urination, severe weight loss, and death depending on the amount consumed, as well as fetal malformation and abortion in pregnant mares

black saddler a person who specializes in making items of saddlery

blacksmith *n.* a person who shoes horses as a profession; may make and fit the shoes on or may use ready-made ones; farrier; smith; smithy

bladder *n.* a sac of membranous body tissue that inflates to hold liquids; especially the urinary bladder in the pelvic cavity which holds urine

blank *n.* in hunting, a covert without a fox in it

blanket *n.* a type of color marking of the Appaloosa that features a white back or rump having spots of any color

blanket *n.* a cover that is strapped on to a horse for protection from cold weather; a saddle blanket is a pad that is put on a horse under the saddle to protect the back

blastocyst *n. see* **blastula**

blastula *n.* an embryo at the early stage of development when it comprises one or several cell layers (blastoderms) surrounding a hollow sphere (blastocele)

blaze *n.* a wide white mark on the face running from between the eyes down to the muzzle and possibly including one or both lips

bleb *n.* a blister or fluid-filled sac under the skin — **blebby** *adj.*

bleed *vi.* to lose blood

bleeder *n.* a horse with one of several blood disorders manifested by bleeding from one or both nostrils; common in racehorses due to strain; may also be caused by an ulcerative infection of the guttural pouch

Blenkinsop shoe a thin broad-webbed shoe to counteract stumbling and slipping; at the toe of the front shoe, half of its width is turned up at an angle of 22 degrees; heels are tapered; the hind shoe is similar, except that it is not rolled but has two toe clips

blepharitis *n.* inflammation of the eyelids; may be caused by an injury or bacterial infection

blepharospasm *n.* spasm of the eyelids caused by a pathology of the eyeball

blind *adj.* without sight — **blindness** *n.*

blind boil a pus-filled eruption on the skin that does not form a core and may not burst

blind bucker a horse that bucks "blindly" when ridden, heading into anything

blind country in hunting, terrain unsuitable for horses' footing

blinders *n.pl.* a pair of leather flaps on a bridle that prevent a horse from seeing peripherally; also called blinkers

blindfold *vt.* to cover a horse's eyes as a method of restraint for such purposes as leading the horse near or through a fire, for doctoring, etc. — *n.*

blind spavin arthritis of the joint surfaces of the hock, but without visible signs of spavin; rarely causes lameness; occult spavin

blind staggers a condition caused by eating plants rich in selenium, such as milk vetch; characterized by marked behavioral changes: the horse may walk into trees and fences, act depressed, and be oblivious to other animals

blinkers *n.pl. see* **blinders**

blister *n.* a raised patch of skin filled with watery fluid — *vt.* to treat (an ailment, as e.g. a sprained ligament) by applying an ointment which stimulates the circulation, raises a blister and thereby promotes healing — *vi.* to form a blister

blister beetle an insect that may be black, gray, green or striped and is sometimes found in alfalfa hay; inflames the intestines when ingested and can be fatal to horses; name derives from the blistering effects of the beetle's juices when applied to the skin; they contain the chemical cantharidin; meloid; cantharis

bloat *n.* a gassy swelling of the abdomen — *vt., vi.* to swell or puff up, as caused by an abnormal condition, or deliberately by the horse when being girthed — **bloated** *adj.*

block *n.* an obstruction of normal inside body function, such as a heart block or the interruption of nerve impulses by means of anesthesia or pressure

blood *n.* 1. the fluid, usually red, circulating in the heart, arteries and veins; it carries oxygen and cell-building material to, and carbon dioxide and waste matter from, the body tissues; the amount of blood in a horse's body comprises about one-eighteenth of total body weight 2. descent from purebred stock

blood bay a color between the light tan of a sandy bay and seal brown of a mahogany bay

blood blister the formation of a blood clot when there is a break in a blood vessel; usually caused by an injury

blood-brain barrier the brain's barrier to diffusion of foreign substances, such as drugs, from the bloodstream into the brain and spinal cord

blood chemistry profile several tests conducted simultaneously to classify and compare the quantity of enzymes and other chemicals in the blood

blooded *adj.* of fine stock or breed; thoroughbred; purebred

blood gases gases dissolved in the blood, such as oxygen and carbon dioxide

blood glucose simple sugar circulating in the blood stream

blood lactate the level of lactic acid in the blood; as lactic acid is a by-product of strenuous exercise, the assessment of this level is used to indicate fitness or fatigue; **serum lactate**

blood mark a patch of red-colored hairs on a grey coat that can, with age, extend over an ever increasing area; very rare

blood pressure the pressure of blood against the inner walls of blood vessels, especially the arteries

blood spavin the normal saphenous vein over the inside of the hock, which if enlarged is considered a blemish but not an unsoundness

blood-stock *n.* purebred horses

blood urea nitrogen (BUN) a test to determine the adequacy of kidney function by using the blood level of urea nitrogen

bloodworms *n. see* **strongyle**

bloom *n.* a horseman's term which describes a very healthy looking horse

blow *vi.* to produce a noise by strong expiration; trumpet

blow a stirrup to lose a stirrup; if this happens in a rodeo contest, the rider is disqualified

blow away in hunting, to signal the hounds to chase a fox by blowing on the hunting horn in a certain way

blowfly *n.* a fly that breeds in wounds, carrion, and rotting garbage; seldom poses a problem for healthy horses but can be bothersome to them

blow up 1. to start bucking 2. in dressage or shows, to break from the pace at which the horse is meant to be going, or generally to misbehave

blue eye *see* **glass eye; wall eye**

blue nose disease *see* **photosensitization**

blue ribbon the first prize in a competition

bluff *n.* a head covering with leather eye sockets used to calm an ill-tempered horse

bobtail disease *see* **alkali disease**

body language the nonverbal communication used by a rider to guide a mount — *see also* **aid**

body rope a way of tying a rope which sends the rope around the horse's girth (tied in a non-slip knot), then out between the forelegs and through the halter ring

Boerperd *n.* a South African breed developed by the Boers and used in the Boer Wars; today used on farms and for riding, especially endurance riding; often 5-gaited; 13.3–15.3 h.h.; Boer Pony

Boer Pony *see* **Boerperd**

bog rider a cowboy who rescues cattle caught in mud or bog

bog spavin a soft swelling caused by inflammation of the bursa in the joint capsule at the front and sides of the hock; caused by faulty foot conformation (such as a straight, upright hock) or stress on the hock from sudden, sharp movement; does not ususally cause lameness

boil *n.* a pus-filled eruption on the skin; a **blind boil** is one that does not form a core and may not burst; furuncle

boil over to start bucking; blow up

bolt *vi.* to run away — **bolter** *n.* a horse given to running away

bolt a fox a hunting, to make a fox leave a drain or an earth

bolt food *vt.* to eat too rapidly; may cause indigestion

bolus *n.* 1. a lump or mass of chewed food 2. a large pill

bond[1] *n.* a close relationship between horses which can have definite preferences for particular pasturemates, or between mare and foal, referred to right after foaling as **bonding**, or between horse and human — *vi.*

bond[2] *vt.* to apply a substance, which hardens after application, to a hoof which is damaged by cracks, etc., to prevent it from getting worse

bonding *n.* process by which a mare and newborn foal develop a close relationship

bone *n.* material which forms the skeleton of the body; the horse has an average of 210 bones; **bony** *adj.* thin; **good bone** a desirable measurement of the circumference of bone right below the knee or hock; **light bone** a smaller than desirable measurement of the same bone

bone in the ground in hunting, hard terrain in cold weather

bone marrow soft tissue inside long bones in which blood cells form

bone spavin an arthritic bone enlargement that can be felt through the skin in and around the hock joint; often caused by sickle- and cow-hocks or by stress on the hock from activities like polo, calf-roping and racing, especially in young horses

bonnet *n.* a facial color pattern in which white covers the entire face

bookmaker *n.* a person licensed to accept bets placed by others on horses

booster shot an additional immunizing injection, following the original one

boot *n.* 1. a white hair marking of the leg extending from the hoof to about halfway between hoof and knee or hock 2. a protection for the hoof made of leather, rubber, felt, or plastic, of which there are many kinds for different purposes

boot jack a device made of wood or metal used to pull off riding boots; one end is raised and carved out to hold the heel of the boot while the other end supports the other foot while pulling

boots and saddle a cavalry bugle call used as the first signal for mounted drill or other mounted formation

boracic acid *see* **boric acid**

borborygmus *n, pl.* **-mi** normal abdominal or bowel noise

bordering *n.* a facial marking in which there is a roan color bordering a pure white mark; the skin of the bordered area is black while that of the white area is pink

boredom *n.* frustration over lack of activity or freedom to graze which leads to restlessness and can engender bad habits, such as cribbing and pawing — **bored** *adj.*

boric acid a compound used as a mild antiseptic, espec. for eyes; boracic acid

boring *n.* a bad habit wherein a horse under saddle lowers the head, arching the neck as much as possible, trying to resist the bit and increase speed; the rider should check this by a "pull and give" rein action and use of legs — **bore** *vi.*

borium *n.* steel tubing that is heated by a farrier to be sectioned into small knobs or flakes and applied to the ground surface of horseshoes to increase traction in slippery winter conditions or on pavement and also to increase durability of the shoes

borna disease a contagious viral disease, meningo-encephalomyelitis, which develops suddenly; characterized by fatigue and intestinal disorders, with dribbling and clapping of the jaws; constipation; and paralysis of the hind limbs, tail, tongue and muscles that control chewing; mortality is high

Bornu *n.* an African breed (Chad and Nigeria) used chiefly under saddle; gray with black legs, mane, and tail; —height varies

bosal *n.* specifically, the noseband of the hackamore bridle; more generally, a type of hackamore having a braided rawhide noseband attached to a large knot under the horse's chin

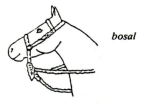

bosal

Bosnian *n.* a mountain pony breed from Yugoslavia where it is used for farm work and mountain transport; 12.3–15 h.h.

bot egg knife an implement for scraping bot eggs off a horse; the tiny yellow eggs cannot successfully be brushed off, but the knife, which is available in various designs is highly effective

bot egg knife

botfly *n.* one of a number of related flies resembling small bumblebees, whose larvae are parasitic in horses —*see also Gastrophilus equi, Gastrophilus hemorrhoidalis, Gastrophilus nasalis; Gastrophilus pecorum*

bots *n.pl.* the larvae of botflies, of which there are several species. The female botfly lays eggs on the horse's hair, usually on the legs but sometimes on the hairs of the muzzle and cheeks; the eggs look like tiny, yellowish/white specks that resemble pollen (removable with a bot knife). These hatch larvae which can be licked and ingested into the stomach where they grow; after 8–10 months they pass out of the horse, burrow in the soil and emerge a month later as a fly; bot maggots cause gastritis, perforation of the stomach and rectal hemorrhage; —*see also Gastrophilus equi*

bottom line the line of pedigree in which the dam of a horse is described; the top line describes the sire

botulism *n.* a lethal forage poisoning caused by *Clostridium botulinum* bacteria found in barnyard soil and moldy feed or rotting, protein-rich organic matter; horses are susceptible and, when poisoned, symptoms are difficulty in swallowing with accompanying drooling from the mouth and spillage of food and water, tongue hanging out, weakness and muscle tremors, and finally paralysis of respiratory muscles resulting in death in advanced cases; an antitoxin is effective if given in time —*see also* **shaker-foal syndrome**

Boulonnais *n.* a heavy French draft breed; about 16–16.3 h.h.

boundary rider a ranch worker who rides and checks the fencing on the huge Australian cattle and sheep properties to find holes and repair them

bowed tendon a warm swelling, or bow, from oozing, inflammatory fluid and capillary hemorrhage resulting from the stretching and tearing of tissue fibers comprising the superficial flexor tendon behind the cannon bone in the leg; caused by insufficient or delayed lift of the pastern with consequent overdorsiflexion of the fetlock, which strains the tendon and tears it. Common culprits are: excessive weight or improperly applied weight, such as when leaning into a sharp turn; jumping; slipping; going on overly soft, deep footing; long-toe/low-heel trimming. Uncommon in the hind leg.

bowlegs *n.pl.* lateral deviation of the hocks in which they are set outward, with the toes turned in (pigeon-toed); often causes a twisting motion of the hock as the foot meets the ground, with the resultant tendency to develop bog spavin and thoroughpin; bandy legs —**bowlegged** *adj.*

bow tie a timed playday event in which a contestant rides around five barrels set in a bow-tie pattern

box muzzle a leather or plastic covering for a horse's muzzle shaped like a round box (or bucket) which attaches to a halter; prevents biting, coprophagy, etc.; there is also a woven-wire type

Brabant *n.* a Belgian draft breed with short back and short, feathered legs; docile and very heavy and powerful; of ancient heritage. There has been little infusion of other blood through the centuries, so these horses breed true to type and are still bred in large numbers in their native land; many have been exported to America and elsewhere; 15.3–17 h.h.

brace[1] *n.* 1. a support for a broken limb 2. a mild counterirritant applied to the skin to stimulate circulation

brace[2] *n.* 1. in hunting, a pair (a — of foxes) 2. in polo, the position from which a stroke is played

brachial *adj.* relating to the foreleg

brachialis *n.* a muscle that flexes the elbow joint

brachiocephalicus *n.* a muscle, the longest in the equine body, that extends from the forearm over the shoulder, along the side of the neck, and up to the head; controls forward motion of the foreleg

brachium *n.* the area in the foreleg from shoulder to elbow

brachydonty *n.* abnormal shortness of teeth; a possible indication of cribbing

brachy gnathia *see* **parrot mouth**

bracken fern a poisonous, coarse plant, *Pteridium aquilinum,* commonly found in wet, temperate areas; if ingested continually it causes acute vitamin B deficiency with usually fatal results; the poisoning is characterized by incoordination, staggering, and muscle tremors

brackish *adj.* mildly salty, referring to water, as in marshes near the sea; the French Camargue horses live in this kind of area —**brackishness** *n.*

bradycardia *n.* abnormally slow heartbeat

braid *vt.* to interweave three strands of hair, as the mane —**plait** *n.*

braiding comb a grooming device which facilitates even parting of the hair

braiding comb

brain *n.* the mass of nerve tissue in the cranium forming an extension of the spinal cord; the **brain stem** is the portion of the brain connecting it with the spinal cord; the horse's brain is about 5½ × 4 inches and weighs about 24 oz.

bran *n.* the skin or husk of grains of wheat, rye, oats, etc. separated in milling; **bran mash** is made by mixing 2–3 lbs. of bran with boiling water and is given to horses as a mild laxative and aid to digestion

branch *n.* the area of a horseshoe that encompasses the nail holes on either side

brand *vt.* to permanently mark (a horse) for identification; there are two kinds of branding: **fire branding,** which is applied with a red-hot branding iron, and **freeze branding,** which is applied with a frozen branding iron —*n. see* **tattoo**

bran disease *see* **big head disease**

break *vt.* 1. to tame and train (a horse);

the term originated in the days when rough methods were used for quick results, as opposed to methods used today   2. to move into a gait other than the directed one

break down to lacerate the suspensory ligament or fracture a sesamoid bone, which results in the back of the fetlock dropping to the ground

breaking bit a bit used when breaking young horses, consisting of a large round bar with attached small movable pendants in the center

breaking the barrier in rodeo calf-roping, the roper and his horse wait behind a barrier for the calf to be let out of its chute; if they start too soon, they "break the barrier," be it a flimsy rope or a beam of light

break maiden a horse or rider winning a race for the first time

breakover *n.* the phase of a horse's stride when the heel lifts and the hoof pivots at the toe and leaves the ground — *vi.*

breast *n.* a muscle mass between the forelegs covering the front of the chest

breastband *n.* a device of leather or nylon used across a horse's chest, which attaches to the saddle and girth to prevent the saddle from slip- *breastband* ping back, or used just for show; breastplate; breast collar

breastbone *n.* see **sternum**

breast collar *see* **breastband**

breastplate *see* **breastband**

breathe *vi.* to inhale and exhale; respirate. Normal adult respiration rate at rest is 12–20 breaths per minute; increases when exercising and in certain illnesses. Young horses have a faster rate, the younger, the faster.

Horses do not breathe through their mouths. — **breath** *n.*

breech birth a birth in which the rump or hind feet of the foal are presented first instead of the normal delivery of forefeet and head first — *see also* **dystocia**

breeching *n.* a strap that goes around the buttocks of the horse and forms part of the harness; also one that attaches to a pack saddle

breed *n.* a substantial number of horses having common ancestors and characteristics that distinguish them from other horses and have the power to almost certainly transmit those characteristics to their progeny; there are about 207 distinct breeds, Russia being the country having the largest number, at least 27 — *vt.* to produce (offspring) — *vi.* to reproduce

breeder's bag a bag to collect semen which is placed over a stallion's penis before he mounts the mare

breeding hobbles hobbles used on a mare's hind legs to prevent her from kicking the stallion when mounted

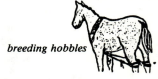

breeding hobbles

breeding roll a roll used between stallion and mare at the time of breeding to prevent an excessively deep or injurious penetration

breeding stitch a suture placed at the upper end of a mare's vulva opening to prevent tearing

breeze *vt.* to work (a horse) at a fairly fast pace — *vi.* to gallop

breeze in in racing, to win very easily

Breton *n.* a French draft breed bred in Brittany, dating to 2000 B.C.; a strong and energetic worker, used on farms and somtimes for pulling coaches;

matures quickly and is used in France for meat. In 1909 this breed was divided into three sub-types: the Corlay, Postier, and Grande Breton; 15–16.1 h.h.

brick wall in jumping, an obstacle made of boxes to resemble bricks

bridle *n.* a head harness used to control and guide a horse when riding or driving; consists of a headstall and reins with a bit or, as in a hackamore bridle, without a bit

bridle bracket a circular wall mounting for hanging up a bridle

bridle butt the part of a cow- *bridle* hide cut from either side of *bracket* the spine from shoulder to tail and sold in pairs for high quality leather reins

bridle path 1. a style of mane wherein a section of mane from the poll down is roached to form a path for the headstall 2. a path for horseback riding

bridle-wise *adj.* trained to neck-rein

bridoon *n.* a snaffle bit used in combination with a curb bit and used with a double pair of reins which allows the rider a choice of control

Brietal sodium trade name for methohexitone sodium

brisket *n.* the breast; lies between the forearms and extends immediately behind and in front of them

British Warm Blood a breed developed in Britain in the 1970s with European imports and Thoroughbreds for sports purposes. Does not breed true to type because of the variety of crosses, but the British Warm-Blood Society was founded at the end of the 1970s and these horses can be registered provided they are at least 50 percent European warm-blood types. They make very fine competitors in dressage, eventing, and show-jumping; 15.3–16.3 h.h.

broad ligament the membrane in which the uterus is suspended and which contains its blood supply

broken *adj.* (*colloq.*) (of a horse) tamed and trained — **broke** (*colloq.*) — **green broke** (*colloq.*) partially broken

broken axis non-alignment of pastern with hoof wall; often caused by improper shoeing or trimming; **broken in angle**

broken knee a condition in which the skin over the knee is being or has been broken

broken lines an exercise at a walk or trot ridden in a straight line, then around in a sharp turn, without changing stride, to continue in a straight line in another direction, making a zig-zag pattern

broken-neck *adj.* having an abrupt bend in the neck at the wrong place instead of bending uniformly

broken winded *see* **heaves**

brome *n.* any of various tall grasses among which some types are weeds but others may be used for hay; also bromegrass

bronchi *n.pl.* tubes extending from the trachea (windpipe) into both lungs; the "branches" of the respiratory "tree"; bronchial tubes — **bronchial** *adj.*

bronchioles *n.* the smallest divisions of the bronchi

bronchiolitis *n.* lung inflammation starting with inflamed bronchioles that become filled with mucus, causing painful and difficult respiration

bronchitis *n.* inflammation of the bronchi

bronchodilator *n.* a medication that dilates the bronchial tubes

bronchopneumonia *n.* inflammation of the bronchial tubes and lungs

bronchospasm *n.* a spasm of the muscles surrounding the bronchioles

bronchus *n., pl.* **-chi** *see* **bronchi**

bronco *n.* a wild, unbroken, or partially tamed horse

bronco-busting *n.* 1. the breaking of broncos 2. the riding of bucking broncos in a rodeo; **bronco-buster** a person who breaks broncos

bronc riding a rodeo event wherein a bronco is ridden with only a wide leather band around his girth from which a leather handhold protrudes

bronc saddle a saddle, used in rodeo saddle bronc riding, which lacks a horn and has narrow oxbow stirrups with leathers set well forward and swinging freely to allow the rider to get his feet up to the bronco's shoulders

brood mare a female horse used for breeding

broomtail *n.* a Western term for an inferior horse

brougham *n.* a closed, 4-wheeled carriage with an outside driver's seat, named after the English politician Lord Brougham and originally built in 1839

browband *n. see* **headband**

brown *adj.* a color often mistaken for black; the difference is in the flanks and muzzle, both of which are brown in a horse of this color

browse *vi.* to nibble at tree leaves or to graze

brucella abortus a rare abortion caused by the brucella genus of bacteria

brucellosis *n.* a bacterial (*Brucella*) disease of the ligament extending from poll to withers; **bangs** —*see also* **poll evil, fistulous withers**

bruise *n.* a contusion on the body surface, tissue, hoof, etc. — *vt.*

Brumby *n.* an Australian wild horse that multiplied from imported horses around 1851. Due to interbreeding and poor grazing environment, these horses deteriorated in quality. Because of their poor quality and typically intractable character, as well as their posing a nuisance to farmers, large numbers were culled and few remain today.

Brumby runner an Australian bush horseman who captures wild horses

brush *n.* 1. an implement for grooming; usually three kinds are used for the body: a dandy brush, with coarse, stiff bristles for removing surface mud and dirt; a body brush, with semi-stiff bristles for cleaning the coat thoroughly; and a finishing brush, with soft bristles for final, gentle, all-over use — *vt.* to use a brush 2. in hunting, the tail of the fox

brush fence a jumping obstacle composed, either artificially or naturally, of brushwood or some sort of plant

brush fence

brush oxer a brush fence with posts and rails on either side

brush picker *see* **bit burr**

brushing *n.* a faulty way of going in which the inside edge of a foot in motion brushes against the inside of the opposite fetlock, causing cuts and abrasions; may occur with either hind- or forelegs

brushing boots boots that fasten on the outside and protect the inside of the fetlock; made of rubber, felt or leather; galloping boots

brushing boots

buccal *n.* the inner surface of the cheek

buccinator muscle a cheek muscle

Bucephalus *n.* the famous war-horse owned by Alexander the Great, who held the stallion in such high regard that he built the city of Bucephala (Jalapur) in India in his honor

buck *vi.* to leap into the air with all

feet off the ground, head down, back arched; pitch —*n*.

buckaroo *n*. 1. a cowboy 2. a broncobuster

buckboard *n*. an open carriage with 4 wheels and seats that rest on a flexible wood flooring, the ends of which are fastened directly to the axles

bucked knee a slightly bent knee due to scar tissue or contraction of ligaments behind the knee joint

bucked shin an incomplete shear fracture, or several fractures, of the cannon bone in young horses (chiefly racehorses) incurred by heavy work; new bone forms but pain and warmth in the area signal the start of shear fracture of the new, undeveloped bone; if work is not then reduced, bucked shins will result forming a periostitis at the front of the bone; also called metacarpal periostitis; sore shin

bucket elimination a mounted game in which competitors, in single file, jump over a successively decreasing line of buckets or cans; touching the bucket or refusal eliminates the competitor; it continues until all riders are eliminated or only one bucket remains; in the latter case the remaining competitors continue till one winner is left

buck eye a protruding eye

bucks *n.pl.* wooden crosspieces that form part of a pack saddle

buckskin *n*. a coloration that is yellow with black points; often used synonymously with dun but differing exactly in primitive markings (dorsal and zebra strips), the dun having them and the buckskin having none; shade variations include dusty buckskin (brownish cast to the yellow color), dark buckskin (black hairs with yellow ones), silver buckskin (cream) —*adj*.

buck tooth *see* **parrot mouth**

buddy pad a pad that attaches to the cantle of a saddle for use by a second rider when riding double

Budyonny *n*. a Russian breed of very good conformation, used in competitive sports; originally bred in the 1920s for the cavalry with crosses of local breeds with Thoroughbreds; registry established in 1949; 15.2–16.1 h.h.

buffing *n*. a less serious form of brushing in which the horn of the inside of the hoof just below the coronet is struck by the shoe of the opposite foot; horses with low, close action can be prone to this

bug-eyed *adj*. having eyeballs that bulge out unattractively beyond the upper orbital rim of the eye; not to be confused with prominent bone orbits themselves, characteristic, for example, of the Arabian

buggy *n*. a light, two- or four-wheeled carriage, usually drawn by one horse

build *n*. the exterior structure of the body

bulbourethral gland an accessory sex gland of the stallion

bulbs *n.pl.* the round cushions of the heel of the foot

bulla *n*. a large blister

bulldogging *n*. a rodeo event so named because the originator, a cowboy named Bill Picket, noticed that bulldogs often subdued their opponents by chewing their ears, so he always bit the ear of the steer he was wrestling —*see also* **steer wrestling**

bulldogging horse a horse used for steer wrestling

bulldog mouth *see* **undershot jaw**

bullfight *n*. an event popular in Spain, Portugal, South America and Mexico in which a matador (bullfighter) provokes a bull in various ways until it is subdued and, in Spain, killed with a sword; although the event is chiefly between man and bull, ridden horses do take a sideline part in it; they are heavily padded to protect them from the bull's horns

bullfighting clown in rodeo, a clown who gets between a bull and a downed bull rider

bullfinch *n.* in hunting, a type of jump comprising a dense hedge too high to be jumped, thus forcing horse and rider to go through it

bulling *n.* a test wherein a horse is taken against a wall and threatened with something, such as a stick, to see if he is a grunter — *see also* **grunting**

bull-nosed foot a hoof whose toe ends at an abrupt angle; may be caused by improper trimming or shoeing, heredity, or excessive wear at the toe from poor conformation or lameness; dubbed foot; dumped foot

bull riding a rodeo event in which the competitor rides a bucking bull bareback with only a rope around the bull which he holds with one hand. The rider must not touch himself, the animal or equipment with his free hand; he is not required to spur but can add points if he does; he must stay on for eight seconds to qualify.

bull rope in rodeo, a loose rope with a bell that goes around the bull and is held by the rider with one hand; it is only the rider's hold that keeps it in place; as soon as he lets go of the rope, it falls to the ground, pulled off by the weight of the heavy bell

bumper *n.* 1. an amateur race rider 2. an amateur race

BUN *see* **blood urea nitrogen**

bur, burr *n.* 1. a round instrument with spikes used in certain operations, such as the Hobday operation 2. the prickly seedcase or fruit of certain weeds, which can get caught up in and tangle a horse's mane or tail

Burguete *n.* a Spanish breed; no further information available

Burmese *n.* a hardy pony breed indigenous to Burma, used for riding and as a pack pony; has a bad character; about 13 h.h.; **Shan**

bursa *n.* fluid-filled sac surrounding joints, ligaments, tendons — **bursal** *adj.*

bursatti *n.* a skin disease found in India and characterized by fibrous tumors and ulceration of the covering skin; usually occurs in rainy seasons and is evidently caused by habronema worms

bursitis *n.* a painful inflammation of an injured bursa. Simple bursitis can become infected, which makes the bursa break and drain; it may then form a fistula which refuses to heal. There are many types of bursitis including fistula of the withers, poll evil, shoe boil, capped hock, car bruise, navicular disease, whirlbone lameness and inter-tubercular bursitis.

burst *n.* in hunting, a point at which hounds chase away quickly after the fox

bush *vt.* at an auction, to obtain a better price for a horse than that originally bid by discovering flaws that were not revealed by the auctioneer

bush track an unofficial race meeting

Butazolidin *n.* a trade name for phenylbutazone, an anti-inflammatory drug for relief of pain connected with arthritis, bursitis, etc.; bute (colloq.)

bute *n.* *see* **Butazolidin**

butorphanol *n.* an analgesic

butt *n.* 1. the thick end of something, like the handle of a whip 2. (slang) the buttocks

buttock *n.* either of the rounded parts behind the hip above the hind leg; rump

buttress *n.* the thickened part at the heel of the hoof wall

buttress foot a form of low ringbone in which the hoof takes the shape of a pyramid; pyramiditis, pyramidal disease

Buxton bit a driving bit with a bent shank

buzkashi *n.* an equestrian sport popular in Turkey and Afghanistan in which the skin of a goat or calf is filled with sand and soaked in water overnight, after which it weighs about 65–85 lbs; it is put in a marked circle on the playing field whereupon one of a number of fearless mounted competitors grabs it and tries to gallop off with it around a post and back to the circle while other riders try ferociously to snatch it away; a very dangerous game; the horses used are very valuable

bye-day *n.* in hunting, an extra meet held either during holidays or to make up for one lost due to bad weather or other circumstances

Byerley Turk one of the three foundation sires of the English Thoroughbred breed, named for his owner, a British Army officer, who captured him from a Turk in battle in Hungary in 1686, then took him to Ireland where he rode him in the battle of Boyne. After that he was taken to England where he stood at stud.

– C –

cab horse disease a ringbone enlargement on the first phalanx caused by working on hard street surfaces; lameness precedes the enlargement

cable headsetter a kind of headstall attached to a tie-down used to obtain a desirable headset

cabriolet *n.* a hooded, one-horse, two-wheeled carriage seating two with a rear platform for a groom

cachexia *n.* a state of emaciation

cade *n.* a foal reared by a human

cadence *n.* in dressage, the rhythmic movement of a horse

Caesarean section a surgical operation for removal of a fetus when it cannot be born in the normal manner

Calabrese *n.* an Italian breed developed in the 19th century for use as a riding horse; today, after much cross-breeding, there are few purebreds remaining; 15.3–16.1 h.h.

calash *n.* 1. a light carriage with low wheels and folding top 2. a folding carriage top

calcaneo-cuboid ligament a ligament at the back of the hock which unites the point of hock with the back of the cannon bone

calcaneus, -um *n.* the tarsal bone which forms the point of the hock —**calcaneal** *adj.*

calciferol *n.* a crystalline alcohol

calcification *n.* the hardening of body tissue due to calcium deposits —**calcify** *vi., vt.* to harden by deposit of calcium salts

calcium *n.* a chemical element normally present in body tissues, including bones, teeth, blood plasma, etc.; calcium and phosphorous are the chief minerals in bone —**calcareous** *adj.* having calcium

calculus *n.* a mass or "stone" in the body, such as a kidney stone

calf horse a specially trained horse used for calf roping

calf knees a conformation defect wherein the knees are set too far back

calf roping one of the standard events in rodeo, in which the rider ropes a calf with a 25 ft. lariat and then swiftly dismounts to tie the calf by three legs; the horse must get the rider close enough to the calf to rope the calf and then keep the rope taut until the rider signals the horse to release it

Calgary Stampede Canada's top rodeo, held every year in July; in addition to the usual rodeo events such as bronc and bull riding, steer wrestling, etc., there are the exciting chuckwagon races, Indian dancing, Thoroughbred racing, and a musical ride of the Royal Canadian Mounted Police

California head set a horse's manner of holding the head erect when being ridden

California reins closed reins, about eight feet long from bit end to bit end, with a romal; often these reins have buttons, barrels or knots which are convenient for gripping and give better spade-bit balance

calk *n.*, *usu. pl.* a metal projection from the bottom of a horseshoe to provide traction — *vt.* 1. to furnish with calks 2. to accidentally inflict self injury with a calk

calks

calling *n.* in polo, commands in play by the captain or member of the team

call over in racing, the setting by bookmakers of ante-post prices for betting on certain races; the odds against the horses are called over and changed in accordance with the betting

callus *n.* 1. new bone which develops in soft tissues between ends of a fractured bone 2. a hard thickened area of the skin

calomel (mercury subchloride) a medication used internally as a purgative or externally, as for thrush

calorie, calory *n.* a measurement of energy content of foods when oxidized in the body

Camargue *n.* a French breed that gets its name from the Camargue area of Southern France, in the Rhône delta, which is its home. The hardy, agile horses of this breed do not have good conformation but are interesting for their unusual qualities. They are called the "white horses of the sea" because they are always white in maturity and thrive on tough grass and salt water; they are often used to work the well known black bulls of the area for the bullring. Rarely exceed 15 h.h.

Camarillo *n.* an Albino horse with black eyes

cambendazole *n.* generic name for a dewormer

camera patrol equipment for filming a horse race; deters illegalities

camouflage *vt.*, *vi.* to conceal; during wars horses have sometimes been camouflaged with paint; dishonest horsetraders may sometimes camouflage the age of a horse by creating false infundibula — *see also* **bishoping** *n.*

Campagne School in dressage, a level below haute école; lower school

camp drafting an Australian stockman's sport often staged at rodeos and major shows, or as an independent event. The rider separates a large bullock from a group of cattle and drives it at high speed over a course marked by poles or oildrums to a designated place called "the yards."

camped *adj.* having a stance in which the forelegs are stretched straight forward and the rear legs straight back; a horse may take such a position briefly to stretch its muscles or be trained to pose in this way on command; otherwise, if a horse does so at length of its own accord, a pathological problem probably exists — **camp** *vt.*, *vi.* stretched

Campolino *n.* a Brazilian breed developed in the late 19th century by crossing the native Crioulo with Criollo,

Andalusian, Thoroughbred, and Percheron stock

campylobacter *n.* a gram negative bacteria; subspecies include *C. fetus intestinalis*, causing abortion, and *C. fetus jejuni* (*Vibrio hepaticus*) causing diarrhea.

Canadian pox *see* **acne**

canas *n.* an old riding sport in Spain introduced by the Arabs; riders carrying leather shields threw spears at one another

cancer *n.* a malignant growth or tumor

Candida albicans a fungus that may cause uterine or vaginal infection, or infect a foal's tongue; manifested by whitish coating of the affected area

canine *n.* any of four small pointed teeth that develop in the male horse at five years of age just behind the corner incisors; mares may rarely have two very small ones

canker *n.* ulceration of the sole and frog caused by malfunction and growth loss of the horn with moist, fetid discharge

cannon *n.* the bone between knee and fetlock in the foreleg and between hock and fetlock in the hind leg; does not grow longer after birth

cannula *n.* an instrument for insertion into a body channel —**cannular** *adj.* —**cannulate** *vt.*

canter *n.* a three-beat gait resembling a slow gallop; originally called the Canterbury gallop in allusion to the easy pace of pilgrims riding to the shrine of Thomas à Becket in Canterbury, England —*see also* **collected canter; disunited canter; counter canter** — *vi.*

cantharis *n., pl.* **-tharides** 1. blister beetle; Spanish fly 2. an extract from the blister beetle, also called **cantharidin**, which is used for blistering; if ingested, it inflames the intestines with sometimes fatal results

canthus *n., pl.* **-thi** either corner of the eye where upper and lower lids meet

cantle *n.* the rear part of a saddle that projects upward

cantle bag a kidney-shaped, zippered bag with two rings to fasten onto the cantle of a Western saddle

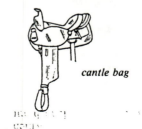

cantle bag

cantle-boarding *n.* a rodeo term describing the action of a saddle-bronc rider whose legs swing back so far that the spurs strike the saddle's cantle

cantle saddle a small saddle to carry a child behind the front rider; it forms to the cantle of a Western saddle

cap *n.* 1. a hard, velvet-covered piece of rider's headwear —*see also* **helmet** 2. a horse's headwear attachable to halter or bridle; horse cap; can serve as a cooling cap when soaked with water or repellent cap when sprayed with water-based fly repellent 3. fee paid by a guest for the privilege of hunting at a meet; capping fee

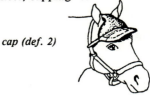

cap (def. 2)

capel *n.* 1. a swelling at the back of the hock or point of elbow; capulet 2. a farm horse used in medieval times

caper *vi.* to buck playfully, as seen particularly in young horses — *n.*

capillary permeability the ability of fluids and nutriments to pass through the walls of capillaries into body tissues

capillary refill time the time it takes for blood to return to the gums after pressure is momentarily applied; normally one or two seconds; longer time may indicate low blood pressure, shock or dehydration

capped elbow a round, soft, fluid-filled swelling or bursitis on the elbow, which later hardens; caused by irritation from a front shoe pressing on the elbow when the horse is lying down or from the shoe on the affected leg hitting the elbow when, for example, stamping at flies or from excessively high action; shoe boil

capped hock a bursitis or swelling on the point of the hock caused from bruising; this is often done on the tailgate of a trailer —*see also* **bursitis**

capped knee *see* **big knee**

capping fee a fee for the privilege of hunting paid by a guest when arriving at a meet; cap

Ca-P ratio calcium-phosphorus ratio

capriole *n.* in dressage, an exercise wherein the horse springs high above the ground and kicks out its hind legs

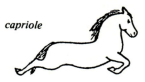

capriole

capsularis *n.* a muscle that flexes the shoulder joint

capsule *n.* a covering, as of a body organ

capsulitis *n.* inflammation of a joint capsule

captan *n.* a fungicide used to treat ringworm

carbachol *n.* medicinal compound with a faint fishy odor used for treatment of mild colic, etc.

carbamate *n.* a synthetic insecticide

created from carbamic acid

carbohydrate *n.* any of certain compounds comprising carbon, hydrogen, and oxygen which form the major part of animal nutrition, supplying energy to the body; examples include sugar, starch, and cellulose

carbolic acid a strong antiseptic solution produced from coaltar; rarely used now as it tends to penetrate the skin and mucous membranes; phenol

carbon bisulphide an anthelmintic for botfly larvae; it is very toxic and should be administered professionally and with much caution; also **carbon disulphide**

car bruise bursitis at the pin bones, the bony prominences of the rump

carbuncle *n.* a localized, painful infection of the tissue beneath the skin, discharging pus through several openings —**carbuncular** *adj.*

carcass *n.* the dead body of an animal

carcinogen *n.* a cancer producing substance —**carcinogenic** *adj.*

carcinoma *n.* a malignant tumor of the epithelium —**carcinomatous** *adj.*

carcinomatosis *n.* a condition of widespread growth of carcinomatous tumors

cardia *n.* the one-way valve at the entrance to the stomach that prevents reflux

cardiac *adj.* of or relating to the heart

cardiac muscle the heart muscle, capable of independent activity without outside stimulus

cardioactive glycoside a heart stimulant found in plants

cardiogram *n.* a recording made by a cardiograph; **electrocardiogram**

cardiograph *n.* an instrument used to record a cardiogram —**cardiography** *n.* the process of making a cardiogram; —*see also* **electrocardiograph; electrocardiography**

cardiopulmonary *adj.* of or relating to the heart and lungs

cardiovascular *adj.* of or relating to the heart and blood vessels

caries *n.* dental decay; although the equine tooth is usually hard enough to resist bacterial invasion, it does sometimes become subject to decay

carotene, carotin *n.* hydrocarbon found in plants and converted in the liver to vitamin A; particularly concentrated in carrots

carotid artery a large artery extending along the windpipe at the underside of the neck and supplying blood to the head

carousel, carrousel *n.* a musical ride involving a group of riders performing equine dance routines together, usually in period costume

carpal *adj.* of the carpus or knee

carpal joint the knee

carpal sheath a membrane covering the flexor tendons in the carpal canal, which is a tunnel of bone and tissue extending along the back of the carpus

Carpathian *n.* a breed that takes its name from the Carpathian mountains of Eastern Europe, where it originated, although today it is thought of as a Polish breed; about 12.3 h.h.

carpitis *n.* inflammation of the knee joint caused by concussion associated with racing, polo, jumping, etc.; also caused by another horse's kick or a horse hitting his knee by pawing at something solid like a stable door; knee spavin, Cherry's disease

carpus *n.* knee joint; corresponds with the human wrist rather than knee since it applies only to the foreleg

carrier *n.* an individual that carries diesease-producing organisms without showing evidence of having the disease

carron oil linseed oil and lime water mixed in equal parts; used for burns

carrot *n.* a root vegetable, orange-red in color; horses love it and, being rich in vitamin A, it is good for them; should be fed in pieces to avoid choking

cart *n.* 1. any two-wheeled vehicle drawn by a horse 2. a wagon

carted *adj.* concerning a rider on a runaway horse

Carthusian *n.* a Spanish breed developed from Andalusian stock by Carthusian monks in Seville; about 15.3 h.h.

cartilage *n.* gristle; semi-hard, fibrous tissue covering some bones, particularly joints (**articular cartilage**) — *see also* **lateral cartilage**

caruncle *n.* a pea-like, soft structure in the lower corner of the eye

cascara *n.* a laxative derived from tree bark

caseation *n.* degeneration of tissue into a substance that resembles cheese as a result of tuberculosis — **caseate** *vi.*

casein *n.* a major protein component of milk

Caslick's operation partial stitching of a mare's vaginal lips

Caspian *n.* an all-purpose pony breed of ancient heritage indigenous to Iran; has been exported to America, Britain, and Australia and is used for driving competitions, but its gentle nature makes it an ideal children's mount; 10–12 h.h.

cast[1] *vt.* to force (a horse) into a reclining position using tranquilizers; to force (a horse) to lie immobile either by flexing its hind legs and setting it down before the horse is put on its side, or by pulling all four legs until the horse falls over, a method rarely used now as it can be injurious to the horse — *adj.* lying down and unable to safely get up without help

cast[2] *vt.* in hunting to order (hounds)

by voice and horn to spread out and search for the scent of the fox; they may also cast themselves over ground that is not negotiable by horse and rider

cast³ *n.* a casing made of material that hardens after it is formed; used to immobilize the site of an injury

cast⁴ *n.* shade, as in relation to coat color

castor bean plant a plant whose seeds are deadly to a horse if as few as seven are ingested

castor oil a foul-tasting liquid occasionally administered to foals up to 12 hours old to promote the passage of meconium

castrate *vt.* to surgically remove both testicles of (a male horse); geld; sterilize — **castration** *n.* — **castrated** *adj.*

catabolism *n.* the process by which living tissue is converted into waste matter

catalysis *n.* the increase or decrease of the rate of chemical reaction by means of adding a substance which itself does not thereby chemically change — **catalytic** *adj.* — **catalytically** *adv.* — **catalyst** *n.* an agent in catalysis

cataplasm *n.* a soothing poultice to reduce swelling

cataplexy *n.* a disorder that causes a horse that is totally awake to suddenly and briefly enter into a state of sleep wherein muscle paralysis occurs and the horse suddenly becomes limp and collapses; usually lasts only a few seconds

cataract *n.* an opacity of the lens of the eye; may be extremely small or may cover the whole lens; may be congenital or caused by injury — *see also* **phacofragmentation**

catarrh *n.* a contagious viral infection of the mucous membranes of the nose and or throat; characterized by an elevated temperature and nasal discharge; in its simple form, lasts about 4-5 days — **catarrhal, catarrhous** *adj.*

catch-as-catch-can a rodeo term describing the allowance given a calf roper to catch the animal in any manner he chooses, provided he turns the rope loose when throwing the loop and the rope holds the calf until he reaches it

catch hold in hunting, the collection of hounds by the huntsman to take them forward in response to a voiced signal that the fox is seen

catching a whip a coachman's skillfull toss of the thong of his driving whip around the crop

catch pigeons in racing, a term for sprinters

catchweight *adj.* in racing, having no set rules on the weights carried by racehorses; this no longer applies today, except in a race between only two horses — *adv.*

catecholamine *n.* a compound, such as dopamine or adrenaline, that is a secretion of the adrenal gland and affects the sympathetic nervous system

catgut *n.* a tough, threadlike material made from the intestines of sheep, horses, etc., and used for suturing wounds

cat hairs long, individual hairs that appear on a horse's coat after clipping

cathartic *n.* a laxative

catheter *n.* a tube inserted into natural orifices of the body for withdrawal of fluid, especially urine — **catheterization** *n.* insertion of such a tube

CAT scan *see* **computerized tomography**

cauda *n.* tail — **caudal** *adj.* — **caudally** *adv.* — **caudate, -ed.** *adj.* having a tail

caudal teeth the lower cheek teeth

caustic *adj.* causing burns (said of chemicals)

cauterize *vt.* to burn (tissue) with a caustic substance or an electric instrument (*see* **electrocautery**) to seal blood vessels or for other curative purposes —**cauterization** *n.*

cautery *n.* 1. an instrument or agent for cauterization 2. the procedure of cauterizing; firing

cavalcade *n.* a procession of riders

cavaletti *n.* a series of usu. round wooden poles each extending between wooden crisscrosses and elevated about six to eight inches above the ground and spaced at set intervals; the horse is either lunged or ridden over the poles, which provides good training and develops balance

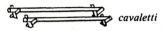 *cavaletti*

cavalier *n.* a horseman, chiefly one who is armed

cavalry *n.* a military unit originally comprising only horses and riders, though today a horse cavalry may be mechanized; the Assyrians were the first people to use cavalry horses and horse-drawn chariots in battle

cavesson *n.* a separate noseband running horizontally across the nose between the bit and the beginning of the cheekbones; it is held in place by its own headband and cheekstrap and is used as an attachment for a standing martingale and to prevent the horse from opening its mouth

cavity *n.* 1. a natural hollow area in the body 2. a dental hollow usually caused by decay

cavvy *n.* a collection of horses

Cayuse *n.* 1. an Indian horse descended from Spanish horses brought into Mexico by the first Spanish settlers in the 16th century. The Spanish Barb was crossed with the French Norman Cobb out of Canada and became known as the Cayuse. 2. a horse of nondescript breeding

cecum *n.* the pouchlike beginning of the large intestine —**cecal** *adj.*

cell *n.* a microscopic complex unit of protoplasm containing a nucleus and cytoplasm and enclosed by a membrane

cell-mediated immunity immunizing bodies attached to cell surfaces

cellulase *n.* an enzyme produced by intestinal flora

cellulitis *n.* inflammation of connective tissues

cellulose *n.* a plant fiber

CEM contagious equine metritis

cement, cementum *n.* the outer layer of the root of a tooth that connects it to the jawbone

cementoma *n.* a tumor of the dental cement-producing cells

centaur *n.* in Greek mythology, a creature with a horse's body and a man's head

center fire a Western saddle with a cinch hung from center

centesis *n. see* **abdominocentesis**

central nervous system (CNS) the part of the nervous system which supervises and coordinates all the activities of the body; consists of the brain and spinal cord

centrifuge *n.* a laboratory machine which spins to separate parts of a whole, such as cells from plasma in blood tests, by centrifugal force —*see also* **hematocrit**

centrosome *n.* a minute substance, like a dot, near the nucleus of a body cell considered responsible for the reproductive division of the cell

centrum *n.* the central body of a vertebra

cephalic *adj.* pertaining to the head

cerebellum *n.* the part of the brain behind and below the cerebrum which controls muscular movement and coordination —**cerebellar** *adj.*

cerebral *adj.* pertaining to the cerebrum

cerebral cortex the outer layer of nerve cells covering the brain

cerebral edema abnormal collection of fluid in the brain tissues

cerebral hemorrhage bleeding in the brain

cerebral motor cortex the part of the brain that controls motor function

cerebral vascular accident impairment of the blood supply to the brain, either by an aneurysm or embolism; stroke; signs include loss of coordination, lurching, crashing, and finally death

cerebrospinal nerve a nerve which originates in the brain or spinal cord

cerebrum *n.* the main part of the brain —**cerebral** *adj.*

certainty *n.* in racing, a horse regarded as a sure winner in a particular race

cerumen *n.* earwax

cervic *n., pl.* —**vices** 1. the neck 2. the neck-like part of an organ, as of the uterus —**cervical** *adj.*

cervical *adj.* relating to the cervix

cervicalis ascendens muscle muscle which extends the neck

cervical stenotic myelopathy damage to the spinal cord in the neck

cervical vertebral malformation (CVM) a spinal disorder of the neck vertebrae in which a young horse's neck bones grow abnormally in such a way as to cause compression of the spinal cord, resulting in wobbles; thought to be caused by dietary deficiency; more common in male Thoroughbreds, usually before the age of two; surgical correction can be successful, or partially so, in some cases

cervicitis *n.* inflammation of the vaginal cervix

cervicovaginal *adj.* pertaining to the vaginal cervix and vagina

cesarean (caesarean, cesarian) section the surgical removal of a fetus from the mare

cestode *n.* any of the Cestoda class of parasitic flatworms; tapeworm

CF test complement fixation test

Chadwick spring a V-shaped steel spring fitted to the bottom of the foot to keep pressure on the bars of the foot

chafe *vt.* to rub until sore —*n.* a sore caused by rubbing —*see also* **gall**; **chafe at the bit** to irritably champ at the bit

chaff *n.* 1. husks of grain separated by threshing or winnowing 2. chopped straw, usually mixed with chopped hay and used for fodder

chain twitch *see* **twitch**

chair a difficult obstacle jumped on the Grand National steeplechase course at Aintree, England; an open six-foot ditch with a five-foot, two-inch fence on the other side; located in front of the stands

chaise *n.* a light two- or four-wheeled carriage drawn by one or two horses

chalk *n.* calcium carbonate; used with other ingredients to treat diarrhea

chalk horse in Thoroughbred racing, the favorite horse

chamber *n.* 1. a hollow area in the body —*see also* **counting chamber**

chambon martingale a headsetting device consisting of a cord on either side of the head, running from the bit ring, up through a pulley at the poll strap, down to a point where the two cords

chambon martingale

join into a single strap continuing to the girth; encourages the horse to raise the root of his neck and stretch the top of the neck; it can have adverse effects and should be carefully used only by a knowledgeable person

chamfrain *n.* armor for a horse's head used in medieval times

champ at the bit to restlessly or irritably chew on the bit

change *vi.* in hunting, to stop following the scent of one fox to follow that of another (said of dogs)

change of hand a rider's action on the rein which cues the horse to change direction

change of rein *see* **change of hand**

chaparajos *n.pl.* *see* **chaps**

Chapman Horse *see* **Cleveland Bay**

chaps *n.pl.* (a short form of **chaparajos**) over-trousers used in Western riding attire and originating as a protection against brush and thorns as well as against cold, wind, and rain

charabanc, char-a-banc *n.* a type of four-wheeled, open carriage with transverse seats facing forward; there are various designs

character *n.* the nature of a horse, which governs its behavior; partly inherited and partly the result of environmental influences; specific breeds are associated with particular kinds of character

charge *vt.* to attack or threateningly move toward another horse or person — *vi.*

Charollais Half-Breed a French halfbreed used chiefly as a hunter; 15-16.2 h.h.

charriada *n.* rodeo

charro *n.* a Mexican cowboy who competes in charriadas in colorful costume, as opposed to the vaquero who is a working cowboy

chaser *see* **staplechaser**

chaugan *n.* the mallet used in polo (from the Persian word meaning the same)

check *n.* in hunting, a halt when hounds lose the scent and the field waits for them to recover it — *vt.* to pull in with the reins

check ligament a band of tissue that connects a tendon to a bone, enabling the tendon to provide support without muscular effort, as those in the legs that lock and enable a horse to sleep standing up

check rein 1. a harness branch rein connecting the driving rein of one horse of a team with the bit of another horse 2. in a bitting rig, an overhead or side rein running from the bit back to the harness or surcingle causing the horse to set its head or carry it in what is considered the correct position

cheek strap the bridle strap that runs down the side of the cheek to hold either bit or noseband; **cheekpiece**

cheek teeth the 24 premolars or molars located behind the bars

Chef d'Équipe the manager of an equestrian team who makes the arrangements for a national team competing abroad

chemoreceptor *n.* any sense organ that responds to chemical substances or to chemical changes in the blood; e.g., organs of taste and smell — **chemoreceptive** *adj.*

chemotherapy *n.* the administration of chemical drugs to treat disease — **chemotherapeutic** *adj.* — **chemotherapeutically** *adv.*

cherries *n.pl.* *see* **roller mouth**

Cherry's disease *see* **carpitis**

chest *n.* the area encased by the ribs, from between the forelegs to the flanks

chestnut[1] *n.* a horse whose color is one of a large number of reddish shades, especially liver chestnut (darkest red), chestnut (medium red), and sorrel (light red). The term sorrel is not used in describing certain breeds such as Arabian, Morgan, or Suffolk, whereas the light red Quarter Horse is termed sorrel colored. Chocolate chestnut is rare and points are brown. Spanish terms that describe distinctions in chestnuts are *tostado, alazan, ruano* — *adj.*

chestnut[2] *n.* a small knob-like callus on the inside of the leg, above the knee in the foreleg and below the hock in the hind leg; thought to be a vestigial toe and may be considered a piece of hoof material; name derived from a leaf stalk of the chestnut tree when pulled off, which looks like a horse's tiny hock and shod foot; sometimes called night eye or mallender

chew *vt., vi.* when eating, to move the lower jaw from side to side to crush food between upper and lower molars

Cheyne Strokes breathing a respiratory irregularity wherein breathing increases, quickens and becomes intense, then gradually subsides, even to the point of temporarily stopping

Chickasaw *n.* a type of horse named after the Chickasaw Indians, who allegedly obtained them from Spanish settlers in the 16th century, probably around 1540; at that time these horses were considered a breed and were described as being about 13.2 h.h. and of muscular conformation

chicken coop in jumping, a type of hurdle

Chifney bit an almost circular bit with a straight or curved mouthpiece, usually used for leading to correct rearing but often used with yearlings to accustom them to bits; designed by Englishman Samuel Chifney who lived 1753–1807

Chifney bit

chime *n.* in hunting, the howling of hounds when on the line of the quarry

Chincoteague *n.* an American pony breed that, with similar Assateague ponies, inhabit the islands of Chincoteague and Assateague, two small islands off the coast of Maryland and Virginia; descended from shipwrecked Spanish horses that swam to Chincoteague island in the 17th century; each summer the Chincoteague Fire Department has a fundraising day when they first transport their own horses by boat to Assateague Island where ponies there are rounded up and swum to Chincoteague; the next day ponies from both islands are selectively auctioned; the ponies are hardy and, although initially wild, quickly become gentle and docile with proper treatment; about 12 h.h.

Chinese Pony a type, rather than a breed, of pony indigenous to China; frequent breeding with wild Mongolian ponies makes them similar to the latter; hardy and sure-footed; mostly dun colored; conformation is poor; 12–13.2 h.h.

chinks *n.pl.* a cowboy's shortened version of chaps

chip *n. see* **osteophyte**

chiropractic treatment manipulative treatment of body joints

chloral hydrate a crystalline compound used well diluted as a sedative and for reduction of pain

chloramphenicol *n.* an antibiotic

chlorhexidine hydrochloride a strong antiseptic; trade name Hibitane

chloroform *n.* an inhaled anesthetic

chlorpromazine *n.* a tranquilizer; trade name Thorazine

chlortetracycline *n.* an antibiotic

choke *vt.* to clog (a horse's) throat or esophagus — *vi.* to become clogged there — *n.* a condition caused by a bolus of food or some other object, like a piece of wood, lodging in the gullet or esophagus; symptoms include convulsive swallowing movements with arched neck, green or brown nasal discharge and saliva dribbling from the mouth; the horse may have a distraught expression and may stand near a water supply swilling water through the mouth without swallowing

chokecherry *n.* a wild cherry tree, *Prunus virginiana*, indigenous to North America, which produces a toxin containing cyanide which affects the horse's respiratory system; without immediate medical attention, death can occur within as short a time as one hour after ingestion

choking up *see* **tongue swallowing**

Chola *n.* a Peruvian all-purpose breed that is usually dun-colored; about 14 h.h.

cholagogue *n.* a medication which increases the flow of bile from the liver

cholesterol *n.* a chemical component of animal fats and oils

choline *n.* a B-complex vitamin found in animal and vegetable tissues

cholinesterase *n.* an enzyme responsible for deactivating the chemical which jumps nerve impulses from one junction to the next

chondritis *n.* inflammation of cartilage

chondroblast *n.* a cartilage-producing cell

chondrocyte *n.* a cartilage cell

chondroid *adj.* similar to cartilage

chondroma *n.* a tumor composed of cartilage; benign but can multiply and spread

chondrosarcoma *n.* a malignant tumor composed of cartilage

chop a fox in hunting, to kill a fox before he runs and is chased

chord *n.* in the body, a ligament, tendon, or band of fibrous tissue

chorion *n.* a membrane which surrounds a fetus within the womb —**chorionic** *adj.*

chorioptic mange a disease of the skin on the legs caused by mites, often with

a secondary infection having a greasy, fetid exudate; the skin is red, moist and hot and later thickens and wrinkles; dirty conditions, particularly in wet weather, contribute to the disease, which is now rare; grease, seborrhea; scratches

choroid *n.* a membrane of the eyeball

chromatin *n.* that part of the cell nucleus which stains easily for microscopic examination; normally present in females but not in males

chromatograph *vt.* to separate by chromatography —**chromatographic** *adj.* —**chromatographically** *adv.*

chromatography *n.* analysis by separating different substances in a solution as they produce bands of color in the process; it is a method used for testing for dope in saliva and urine samples

chromosome *n.* any of the microscopic structures in the nucleus of a cell which carry the hereditary genes; each cell has a constant number of chromosomes set in pairs; the horse has 64 chromosomes or 32 pairs —**chromosomal** *adj.*

chronic *adj.* lasting a long time; opposite of acute

chukker, chukka *n.* in polo, a 7½ minute period of play; because there is a need for changing horses due to the constant speed at which the game is played, the game must be divided into such periods

chute *n.* in rodeo, an enclosure that confines a bull or calf before he is let out into the ring

chyle *n.* fat absorbed from partially digested food

chylothorax *n.* chyle in the chest cavity

cicatrix *n.* a scar or scar tissue

CID combined immuno deficiency

ciliary body a ring of pigmented tissue

of the eye which lies upon the inner surface of the choroid layer and encircles the inner surface of the eyeball

cilium *n.* (usu. pl., **cilia**) 1. an eyelash 2. a minute hairlike structure in any of various body tissues — **ciliary** *adj.*

cimetidine *n.* a drug used to treat ulcers in foals; trade name Tagamet

cinch *n.* the Western term for girth

cinch binder a cowboy term used to describe a horse who bucks, rears and loses balance, falling over backward; it derives from the objection of some horses to being firmly cinched

circadian rhythm a horse's daily biological cycle or biorhythm

circuit rider a Protestant preacher who traveled on horseback in the 18th and 19th centuries into the American frontier preaching to groups wherever he could

circulation *n.* the flow of blood from the heart to all parts of the body, through veins and arteries, and its return

circus horses show horses that perform in a circus consisting of three types: Liberty horses, haute école horses ridden and performing dressage movements, and Rosinbacks

cirit *n.* an ancient but still preserved Turkish game played on horseback, which involves riders throwing lances to each other as they gallop in opposite directions

cirrhosis *n.* an inflammatory liver disease wherein the cells are replaced by fibrous tissue, hardening the liver; caused by chronic poisoning or hepatitis, etc.; characterized by impaired metabolic and digestive function of the liver

cisterna *n.* a space in the body in which lymph or other fluid collects; ex. **cisterna magna** the space at the base of the skull

citric ointment a strong ointment effective, in diluted form, in the treatment of cracked heels and other inflammatory skin conditions; nitrate of mercury

CK creatine kinase

claiming race a race in which the owner of a competing horse states its value before the race, indicating that the horse may be claimed or bought after the race for that price

Clamoxyl *n.* trade name for amoxicillin trihydrate

clamp *n.* a surgical device used to arrest bleeding — *vt.*

clamp the tail to depress the tail

Clarence *n.* a closed, four-wheeled English carriage that originated in 1842; had four passenger seats and one driver's seat outside; later was superseded by the Surrey Clarence with a rear platform for a footman

classical seat *see* seat

Classics *n.pl.* races which, in the U.S.A., consist of the Kentucky Derby at Churchill Downs (1¼ mi.), the Preakness Stakes in Pimlico, Maryland (1 3/16 mi.), the Belmont Stakes in New York (1½ mi.), and the Coaching Club American Oaks, Belmont, New York (1½ mi., for fillies only)

claybank dun *see* dun

clean bred pure bred

clean ground in hunting, land that is not foiled

clear round a show-jumping or cross-country round which is accomplished without jumping or time faults

cleft *n.* 1. a split or crevice 2. a depression between two parts; e.g., the cleft in the foot that lies between the two sides of the heel

cleft palate an uncommon birth deformity wherein there is a split from front to back along the middle of the palate; caused by prenatal failure of

the two sections of the palate to join completely at the center

clenbuterol hydrochloride an agent used as a bronchodilator to relieve trauma from chronic obstructive pulmonary disease

Cleveland Bay an old English breed that originated in the Cleveland district of Yorkshire; known as Chapman Horses in the 17th and 18th centuries because salesmen called chapmen used them to transport their wares; very good all-purpose horses with an excellent temperament and intelligence; as the name implies, the color is always bay, with no white markings except on the face; tractable and strong, they make excellent carriages horses but are also popular for sports; 16–16.2 h.h.

clinch, clench *n.* the end of a nail used by the farrier and bent down over the hoof wall to hold the shoe on — *vt.* to fasten by this means

clinoptilolite *n.* a neutralizing agent used to absorb ammonia fumes in stalls; Sweet PDZ

clip[1] *n.* a protrusion of the outside of a shoe which lies on the hoof and helps to hold the shoe on; side clip

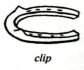

clip

clip[2] *vt.* to shave (a horse's coat). There are three principle styles: the full clip (entire coat removed), the hunter clip (hair left on legs up to elbows and thighs and on the saddle area), and the trace clip (hair removed from belly, between thighs and forearms, across chest, and underside of neck) — *n.*

clitoral sinuses pockets between folds surrounding the mare's clitoris

clitoris *n.* the small part of the external genitals of the mare, located just within the vulva at the base of the vagina; contains erectile tissue and is exposed during "winking" of the vulva

when the mare is in estrus

cloak fly *see* **tabanid fly**

clonic convulsion *see* **convulsion**

cloprostenol *n.* synthetic prostaglandin

close coupled short, strong and well muscled; usually refers to the back where it is considered an advantage

closed arthritis a form of arthritis that is usually caused by bruising or wrenching; acute cases affect the hock, fetlock, pastern, stifle, knee, shoulder, or hip. Cases often develop suddenly with swelling of the joints, which become hot and painful and seemingly filled with fluid. Fever, and rapid respirations may occur; this may continue for a few days before the swelling gradually goes down; or the swelling may increase, then discharge exudate. If the swelling remains closed, this fluid may be absorbed but if not totally absorbed, the joint remains swollen and somewhat stiff, and the condition becomes chronic, as in bog spavin and articular windgalls; these cases are not painful and lameness is rare; sometimes called serous arthritis.

closed registry a registry in which may be recorded only foals from parents who are both registered in the same registry

clostridium *n.* spore-bearing, anaerobic bacteria, of which there are 205 species, that cause various diseases, such as tetanus, botulism and gas gangrene; some normally inhabit soil and feces — **clostridial** *adj.*

clostridium enteritis intestinal inflammation caused by clostridium bacteria

clot *n.* coagulation of blood or lymph — *vi.*

cloud *n.* a dark mark on a horse's face

cloverleaf barrels a timed playday event which involves running around three barrels in a cloverleaf pattern

club foot a foot that is very upright and associated with a short toe and long, often contracted heel; susceptible to suspensory ligament trouble; often causes a rough gait; **boxy foot; donkey or mule foot**

club foot

cluck *n.* a sound made by a rider asking the horse to move faster — *vi.*

Clydesdale *n.* a very large breed originally developed in Scotland in the late 18th century when native mares were crossed with large, imported Flemish stallions and bred mainly in the area of Clydesdale; then in the mid–19th century Scottish breeders, particularly in the Clyde Valley of Lanarkshire, used very good English stock to establish the Clydesdale as a breed and the Clydesdale Society was established in 1877; today high-priced Clydesdales are used mainly for showing and cross-breeding; lesser quality ones are used for agricultural work; like the Shire, this horse has abundant, silky feather and typically white stockings and face; 16.3–18 h.h.

coach dog a dog trained to run under a traveling coach just behind the horse, probably to guard against highwaymen

coaching marathon a marathon for four horse-drawn coaches originating in England in 1909 at the Royal International Horse Show; the coaches depart at short intervals from each other; points are awarded for the horses' condition on return but not for speed, although there is a set time in which the marathon must be completed

coaching whip *see* whip

coachman's elbow a coachman's salute, given or returned with the whip raised to face level so that the elbow is raised

coastal ataxia poisoning from ingestion of large quantities of a plant called gomphrena celosioides that grows in Australia; results are lack of coordination, dullness, appetite loss, and body swaying; **gomphrena poisoning**

coastal hay hay derived from Bermuda grass

coat *n.* the hair covering a horse's body

cob *n.* a type of horse rather than a breed; short-legged, compact, and strong with much bone; very tractable; a maximum height of 15.1 h.h.

cocaine *n.* a drug obtained from coca leaves; used as a local anesthetic or as a stimulating dope when given orally

coccidia *n.* an order of sporozoans; intestinal parasites; **coccidiosis** is a disease caused by coccidia

coccidioidomycosis *n.* a fungal infection that in its primary form attacks the lungs when the fungal spores are inhaled; the secondary form attacks the viscera, central nervous system, lungs, etc.

coccus *n.* a round bacterial cell; e.g., streptococcus

coccygeus muscle the muscle that clamps the tail or swishes it

coccyx *n.* a bone at the rear end of the vertebral column — **coccygeal** *adj.*

cocked ankles fetlocks that are bent forward, usually the hind ones

cock-eyed stirrup irons irons that have the slot slanted and the bottoms sloped rearward to encourage inward slope of the foot and lowered heel

cockeyes, cocks eyes metal eyes on a harness that hook the traces to the bars

cock fences in hunting, low-cut thorn fences

cockhorse *n.* a supplementary horse used to help pull a stagecoach up a steep hill; ridden by a **cockhorse boy**

and connected just ahead of the lead horses

cocking cart a tandem drive, two-wheeled cart popularly used in the 19th century for transporting fighting game cocks

cocktail *n.* a potential racehorse but not a Thoroughbred

codeine *n.* a drug from opium used to relieve pain and in cough medicines

co-favorite *n.* in racing, one of two or more horses equally favored to win and given the same shortest price in the betting odds

coffee housing in hunting, undesirable chatting at the covert

coffin *n.* a cross-country fence made up of two sets of post and rails separated by a ditch

coffin bone the end bone of the leg; shaped like a miniature hoof and encased within the hoof forming its internal bony foundation; situated mainly towards the hoof's anterior and lateral parts, it is connected to the hoof wall by sensitive laminae attached to it and interlocking with insensitive laminae attached to the horn wall; in founder, the coffin bone tips down, causing the sole to drop down and separate from the wall; third phalanx, pedal bone

Coggins test a test given to detect antibodies against equine infectious anemia virus; agar gel immuno-diffusion test

coital exanthema a contagious disease characterized by small ulcers on the vulva and vagina of a mare or the penis of a stallion; transmitted by coitus, insects, or personnel handling the horses; infection may result in loss of appetite, rise in temperature, and general malaise

coitus *n.* sexual intercourse —**coital** *adj.*

cold *n.* a catarrhal disorder of the upper respiratory tract

cold abscess a slowly developing localized collection of pus

cold back an attitude typical of a horse that has not been properly broken to the saddle or has been saddled with an ill-fitting saddle causing pain or that has been mistreated sometime in its training. A horse with a cold back will bolt, plunge, rear, or buck in reaction to the sudden weight of a saddle on its back or the tightening of the girth. —*see also* **spondylosis deformans**

cold-blood *n.* a heavy draft breed descended from the large forest horses of northern Europe that survived the Ice Age and were domesticated about 3,000 years ago; progenitors of today's heavy draft breeds; the term has nothing to do with blood temperature but rather refers to the breed's calm and passive temperament —**cold blooded** *adj.*

cold-jawed *adj.* hard mouthed

cold lameness inability to move normally on first starting exercise

cold line in hunting, a quarry's scent that is faint

cold scenting in hunting, terrain likely to sustain little scent

cold shoe a ready-made or keg shoe

cold shoeing the process of shaping a shoe to fit with hammer and anvil without the use of heat

colibacillosis *n.* disease caused by *Escherichia coli* bacteria

colic *n.* a painful, sometimes fatal, stomach ailment having various causes, among which are insufficient intake of water resulting in impaction of ingested food, drinking very cold water when overheated from work, irregular feeding or sudden change of feed or overeating (**alimentary colic**), ingestion of sand (**sand colic**) or other foreign matter, and parasites (**verminous colic**). Spasmodic colic is caused

by excessive activity of the gut, which results in a spasm and sometimes diarrhea; **twist colic** (volvulus) occurs when an acutely obstructed intestine becomes twisted; **tympanitic colic** is caused by gas accumulation from fermented food. Colic is characterized by the horse's kicking at his belly; reluctant to stand, the horse lies down for long intervals. Also sometimes called gripes, fret, bellyache — *vi.* to colic

coliform *adj.* relating to the aerobic bacillus normally residing in the colon

colitis *n.* inflammation of the colon, a severe disorder characterized by fever, acute pain, diarrhea; fatal when hemorrhage in the colonic wall occurs

collapse *vi.* 1. to suddenly fail in health, usually from heart trouble 2. to suddenly fall down, as from exhaustion or a blow, etc.

collapsed temperature a body temperature that is much lower than normal; signals death

collar *n.* part of a harness made of thickly padded leather, worn around the base of the horse's neck, to which the hames are attached

collar work any driving work requiring strain on the collar, as pulling uphill

collateral cartilages two cartilages inside the hoof, attached to and projecting up from the coffin bone

collect *vt.* to tighten the reins and simultaneously and steadily apply leg pressure so as to make a horse bring its hocks well under its body, resulting in proper balance — **collected** *adj.* — **collection** *n.*

collected canter a slow canter with impulsion, flexed head-set, and low quarters

collecting ring a ring next to a show- or jumping ring where competitors collect

collection classes at shows, one collective entry of three or more exhibits from one stable

Collier *n.* a draft or pack horse formerly used in the coal mines of Wales

colon *n.* the part of the large intestine that extends from the cecum to the rectum

color breed a breed registered according to certain color qualifications, such as Appaloosa, Albino, Palomino, Pinto; may also be double-registered with another breed, e.g. Palomino-Quarter Horse

colostrum *n.* the first milk a mare produces; it is very thick, bright yellow to orange in color, and contains the protein globulin, which gives the foal immunity against infection in its early days; it is produced during the first 24 hours after birth of the foal; sometimes called first milk

colt *n.* an uncastrated male horse between the ages of one and four years

coma *n.* unconsciousness — **comatose** *adj.*

comanche twitch a type of gag twitch wherein the rope is connected to the D on the near side of the headstall

combination martingale a combined form of a running and standing martingale

combination obstacle in show jumping, an obstacle consisting of two or more seaparate jumps which are numbered and judged as one

combined immunodeficiency (CID) lack of disease fighting capacity in foals

combined training competition a comprehensive test of both horse and rider, consisting of the following three phases: dressage, cross-country, and show jumping; held over a period of one, two, or three days, depending on the competition

combiotic *n.* a brand name for penicillin-streptomycin combination

come a cropper to fall from a horse

come again in racing or hunting, to appear suddenly revived from a tiring condition and regain speed

come-along *n.* a rope tied in such a way as to encourage a foal to lead forward; about 15 feet of rope is used, looped around the back of the legs (about halfway between hocks and root of tail) and up to the front of the croup; the end is run through the halter or can be held by the trainer; tends to propel the foal forward by a pushing action on hindquarters rather than a pulling on the head

comminuted fracture a fracture in which the bone is broken or crushed into pieces; crushed fracture

commissure *n.* tissues that join opposite but corresponding parts, such as the corners of the lips

common dystocia *see* **dystocia**

complement *n.* in immunology, a substance formed in the blood for antigen/antibody reaction; used in complement fixation tests for diagnosis

complement fixation (CF) test a laboratory blood test to determine the presence of antibodies to specific infections

complete blood count the number of various types of cells in a blood sample

complexus muscle the muscle which extends the head and neck or turns them sideways

compound *n.* one substance formed of two or more materials — *vt.* to combine two or more materials into one substance — *adj.* consisting of two or more materials

compound fracture a bone fracture wherein the broken bone has punctured the overlying skin

compress *n.* a poultice applied to relieve inflammation; may be wet or dry, cold or hot

compression plating an orthopedic technique used in surgery of a fractured leg bone involving a plate or plates and screws across the fracture to hold the bone ends together firmly enough to eliminate all motion; this procedure prevents pain and hastens healing with very little unwanted new bone formation — *see also* **plate luting**

computerized tomography a sophisticated X-ray technique that produces detailed images of internal body structures and provides invaluable information for diagnosing equine problems; abbr. CT or CAT scanning

Comtois *n.* a very old French light draft breed; used at one time in the cavalry; since the 19th century has been crossed with other breeds; popularly used in harness and for meat; 14.3–15.3 h.h.

concave *adj.* curved inward, as may describe the side profile of a horse's back — *see also* **sway back**

conceive *vi.* to become in foal — *vt.* to start an embryo in the womb

concentrates *n.pl.* grains, such as oats, corn, barley, that provide a high degree of nourishment in concentrated form

concho *n.* a decoration, usually of silver, used on tack

Concours de Sauts d'Obstacles Internationale, -Officiel *see* **international horse shows**

concussion *n.* a hard blow, usually associated with the head; also associated with the effect on the hooves as they strike the ground, especially at speed

condition *n.* a state of being or health — *vt.* to train into a desired condition of fitness or accustom the individual to new surroundings — **in condition** in a healthy state — **conditioned** *adj.*

condom *n.* a covering put on the stallion's penis before coitus to collect semen

condyle *n.* the rounded portion of a bone, usually at the joint

cones *n.pl.* bodies within the retina of the eye that generate electrical impulses under the influence of light

Conestoga wagon a crude wagon covered with canvas over wooden hoops used by American settlers; covered wagon; prairie schooner

conformation *n.* a horse's build; the form or shape of the body

conformation hunter a hunter, usually a Thoroughbred, who is judged in the show-ring on his conformation and way of going, as well as on performance

congenital *adj.* existing from the time of birth — **congenitally** *adv.*

congestion *n.* an excessive accumulation of blood in an area of the body — **congestive** *adj.* — **congest** *vt.* to cause excessive blood accumulation

conine *n.* an alkaloid

Conium maculatum *see* **poison hemlock**

conjunctiva *n.* the covering mucous membrane of the front part of the eyeball and inner surface of eyelids — **conjunctival** *adj.*

conjunctivitis *n.* inflammation of the conjuctiva; pink eye

Connemara *n.* a pony breed originally indigenous to Ireland but now bred in England as well as other parts of the world; 13–14.2 h.h.

conquistador *n.* one of the Spanish conquerors of Mexico in the 16th century who brought the first horses to the Western Hemisphere since their disappearance millenia before

consolidation *n.* solidification, as of a lung in the case of pneumonia

constipation *n.* infrequent and or difficult evacuation of the bowels with hard, dry feces — **constipated** *adj.* — **constipate** *vt.*

contact *n.* the communication between rider and mount by means of

the reins as well as the rider's legs and seat; if the reins hang loose, the rider does not maintain contact with the horse

contact dermatitis an inflammatory skin reaction to a substance, such as soap or a chemical

contagious *adj.* communicable, relating to: 1. disease 2. bad habits, such as cribbing; horses tend to imitate their pasturemates

contagious acne a skin infection caused by a small parasite and usually confined to areas rubbed by harness or tack; small, painful lesions may extend over most of the body, especially shoulders, back, and sides; transmitted through use of common grooming tools, tack, etc.; American skin disease

contagious equine metritis (CEM) *see* **metritis**

contaminant *n.* an agent which infects — **contaminate** *vt.* to infect — **contamination** *n.*

Continental panel a forward-cut saddle with knee and thigh rolls

contracted heels a condition in which the heels of the hoof are too close together, occurring when the frog does not touch the ground; can be caused by poor shoeing or trimming, particularly paring of the bars

contracted tendon abnormal contraction of a flexor tendon at the back of the leg, which restricts normal mobility of the fetlock and or coffin joint and causes knuckling over at the fetlock; severe cases may force walking on the front of the joint

contractile *adj.* producing contraction

contractile fibrils protein strands within a muscle fiber which shorten the muscle in contraction

contractile proteins muscle-tissue proteins that slide together and apart as the muscle contracts and releases

contractility *n.* the ability of tissue to contract from stimulation, as from a muscle

contracture *n.* the shortening of a tendon, or muscle, etc., so that it cannot be normally flexed or straightened, often resulting from scar tissue

contusion *n.* a bruise, the skin being initially unbroken — **contused** *adj.*

convalescence *n.* a period of recovery from surgery or illness

convex *adj.* curved outward

convex back *see* **roach back**

convolution *n.* a twisting or folding of something on itself; e.g., the surface of the brain — **convoluted** *adj.*

convulsion *n.* a violent involuntary muscle spasm; **clonic convulsions** are jerky movements caused by alternating contraction and relaxation of muscles; **tetanic convulsions** are those caused by tetanus

cooler *n.* a covering sheet placed over a horse that is cooling off after a good sweat; has a browband, tie straps, and tail cord and extends from ears to dock

cooler

cool off to walk an overheated horse for gradual cooling after strenuous exercise, which is advisable for good health; often done with a cooler

coon-footed *adj.* having long, sloping pasterns with low fetlocks

copper penny *see* **intrusion**

copper sulphate a blue crystalline substance used in fluid form to reduce proud flesh

coprophagy *n.* the eating of feces — **coprophagous** *adj.*

copulation *n.* mating — **copulate** *vi.*

coraco brachialis a muscle that flexes the shoulder joint and adducts the leg

Coramine *n.* trade name for nikethamide

cord *n.* in the body, a stringlike, rounded structure, such as the umbilical cord, spermatic cord, or spinal cord

cording up *see* **atypical myoglobinuria; set fast; tied up**

corium *n.* 1. the deepest layer of the skin 2. tissue inside the hoof horn which nourishes the coronary band, frog, and pedal bone surface

Corlay *n.* a sub-type of the Breton

corn *n.* a bruise on the sole of the foot; a collection of blood under the sole, caused by the rupture of small blood vessels; becomes visible as a discoloration on the sole, usually between the wall and the bar; usually caused by leaving shoes on too long or by improperly fitted shoes

cornea *n.* the outer transparent coat of the front of the eyeball in front of the pupil and iris

corner incisors the outer pair of incisor teeth

corn fines the residue from corn after being processed

cornify *vi.* to convert to keratin in forming hoof, horn or hair

cornu *n.* a horn-shaped projection of an organ; e.g. the **uterine cornu** near the entrance of the fallopian tubes in the mare

Corona *n.* 1. a type of saddle pad cut to fit the shape of a saddle; has a large, colorful roll around the edge 2. the trade name of a hoof dressing

corona *n.* a crown-like part, such as the upper part of the tooth

coronary *adj.* of the heart

coronary *n.* the upper part of the hoof

adjacent to the foot's hair, sometimes inaccurately called coronet

coronary band the band around the top of the hoof from which the hoof wall grows; has small projections (papillae), each of which corresponds with the upper end of each roof horn tubule and secretes the substance that makes up the horn — *see also* **horn**

coronary band

coronet *n.* a white hair mark forming a band around the foot just above the hoof; partial white bands are usually called right, left or front, according to where they appear; a partial coronet mark at the back of the foot is called a white heel

coronitis *n.* 1. an injury to the coronary band wherein the hoof is twisted or pulled from its coronary seat, such as may happen when a horse has to turn suddenly or catches its foot in a hole or fence; characterized by swelling of the coronary and very painful lameness 2. a horseman's inaccurate term for a condition of the coronary band wherein it has a dry, whitish color due to nutritional insufficiencies, villitis

corpuscle *n.* a cell such as a blood cell

corpus luteum yellow tissue formed in the ovary after the ovum is discharged; if the ovum is fertilized, this tissue secretes the hormone progesterone

corral *n.* an enclosure to contain horses; pen — *vt* to drive into a corral

corrective shoeing the fitting of a special shoe to give relief to a sprained ligament or compensate for faulty hoof or leg conformation

corrective trimming trimming of the hoof to correct faulty hoof or foot conformation or to achieve a certain effect

corrugator supercilii a muscle which raises the upper eyelid

cortex *n.* the external layer of a body

organ; e.g., the adrenal cortex — **cortical** *adj.*

corticosteroid *n.* a hormone normally produced by the adrenal glands; a compound derived from this hormone or synthetically produced for injection

corticotropin, -phin *n.* *see* **ACTH** — **coticotropic, -phic** *adj.*

cortisol *n.* an adrenal hormone that regulates the metabolism of carbohydrates

cortisone *n.* a hormone secreted by the adrenal gland; may be produced synthetically and used as an anti-inflammatory agent

Corynebacterium equi obsolete name for what is now called *Rhodococcus equi,* a bacterium that causes pneumonia in foals; usually fatal

coryza *n.* an acute nasal condition — *see also* **strangles, snotty nose**

costal *adj.* relating to the ribs

costal respirations breathing that causes exaggerated abdominal movements, as in painful abdominal afflictions

Costaricense *n.* *see* **Paso Costaricense**

counter canter a canter performed on the wrong lead in the show-ring; a difficult exercise; counter lead; false canter

counter change in dressage, a change from a traversal in one direction to a traversal in the other direction

counter irritant a substance applied to the skin to cause irritation to counteract a deeper irritation by stimulating the body's healing processes

counter lead *see* **counter canter**

counting chamber a place on a microscope slide used for counting blood cells

coupé *n.* a four-wheeled closed carriage for two passengers and an outside driver

coupling *n.* 1. a region of the lumbar vertebrae joining the last rib to the hip 2. heartbeat arrhythmia in which each heartbeat is followed by a premature contraction (coupled rhythm)

coupling reins harness reins, used for either a pair or team of horses, which connect to the insides of the bits (between pairs) at one end and to the draft reins at the other end; **couple up** to fasten coupling reins

courbette *n.* in dressage, an air above the gound; the horse rears to an almost upright position, then leaps forward several times on its hind legs

course *n.* 1. a track for horse racing 2. in show-jumping and cross-country, a circuit including hurdles to be covered within a time limit 3. — *vt.* in hunting, to pursue by sight instead of by scent

courser *n.* 1. a graceful, spirited or swift horse 2. a war horse

cover *vt.* to mate with (said of a stallion); serve; settle

covered wagon *see* **Conestoga wagon**

covering boots boots put on the hind legs of a mare that is being covered to protect the stallion from being injured by kicks

covert *n.* in hunting, a thicket where a fox may hide

covert hack in hunting, a horse once used to carry a rider to the meet

cowbane *n.* a plant of the parsley family with small white flowers; highly poisonous and, if eaten, causes colic, convulsions, and death

cowboy *n.* 1. a man who herds and tends cattle on ranches, doing his work mainly on horseback 2. a male rider in a rodeo

cowboy seat *see* **seat**

cowboy snaffle a swivel dee-cheek reining bit of which there are various models, some of which have one pair of rein rings at the ends of the shanks, while others have two pairs, one at the mouth and the other at the ends of the shanks

cowgirl *n.* the female counterpart of cowboy

cow-hocks *n.pl.* a hind leg fault wherein the hocks are close together and point toward one another; the feet are widely separated with toes pointing outward

cow hocks

cow horse a horse ridden by a cowboy or cowgirl while working cattle

cow-kick *vi., vt. see* **kick**

cowlick *n.* a whorl

coxa *n.* hip

coxitis *n.* inflammation of the hip joint

coxofemoral *adj.* relating to the hip and thigh

coyote dun *see* **dun**

CP creatine phosphate

crack *n.* a split in the hoof. There are quarter cracks and toe cracks; a crack may start at the coronary band and work down, or at the bottom of the hoof wall and work up, the latter being more common. Cracks are caused by improper or too infrequent shoeing or by dry, shelly hooves which may be congenital, nutritional, or caused by rasping off the moisture-retaining periople. — *vi., vt.*

cracked heel an affliction of the hollow of the pastern wherein the skin becomes red, tender and scaly, developing vesicles that rupture and form cracks

cradle *n. see* **neck cradle**

cranial cavity the area containing the brain

cranial nerves paired nerves originating at the lower surface of the brain and exiting through openings in the skull to various parts of the body

cranial sutures lines of junction of bones composing the skull

craniopathy *n.* any disease of the skull

cranium *n.* the skull — **cranial** *adj.*

crash *vi.* in hunting, to give tongue together on finding a fox (said of hounds)

crease *vt.* to shoot on the poll or crest or near the withers with the purpose of temporarily knocking (a horse) out; this was a method introduced by the French and used by cowboys of the Old West to cut Mustangs out of a wild herd, often killing the horse

creatine *n.* an alkaloid or amino acid in muscle tissue

creatine kinase (CK) an enzyme in skeletal and heart muscle and brain tissue

creatine phosphate (CP) a chemical compound that is an energy source for muscle contraction

creatinine *n.* a chemical in the blood, which is excreted in the urine; excessive amounts are indicative of kidney malfunction

creep feeder a container for supplementary feed for suckling foals

cremaster muscle the muscle that retracts the testicle from the scrotum

cremello *adj.* a cream coat color, almost white, with matching mane and tail and blue eyes — *n.* a horse having this coloration

crepitant rales *see* **rales**

crepitation *n.* 1. the sound made by the edges of a broken bone rubbing against each other   2. the feeling one gets when probing skin under which there is an accumulation of gas   3. the cracking sound of joints — **crepitate** *vi.* — **crepitant** *adj.*

crest *n.* the top of the horse's neck

crib[1] *n.* a manger; a rack or box for fodder

crib[2] *vi.* to habitually bite or chew the crib or feed manger, the wood of a stall or fence, or tree trunks; not only a highly undesirable and destructive habit but also dangerous because wood splinters may be swallowed, leading to digestive disorders; moreover, it is injurious to teeth. When a horse chews and simultaneously swallows air, it is called *wind-sucking.* Cribbing is often imitated by other horses; **cribber** *n.*

cribbing collar *see* **cribbing strap**

cribbing strap a strap used around the throat to curb the habit of cribbing; one of several types is a spiked strap by which expansion of the neck activates prongs through holes

cribbing strap

cricket *n.* a copper roller fitted into the port of a spade or curb bit to entertain the horse's tongue

cricoid cartilage a ring-shaped cartilage of the larynx

cricket

Criollo *n.* a native breed of Latin America that originated with Spanish horses brought over from Spain in the 16th century; after surviving tough environments for several centuries, today's Criollos are a very hardy breed of great endurance and are easy keepers. Paso horses, including Paso Finos and Peruvian Pasos, all have the same ancestry and differ only according to their development and breeders' preferences over time. Argentina has developed its Criollos into excellent ranch workers and, crossed with Thoroughbreds, they are now the well-known Argentine polo pony; 14–15 h.h. — *see also* **Crioulo, Guajira, Llanero, Pasitrotero**

Crioulo *n.* a native breed of Brazil — *see also* **Criollo**

crocus *n.* a plant whose leaves are harmful when ingested, causing abdominal

pain, severe purgation and straining

cronet *n.* the hair at the coronet of the foot growing down over the hoof

crop *n.* a short riding whip with a looped lash

crop eared having small ears; the term derives from a custom long ago of cropping the ears to make them smaller

crossbred *n.* the progeny of a sire registered in one breed association and a dam in another —*adj.* **crossbreed** *vt., vi.*

cross canter a canter in which the horse is on one lead in front and on the other lead behind —*vi.* to canter in this way

crossed oxer a jump consisting of two separated sets of posts and rails slanting in opposite directions

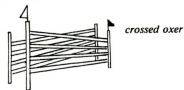
crossed oxer

cross firing the striking of a hind foot against the opposite foreleg or foot

crossing traces a technique used in driving a pair of horses that do not move evenly; the inside trace of one horse is "crossed" or attached to the inside hook of the other horse's bar

crossmatch *vt., vi.* to test a sample of a donor's blood against that of a recipient prior to a blood transfusion to assure compatibility

crossovers *n.* a movement wherein the horse steps sideways by crossing one foot over the other, front over front, rear over rear (**sidepass**), or rear-leg crossovers for the forehand turn and front-leg crossovers for the haunch turn

cross reins a method of holding single reins so that they overlap in the hands across the horse's neck

cross-tie *vt.* to secure (a horse) by means of two lines, one from each side of the halter, to rings set level with his head —*n.*

crotalaria *n.* a poisonous plant sometimes eaten by horses, with fatal results, if there is little or no other forage; rattleweed

crouch *vi.* to bend the limbs low as an animal does when ready to spring; the horse sometimes crouches with only his hindquarters when having his rear under the tail bathed, as if recoiling from the first impact of water there

croup[1] *n.* the top part of a horse's back that lies between the loins and the tail; looking from the side, it is the highest point of the hindquarters; rump

croup[2] *n.* inflammation of the larynx accompanied by coughing, breathing difficulty and sometimes fever

croupade *n.* in dressage, an air above the ground in which the horse rears, then jumps up with hind legs drawn up

crown *n.* the enamel-covered part of a tooth projecting from the gum

crownpiece *n.* a piece of the bridle that goes over the horse's head and attaches to the cheekpiece

cruciate *adj.* shaped like a cross; in regard to the anatomy, a **cruciate ligament** consists of two strong, round bands in the stifle shaped like an X

crude protein in relation to a particular feed, this is the total protein content contained therein, which includes the actual digestible protein used by the horse's body

crupper *n.* a strap that hooks to the cantle of a saddle at one end and at the other end loops around the tail; prevents the saddle from sliding forward; also used as part of a harness

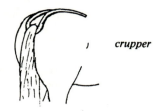

crupper

crush *n.* a narrow enclosure in which a horse can be confined and restricted from movement for rectal or vaginal examination

crushed fracture *see* **comminuted fracture**

cry *n.* in hunting, the sound the hounds make; the **den cry** is made when they chase the fox into his lair; **babbling** is baying unnecessarily; **running mute** means running without baying

cryosurgery *n.* surgery in which tissue or a tumor is destroyed by freezing, usually with liquid nitrogen

crypt *n.* a very small body cavity — **cryptal** *adj.*

cryptococcosis *n.* a fungus infection that is characterized by lesions in the nasal cavity and lips, lungs, and meninges; usually fatal

cryptorchid *n.* a male horse having one or both testicles undescended; rig; ridgling — **cryptorchidism** *n.* the condition thereof

Crystapen *n.* trade name for benzyl-penicillin

CSI Concours de Sauts d'Obstacles Internationale

CSIO Concours de Sauts d'Obstacles Internationale Officiel

CT scan *see* **computerized tomography**

cuboid bone a bone below the point of hock

culicoides *n.* a genus of very small biting flies

cull *n.* an animal that is not up to standard — *vt.* to selectively eliminate an animal from a herd or group, especially one that is not up to standard

culture *n.* an artificially stimulated growth for laboratory testing

culture medium the nutrient material used for cultivating microorganisms in a laboratory

cuneal *adj.* wedge-shaped, as in relation to a body part; cuneiform

cunean tendon a tendon that forks from the main tendon of the hock and extends to the second tarsal bone

cup *n.* infundibulum; the black cavity or mark in the center of the equine tooth which, with age, gradually wears away; used as an indicator of a horse's age up to about 9 years

curare *n.* a paralyzing poison, modified forms of which are used in general anesthesia and to reduce spasms caused by tetanus

curb[1] *n.* an inflammation of the plantar ligament; a semi-circular, hard swelling about four inches below the point of hock; caused by tearing or spraining a ligament; more common in young horses with sickle hocks

curb[2] *vt.* to slow or restrain

curb[3] *n.* an abbreviated form of curb bit or curb strap

curb bit a bit having a solid bar, or mouthpiece, that may be straight, curved, or straight with a port in the middle; at each end is an almost vertical metal bar, or cheekpiece, with a ring at each end, the upper ring to be attached to the cheek strap of the bridle and lower ring to the rein; usually used with a curb chain

curb chain a chain or strap (**curb strap**) which attaches to a bit around the horse's lower jaw; when the reins are pulled, the curb tightens and slows or stops the horse

curb groove the groove of the lower jaw just behind the lower lip

curb strap *see* **curb chain**

curet, curette *n.* a spoon-shaped instrument used for scraping the wall of a body cavity, usually that of the uterus — *vt.* to scrape — **curettage** *n.* the process of curetting

Curly Horse a horse with a curly coat; the Curly Horse Foundation has been founded in America to promote a curly-coated breed that is true to type; this foundation is distinct from the American Bashkir Curly Registry

curricle *n.* an English two-wheeled carriage for two horses abreast — *vt.* to harness two horses to such a carriage with a bar called a curricle bar put across the backs of the two horses

curry *vt.* to groom with a curry comb

currycomb a grooming implement used to remove dirt and scurf from a horse's coat. There are various kinds: (a) flat or roundish back with a hand strap or handle in the middle; (b) a metal spiral design; (c) one that attaches to a water hose to enable washing and currying simultaneously. Currycombs may be made of metal, plastic, or rubber, depending on design — *vt.*

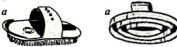
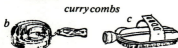

currycombs

Cushing's syndrome a disease caused by excessive hormone production by the adrenal gland; characterized by abnormally long hair, fragile bones, weakness, stupor and abnormal sweating

cushion *n. see* **digital cushion**

cusp *n.* 1. a pointed part of the chewing surface of a tooth 2. a triangular part of a heart valve

cut *n.* 1. to geld or castrate 2. to separate (a selected calf or cattle) from a herd on horseback

cut and set a cruel procedure whereby a tail is surgically cut and set to heal in an artificially upright position; often repeated several times before the desired set is attained; this is sometimes done to fine harness horses, three- and five-gaited Saddlebreds and Hackney ponies; nick

cutaway *n. see* **shadbelly**

cutting *n.* 1. *see* **cut** 2. *see* **brushing**

cutting horse a horse specially trained to cut cattle; a good cutting horse instinctively knows which way the calf will probably turn and turns accordingly without cueing from the rider

CVM cervical vertebral malformation

cyacetazide *n.* a parasiticide used against lungworms

cyanide *n.* a poison which is produced by certain young grasses or wilting leaves; the acid is released when the plant is damaged or decays; ingestion results in convulsions, paralysis, and respiratory failure

cyanosis *n.* a blue coloration of skin membranes, etc.; caused by lack of oxygen which can be due to heart failure or severe pneumonia — **cyanotic** *adj.*

cycle *n.* a bodily change that occurs with regularity, such as the estrus cycle

cyclitis *n. see* **iridocyclitis**

cyst *n.* an abnormal saclike growth in the body filled with fluid or semi-solid material; there are various kinds, such as sebacious, dermoid, and false or spurious — **cystic** *adj.*

cystitis *n.* an inflammation of the bladder

cystoscope *n.* an instrument for diagnostic observation of the interior of the bladder

cytogenetics *n.* the science dealing with cellular heredity, correlating cytology and genetics — **cytogenetic, cytogenetical** *adj.*

cytology *n.* the study of cells — **cytological** *adj.* — **cytologically** *adv.*

cytoplasm *n.* the contents of a cell outside the nucleus, the portion essential to all functions —**cytoplasmic** *adj.*

cytotoxin *n.* an agent used to destroy malignant cells —**cytotoxic** *adj.*

— D —

daily double in racing, a type of bet which, to succeed, must be placed on both winners in two separate races on the same program; if either horse loses, the whole bet is lost

daisy cutting low action at the walk or trot sometimes causing the horse to stumble

Dales *n.* a strong British pony breed of old origins, formerly used as a pack pony; through the years crosses with other breeds improved the Dales and in 1963 the Dales Pony Society was organized; distinguishing characteristics are very strong, large round feet with small silky feathers, action that is very flexed and high, and tremendous energy combined with courage, kindness, and intelligence; 13.2–14.2 h.h.

dally *vt., vi.* to wind a rope around the horn of a Western saddle; in the act of steer roping, the rider ropes the steer and immediately dallies the rope around the saddle horn

dam *n.* the mother of a horse; referred to on a pedigree as the bottom line

dander *n.* tiny flakes from the skin

dandruff *n. see* **pityriasis**

dandy brush a stiff brush used to clean surface dirt and scurf off a horse's coat

Danish Warm-Blood a modern breed of sports horse developed in Denmark from imports of German, British, and Swedish horses; a variety of these horses are registered and make top-class competitors in sport; 15.3–17 h.h.

danthron *n.* a purgative drug which may produce reddish urine; trade names Altan, Istin

Danubian *n.* a half-bred native to Bulgaria; a strong, active horse developed during the 20th century by crossing Nonius stallions with Anglo-Arab mares; characteristics include compact body, strong neck, powerful quarters, deep girth, fairly slender legs; used under saddle and as a draft horse; about 15.2 h.h.

dapples *n.pl.* patterned color variations on a horse, usually about one inch in diameter and usually relating to a gray horse having faint spots (dapples) on a lighter gray coat (*a dapple-gray horse*) —**dappled** *adj.*

Darashouri *n.* an Iranian breed; a spirited saddle horse; 15. h.h.; also called Shirazi

Darbowsko-Tarnowski *n. see* **Malapolski**

dark horse 1. a horse that wins a race unexpectedly 2. a little known contestant regarded as unlikely to win a race

Dartmoor *n.* a British pony breed, native of the Dartmoor area of Devonshire; registry dates back to 1899; up to 12.2 h.h.

dawn horse *see* **Eohippus**

dead heat in racing, a tie for first, second, or third place; when two or more horses come in exactly in line and are thus eligible for the same prize, they are called **dead heat winners** and the prize is divided equally

dead meat in racing, a horse considered by a stable to be a loser

deafness *n.* a partial or total loss of hearing; deaf horses are often docile and easily controlled when ridden —**deaf** *adj.*

dealer's whip a steel-lined whip with a drop thong used by horse dealers

debilitate *vt.* to weaken —**debilitated** *adj.* —**debilitation** *n.*

debridement *n.* the removal or cutting away of contaminated or necrotic tissue from a wound —**debride** *vt.*

deciduous teeth the temporary teeth which begin to erupt in a foal at about one week of age and are all in at about eight months; by five years these have been replaced with permanent teeth; also called milk teeth

declaration *n.* a statement in writing made by a horse owner or his authorized representative, who is often his trainer, at a specified time before a race or competition, stating that a particular horse will compete

decubitus *n.* the act of lying down; **decubitus ulcers** are sores caused by prolonged lying down and may appear on the hip, elbow, or hock; horses do not normally lie down for prolonged periods

dee bit a type of snaffle bit named for the shape of the rings which are like a capital D

dee bit

deep *adj.* in hunting, a term applied to soft or heavy terrain

deep cut in cutting, the separation of a cow from the middle of the herd; in competition, the cutter must make at least one deep cut according to the rules, as opposed to selecting only cows from the edge of the group

deep digital flexor a major propulsion muscle between the knee and fetlock in the foreleg and between the hock and fetlock in the rear leg

deep digital flexor tendon the tendon connecting the deep digital flexor with the coffin bone

deer fly *n.* a smaller relative of the horse fly that breeds in swampy areas and is extremely bothersome to horses, stubbornly clinging on once it alights; the bite is painful and often leaves a blood mark; in the west, the snipe fly is also considered a deer fly

deer fly

defecate *vi.* to evacuate feces from the bowel —**defecation** *n.*

defensin *n.* a protein inside the body's neutrophils (white blood cells) which fights invading bacteria

defervescence *n.* the declining stage or disappearance of a fever

degenerative *adj.* 1. deteriorated 2. causing deterioration —**degeneration** *n.* —**degenerate** *vi.*

degenerative joint disease a type of arthritis caused by stress on the joints; characterized by inflammation, cartilage loss and new bone growth that alters the shape of the joint and decreases its mobility

degenerative myelitis an inflammatory degeneration of the spinal cord

deglutition *n.* swallowing

De Gogue headsetting reins that run from the hands, through the bit rings, up to a poll strap with pulleys, and on down, between the forelegs, to the girth

dehydrate *vt.* to dry out —*vi.* to become dry

dehydration *n.* a condition in which the body has lost too much fluid —**dehydrated** *adj.*

deltoideus muscle that which flexes the shoulder joint and abducts the leg

demineralization *n.* loss of mineral salts from the body

Demi-Sang *n.* a French breed used primarily for harness racing but also used under saddle; about 16.2 h.h.

demodectic mange a mange or skin disease caused by demodectic mites that live in hair follicles and sebaceous glands, resulting in tissue damage

demulcent *n.* a soothing ointment

den cry in hunting, the sound made by hounds as they chase a fox into its lair

dendrite the part of a nerve cell that receives impulses and transmits them to the cell's center

denervate *vt.* to sever or remove (a nerve) to relieve pain — *see also* **neurectomy**

dental *adj.* relating to teeth

dental pulp the soft core of the tooth which contains nerves and blood vessels

dental star a brown dentin which from wear gradually becomes apparent between the cup and front of each permanent incisor, starting with the central incisors at age 8; it starts as a straight line across the tooth, then curves and finally becomes round and dark brown on all the incisors by age 15

dentigerous *adj.* bearing teeth

dentigerous cyst a cyst containing tooth tissue and usually located just below or in front of the ear — *see also* **dermoid cyst**

dentin, dentine *n.* the hard, yellowish-white tissue which surrounds the pulp of the tooth; the exposed dentin is covered by the enamel

dentition *n.* 1. teething   2. the number, quality and arrangement of teeth in the mouth

deoxyribonucleic acid *see* **DNA**

Depo-Medrone *n.* trade name for methylprednisolone acetate

depraved appetite *see* **appetite**

depression[1] 1. a lessening of functional activity   2. a mental state of low spirits manifested in various behavioral ways which can be detected by a discerning horseperson, particularly one who is familiar with the horse involved; one cause can be illness — **depressed** *adj.*

depression[2] *n.* a low area on the surface of the body or of an organ in the body; e.g., *prophet's thumb*

depressor *n.* a muscle that pulls down a part of the body, such as the tail

depressor labii inferioris a muscle that depresses the lower lip

dermacentor albipictus a brown tick which can cause equine piroplasmosis; winter tick

demacentor nitens a yellow-brown tick commonly found in tropical climates; causes equine piroplasmosis; tropical horse tick

dermatitis *n.* inflammation of the skin, of which there are many types; e.g., rainrot

dermatophilus *n.* a microorganism with bacterial and fungal characteristics that causes the infection called dermatophilosis — *see also* **mud fever**

dermatosis *n.* skin disease

dermis *n.* the skin layer under the epidermis

dermoid cyst a type of cyst which is most commonly found in connection with the ovary or testicle but which can develop in other parts of the body; may be as large as a foot in diameter and often contains teeth

desensitize *vt.* to reduce or cure an undesirable behavior in (a horse) by exposing the horse, in slowly increasing stages, to the stimulus which triggers the behavior — **desensitization** *n.*

desmitis *n.* inflammation of a ligament

desmology *n.* the study of ligaments

desmotomy *n.* the cutting of ligaments

desoxycorticosterone acetate (DOCA) a hormone secreted by the adrenal gland; a steroid that affects metabolism of water and electrolytes

destrier *n.* a war horse

destroy *vt.* to kill or slaughter — **destruction** *n.*

deterge *vt.* to cleanse, as a wound

detomidine *n.* a premedication used prior to anesthesia with ketamine,

etc.; also used as a tranquilizer by injection; trade name Domosedan

deutoplasm *n.* the substance in ova that provides food for the embryo — **deutoplasmic** *adj.*

develop *vt., vi.* 1. to cause to grow or to bring something latent into activity or apparent existence 2. to grow

developmental stages phases of a horse's growth and lifespan, identified as follows: conception; embryo (first 40 days); fetus (41st day through birth); foal (birth through six months); weanling (six to twelve months); colt or filly (one to four years); and stallion or mare (four years on, or earlier if a mare is in foal before age 4)

deworm *vt.* to purge of intestinal parasites; worm (def. 2)

dew poisoning weepy irritations on the face and legs caused by contact with certain plants, such as small-headed sneeze-weed, stinging nettles, etc.

dexamethasone *n.* a strong agent for treating inflammation

dextrose *n.* 1. a form of glucose in the body 2. a sweet solution given orally or intravenously to treat shock, blood loss, or dehydration

diabetes *n.* a physical disorder characterized by excessive urinary discharge and constant thirst; there are various types of diabetes

diabetes insipidus a type of diabetes that can be caused by eating moldy hay or oats, by glanders, or by tuberculosis; characterized by a heavy volume of urinary discharge, intense thirst, emaciation and weakness

diabetes mellitus a chronic type of diabetes in which insufficient insulin is produced by the pancreas, thereby causing an excessive amount of sugar in the blood and urine; characterized by intense thirst, hunger and emaciation; rare in horses

diagnosis *n.* the identification of an abnormal condition after examination of symptoms

diagonal *n.* a term in English riding that refers to the rider's posting the trot on the inside of a ring when the diagonal hind leg and foreleg of the horse strike the ground together; when the horse and rider are moving clockwise around the ring, the rider posts in rhythm with the horse's left foreleg and is therefore on the left diagonal — *adj.*

diaphragm *n.* the sheet of muscles separating the chest cavities from the abdomen — **diaphragmatic** *adj.* — **diaphragmatically** *adv.*

diaphragmatic hernia a rupture of the diaphragm

diaphysis *n., pl.* **-ses** the shaft or middle part of a long bone, as distinguished from the growing ends — **diaphyseal, diaphysial** *adj.*

diarrhea *n.* abnormal frequency and looseness of bowel movements — **diarrheal** *adj.*

diarthrosis *n.* a joint (e.g., the hip) which permits free movement in any direction — **diarthrodial** *adj.*

diastema *n.* a distinct gap between two teeth; the gap between the incisors and molars

diastole *n.* the normal, steady and rhythmic dilation of the heart, especially of the ventricles, following the systole (contraction), during which the heart muscle relaxes and the chambers fill with blood — **diastolic** *adj.*

diathermy *n.* medical treatment that involves the application of electromagnetic radiation to heat body tissues so as to promote healing by stimulating circulation

diazepam *n.* a tranquilizer used as an anticonvulsive medication in foals and to control muscle spasms in older horses who have contracted tetanus

Dibencil *n.* trade name for benzamine penicillin

dichlorvos *n.* generic name for one of the agents used to control bots and roundworms

dicoumarin *n.* a substance which forms from fermentation of sweet clover; prevents blood clotting

dictyocaulus *n.* a genus of lungworm

die *vi.* to cease to live; horses usually die convulsively, struggling violently to the end, and may even gallop themselves to death — **death** *n.*

diestrus, dioestrus *n.* the 15-day period in a mare's reproductive cycle when there is no estrus

diethylcarbamazine *n.* generic name for a dewormer effective against lungworms and other tissue parasites

diethylstilbestrol *n. see* **stilbestrol**

differential diagnosis the distinguishing of one disease from another by comparing symptoms and arriving at a definite diagnosis

differentiation *n.* the process of acquiring individual character during the development of an embryo

diffusionist *n.* one who believes that horsemanship was born in one particular center and from that center horse culture spread, or diffused, worldwide

digastricus muscle a muscle which opens the mouth and helps swallowing when jaws are closed

digestible protein in any particular type of feed, the protein that is assimilated by the horse's digestive system

digestion *n.* the body's process of changing ingested food into a form that can be absorbed through the lining of the intestinal tract. The digestive tract takes the following route: mouth–pharynx–esophagus–stomach–small intestine–cecum–large intestine; indigestible residues then exit, in the form of feces, through the rectum and anus — **digest** *vt.* — **digestive** *adj.*

digit *n.* a toe; the term does not apply to present-day horses as such, but millions of years ago the horse had toes rather than hooves; in today's horse it is the part of the leg from the fetlock down to and including the hoof — **digital** *adj.*

digital cushion a firm but spongy wedge-shaped tissue mass of the foot that fills the area between the frog below and the deep digital flexor tendon above; forms the bulbs of the heel

digital extensor tendon a tendon that runs down the front of the cannon bone

digitalis *n.* a medicinal heart stimulant

digital palmar nerve one of the two main nerves in the forefoot on either side of the rear of the pastern

digital pulse the pulse in the digital arteries leading to the foot

digital sheath the membrane that envelops the deep flexor tendon and secretes lubricants that reduce tendon friction

digitigrade *n.* an animal that walks on its toes without heels touching the ground, as the horse does, although the horse's "toes" are called hooves and the toe of the hoof is technically the front section of the hoof (the quarters being the sides). The hooves, millions of years ago, were literally toes; thus the horse can be called a digitigrade — *adj.*

digitoxin *n.* a medication prepared from digitalis

dikkop horse sickness a cardiac form of African horse sickness, characterized by a marked swelling of head and neck and affecting the heart; thick head horse sickness

dilate *vt., vi.* to stretch or expand — **dilation** *n.*

dilator naris lateralis a muscle that dilates the nostrils

diligence *n.* a stagecoach, particularly one formerly used in France

dilute *vt.* to make weaker as by mixing with water or other fluid

dimethyl sulfoxide (DMSO) an anti-

inflammatory agent that is also anti-bacterial and analgesic and is absorbed through the skin

diminazene aceturate a parasiticide

diphenhydramine hydrochloride an antihistamine given internally as well as externally in cream or lotion

diplococcus *n.* round bacteria that occur in groups of two

diploid *adj.* twofold; having the normal set of paired chromosomes (32 in the horse)

dipteran *n.* a two-winged insect of the order Diptera (e.g., flies, mosquitoes, gnats), all of which are pests to horses and can carry disease

dipyrone *n.* generic name for a drug that is used to relieve pain, fever and muscle spasms

direct rein in riding, a method of control which causes a horse to displace its weight from the forehand to the hindquarters; most frequently used in English riding to decrease speed, turn or back; pressure is never increased when used correctly; open rein

Direma *n.* trade name for hydrochlorothiazide

discipline *vt.* to train; to enforce obedience; to control; to punish — *n.* **disciplined** *adj.*

disease *n.* 1. general illness 2. a specific disorder with destructive effects on an organ and having a specific cause and characteristic symptoms

Disex *n.* an extinct, semi-wild breed of small horses with zebra-like markings that inhabited the Pyrenees Mountains until the late 1930s

dish *n.* a concave shape, as applied to an Arabian's profile — **dish-faced** *adj.* — **dished** *adj.* — *see also* **jibbah**

dished hoof, dished foot *see* **flare foot**

dishing *n.* a faulty way of going in some horses, usually pidgeon-toed, wherein one or more feet break over the outside of the toe, swinging inward in an outward arc; paddling

disinfect *vt.* to sterilize or make free of harmful bacteria — **disinfectant** *n.*

disk *n.* a shock-absorbing and connective layer of tough, fibrous tissue between adjacent vertebrae

dislocate *vt.* to displace (a bone) from the proper position at a joint — **dislocation** *n.*

dismount *vi.* to get off a horse

disobedient *adj.* failing to obey the owner's or rider's commands — **disobey** *vt., vi.*

disorder *n.* an ailment or abnormality in health

dispensary *n.* a place or room where medicines are dispensed

disqualify *vt.* to make ineligible, as for participation in a given sport — **disqualification** *n.*

distaff side the female side of descent in a pedigree

distal *adj.* in reference to the anatomy, farthest from the center or place of origin or attachment

distal sesamoid bone navicular bone

distance *n.* a space between two points; in racing, the space that is a certain length back from the finish line; in order to qualify for future heats, a horse must have reached this space by the time the winner completes the course

distemper *n.* *see* **strangles**

distension, -tion *n.* a condition of being inflated or enlarged from within — **distend** *vt.* — **distended** *adj.*

distressed breathing difficulty in breathing; causes include obstructed air passages due to nasal growths, paralysed vocal cords, pneumonia, broken wind, etc.

disunited canter a canter having the following sequence; on a right lead, RH, LF and LH together, RF; on a left lead, LH, RF and RH together, LF

diuresis *n.* an excessive passing of urine

diuretic *n.* an agent that increases the output of urine

diverticulitis *n.* an inflammation of a diverticulum

diverticulum *n., pl.* **-la** a normal or abnormal pouch or sac occurring from a cavity or organ within the body; diverticula only cause problems when inflamed — **diverticulosis** *n.* the presence of many diverticula

dividend *n.* in racing, a pay-off

DMSO (dimethyl sulfoxide) an organic chemical that has a number of medical uses; has anti-inflammatory, antibacterial, and analgesic properties; and is able to penetrate readily through the skin

DNA (deoxyribonucleic acid) protein chains present in cell nuclei which determine individual hereditary characteristics

DNA mapping a method of identification in which horses' chromosomes are matched

dock *n.* the bony portion of the tail that tapers to a point about one-third of the way down the tail — *vt.* to cut off the end of the dock and set it for a high carriage by cutting the tendons, a widely deplored practice; flag

DOCO desoxycorticosterone acetate

dog-cart *n.* a small open trap on usually only two wheels and having two back-to-back seats; so called because it originally had a carrier under the seat for a sportsman's dog

dog-fall *n.* in rodeo steer wrestling, a term referring to the illegal downing of a steer by a steer wrestler when the steer lands with all four feet and head not in the same direction; to qualify, the wrestler must turn the animal over or let it up and throw it down again in the correct manner

dog-sitting posture crouching of the hindquarters with forelegs unbent; this is rare but can be seen in cases of colic or encephalomyelitis — *see also* **crouch**

Dole Gudbrandsdal a Norwegian breed found throughout Scandinavia where they vary in type and size, some being of a heavier type than others and used for haulage and farm work. The introduction of the Thoroughbred and Arab, among others, has developed the lighter type and these are used for riding and for trotting races. Very strong, sure-footed, all-purpose horses with a good temperament. Usually black or brown; 14.2–15.2 h.h. — *see also* **Dole Trotter**

Dole Trotter a Norwegian breed used in harness for trotting races; a modern version of the Dole Gudbrandsdal; also called Norwegian Trotter; about 15 h.h.

doll *n.* a movable barricade on a racecourse to keep horses on course

domesticated *adj.* tamed and used for humans' purposes, as opposed to wild — **domesticate** *vt.*

dominant *adj.* 1. exercising authority or leadership in a herd of horses 2. in genetics, describes a gene that guarantees its traits in the offspring

Domosedan *n.* trade name for detomidine

Don *n.* a very hardy Russian breed that proved its amazing hardiness and courage as a cavalry horse in 1812 in the war against France; originally developed in the steppe country around the rivers Don and Volga where it is still bred and herds run free despite very harsh winter conditions; today they are no longer needed to any significant extent by the cavalry but are used for general-purpose riding, especially in endurance races, or to improve other breeds; 15.1–15.3 h.h.

Dongola *n.* a breed indigenous to Ethiopia and Somalia; used mainly for racing

donkey *n.* (*Equus asinus*) a domesticated ass and relative of the horse family but quite different in appearance; has a large head with a small body, very long ears, a dorsal stripe and stripe across the shoulders; the tail is short-haired with a tufted end; has 62 chromosomes (2 fewer than the horse); the female is called a jenny, the male a jackass; mating with a horse produces a mule

dope¹ *vt.* to drug a horse either to improve or hinder its performance in a race or competition, an illegal act subject to large penalties in any equestrian sport — *n.*

dope² *n.* (*colloq.*) in racing, advance information on contestants, especially concerning condition and speed

dormeuse *n.* a heavy, four-horse, four-wheeled, privately owned carriage used in Europe in the 19th century by travelers who could afford their own transport

dorsal *adj.* of, on, or near the back

dorsal stripe a dark color stripe along the backbone from withers to tail

dose *n.* the measurement of medicine given or taken at one time; a **skin dose** is the amount of radiation at the skin's surface when radiation is used in treating problems such as carpitis — *vt.* to give a dose

double¹ *n.* 1. in show-jumping, a combination obstacle consisting of two separate jumps 2. in hunting, a fence with a ditch on either side

double² *n.* in race betting, a bet made on two horses to win in different races; if the first one wins, the money won plus the original amount bet are put on the second horse; both horses must win or the whole wager loses

double back a spine that is lower than the muscles on either side

double barrel flags a timed playday event in which there are three barrels in line with each other; a competitor rides up to and circles around either the first and second or second and third barrels and returns

double bridle a bridle having two bits, a curb and snaffle, the snaffle in this case being called a bridoon; a double bridle called a Weymouth has an extra set of straps to hold the bridoon; there are two sets of reins; the purpose of a double bridle is to give the rider a choice of using either bit according to what response he wants from the horse

doubletree *n.* in harness for two horses abreast, a crossbar whose ends attach to the singletrees

doubling *n.* pulling a horse's head all the way to one side in order to stop the horse — *vi.*

doubling the horn in hunting, making trilling notes on the horn

doughnut *n.* a roll that is fitted around the pastern to prevent capped elbow or shoe boil; shoe boil ring

dourine *n.* a contagious venereal disease caused by the protozoan *Trypanosoma equiperdum* and transmitted by copulation; characterized by swollen lymph glands and genitalia, patches of oozing skin rash, anemia, and emaciation, paralysis of lymph glands; equine syphilis

dovetail *n.* a dental projection that from wear appears on the rear edge of the top corner incisor at about age 7; by about age 9 it disappears but at age 11 it develops again and remains

draft horse a strong, powerfully built horse bred and used for farm work or pulling heavy loads

drag¹ *n.* in hunting, (a) an artificial scent made by dragging something with a strong smell, such as material impregnated with a fox's urine; or (b) a scent left by an animal; or (c) a hunt over a trail of scent left by an animal; **drag hunt**

drag² *n.* a private horse-drawn coach

drag a field to scatter horse droppings in a field with a harrow

dragman *n.* a driver of harness horses

drag rider a kind of safety rider who trails or drags behind other riders taking part in a competition to deal with any emergencies

draschia *n.* a parasitic worm that infests open wounds and the stomach

draw *vi.* to unsheath the penis or achieve erection — *vt.* 1. to extract, as to draw blood for examination 2. to pull and make tense (*to draw the reins*)

draw a covert in hunting, to look for a fox in a covert, usually by casting hounds in the covert

draw reins reins that run from the girth area, through the rings of a snaffle bit, then to the rider's hands; used to train a horse to lower its head and flex at the poll

dray *n.* a low wagon with removable sides, for carrying heavy loads — *vt.* to haul on a dray — *vi.* to drive a dray

drench *vt.* to administer liquid medicine to a horse orally — *n.*

dressage *n.* a form of refined exhibition riding in which the horse performs certain difficult steps and gaits with perfect balance and extreme lightness, receiving almost invisible aids from the rider; also called high school training or haute école training — **dresseur** *n.* a rider who engages in dressage

drive *vt.* 1. to control and direct the course of (one or more horses) from a wagon, carriage, etc., either for sport, transportation, or agricultural work 2. to herd (cattle) from horseback

driver *n.* a person who drives a harness horse or horses

driving horse a harness horse; a horse trained to pull wheeled vehicles

drool *vi.* to salivate excessively; brought on by overstimulation or irritation of the salivary glands; may be caused by a particular feed constituent having toxic irritants, an oral injury, a foreign substance lodged in the mouth or throat, or abnormality of teeth

drop jump a jump that involves landing on a level lower than the take-off side

dropped elbow *see* **radial nerve paralysis**

dropped (or drop) noseband a noseband (not a cavesson) forming part of a bridle and fitting about three inches above the nostrils; used to increase control and prevent mouth-opening and excessive movement of the tongue

droppings *n.pl.* feces or dung

dropsy *n. see* **anasarca** — **dropsical, dropsied** *adj.* — **dropsically** *adv.*

droshky, drosky *n.* a low, open, four-wheeled Russian carriage

drycoat *n. see* **anhidrosis**

dry gangrene a form of gangrene in which putrefaction has partly or totally stopped due to lack of moisture; may, for example, exist on the end of the ear

dry rales *see* **rales**

dry rot a fungus decay that affects the hoofs

dry single in hunting, a bank with no ditch

dual paternity the recording of two sires for a foal when the dam was covered by two stallions during the estrus in which the foal was conceived

dubbed foot *see* **bull-nosed foot**

duct *n.* a body channel; e.g., a bile duct

ductule a small duct

ductus arteriosus a blood vessel in the fetus connecting the pulmonary artery to the aorta; normally closes within four days of birth

dude *n.* a Western term applied to a paying guest who spends a vacation at a guest ranch called a dude ranch

dude horse a horse used by a guest at a dude ranch

dude ranch a guest ranch where dudes spend vacations

dull *adj.* 1. sluggish and lacking spirit, as symptomatic of illnesses 2. lacking luster, as a horse's coat — **dullness** *n.*

Dulmen *n.* German pony breed of ancient heritage; becoming rare; about 12.3 h.h.

dummy foal syndrome *see* **neonatal maladjustment syndrome**

dumped foot *see* **bull-nosed foot**

dun *adj.* of a coat color that in a general sense is yellow with brown points and is often used synonymously with the term buckskin; the difference can be said to refer to primitive markings (dorsal and zebra stripes), the dun (also called zebra dun) having these and the buckskin having none. Grullo is another type of dun. Various shades of dun may be classified under two general groups, red dun and yellow dun; red dun includes muddy dun (light brownish red or yellow with brown head), red dun (light red with darker red points), orange dun, and apricot dun; yellow dun describes a definite yellow shade; claybank dun generally covers all red and yellow shades but specifically is a lighter or more yellow version of the apricot shade; coyote dun is a mixture of yellow and black hairs; silver dun is cream; dusty dun is yellow with brownish coat; lobo dun is grullo with a mixture of slate-colored hairs and black; lilac dun is a lilac shade with chocolate brown points and amber eyes and a pink or light brown skin. — *n.* a dun-colored horse

dung *n.* excrement; manure; feces; droppings

dung beetle any of several beetles that breed in and eat dung

dung eating *see* coprophagy

duodenum *n.* the first portion of the small intestine, between the stomach and the jejunum — **duodenal** *adj.*

-dupp the second part of a term that represents the second sound the heart makes when it beats; the complete term is lubb-dupp

dura mater the outer and most fibrous of the three membranes covering the brain and spinal cord

dust *vt.* *see* **fan a horse**

dust ball an intestinal calculus composed of vegetable fibers coated with lime salts

dusty dun *see* **dun**

Dutch Draft a heavy Dutch draft breed established as a breed in 1914; an exceedingly massive and muscular horse with smallish head and short, thick, feathered legs; has a willing, docile nature; matures early and lives to be very old; up to 17 h.h.

Dutch Warm-Blood a breed developed in the 1960s and comprising various types focused towards sports, pleasure riding, and driving; 15.3–16.3 h.h.

DVM Doctor of (or Diploma in) Veterinary Medicine

dwell *vi.* 1. a Western term roughly synonymous with the English half halt 2. in hunting, to delay on the line (said of hounds)

dynamics *n.* the study of physical motion; in medicine, the study of body parts or organs in action

dysentery *n.* intestinal inflammation characterized by acute diarrhea — **dysenteric** *adj.*

dysfunction *n.* a condition of a full-term foal that has signs of prematurity

dysphagia *n.* a swallowing impairment, causes include grass sickness, botulism, hooks of the molar teeth, infection of the guttural pouches, hyoid fracture, pneumonia often results from aspiration of food into the windpipe; barium may be used for diagnosis

dysplasia *n.* a faulty growth; e.g., epiphysitis

dyspnea *n.* difficulty in breathing

dystocia *n.* difficulty in giving birth; causes include abnormal size, posi-

tion, etc., of fetus (fetal dystocia); head of fetus bent backward (wry neck); abnormal presentation wherein the foal is backward or upside-down (common dystocia); uterine inertia, i.e. weakness of uterine contractions (maternal dystocia)

dystrophy *n.* a wasting disorder of tissues, especially muscles, that results from poor nutrition

dysuria *n.* difficulty in urinating

Dzhabe *n.* one of two subdivisions of the Kazakh breed

— E —

each way in racing, a term applied to backing a horse to win or finish in the first three races

eagle shoe a rubber horseshoe designed primarily for racing to alleviate foot stress; weighing only about 6 oz., it is composed of three rubber sections called rails; these are fixed to an aluminum plate by short stud-bolts; the toe rail is made of a hard rubber compound, the quarter rails of a softer compound; the plate is nailed to the hoof in the conventional manner

ear *n.* the organ that perceives sound; the inner part of the horse's external ear grows a substantial amount of hair which helps to keep out insects; it is usually clipped on show horses for what is considered a neat look

eardrum *n.* the tightly stretched membrane that separates the external ear from the middle ear and transmits sound; tympanic membrane

early dough stage in the development of grain, the stage in which starch in the kernel starts to solidify into the consistency of dough

early fetal loss (EFL) abortion during gestation between 60 and 110 days

ear mites tiny, sometimes microscopic, parasites that can infect the ear; symptoms of infestation include a tendency for the ear or ears to droop; sensitivity to the touch of the hand or the bridle as it is being put on or removed; a tendency to hold the head to one side, shake it and rub the ears; and a wax

discharged from the ear

ear-stripping massaging a horse's ears from base to end to stimulate circulation when the horse is cold

earth *n.* the lair of a fox — *vi.* to hide in a burrow, as does a fox

earth stopper a person who, in preparation for a fox hunt, blocks the earth of the fox while it is out

earwax *n.* a secretion of the ear canal; cerumen

East Bulgarian a Bulgarian all-purpose breed used for agricultural work as well as under saddle; up to 16 h.h.

Eastern horses horses that are indigenous to or have their origins in the Middle East or Far East. Examples are Arabian, Barb, Turkish, Syrian breeds among others

ecchymoses *n.* bloody exudation into tissues caused by a bruise — ecchymotic

eccrine *adj.* relating to sweat glands

ECG equine chorionic gonadotrophin

echocardiography *n.* an ultrasound technique of recording heart function — echocardiogram *n.* the record thus made — echography *n.* the use of ultrasound in diagnosis

eclampsia *n.* a disorder involving convulsions and coma

ectoderm *n.* the outer tissue of the embryo which eventually forms the skin of the fetus, lining of the intestinal tract, etc. — ectodermal *adj.*

ectoparasite *n.* any parasite that lives

on the external parts of the body (as opposed to an endoparasite); e.g., ticks

ectopia *n.* an abnormal placement of a body part or organ — **ectopic** *adj.*

ectoplasm *n.* the outer layer of a cell

eczema *n.* an inflammatory skin disease that causes itching and scabbiness

edema *n.* swelling or abnormal fluid accumulation in body tissue — **edematous** *adj.*

EDM equine degenerative myelopathy

EEE eastern equine encephalomyelitis; *see* **encephalomyelitis**

eel stripe a dark stripe down the spinal column, extending from the withers to the base of the tail; dorsal stripe

efferent *adj.* leading or carrying away from a central part; e.g., an **efferent nerve** is a nerve that sends impulses from the brain and spinal cord to various parts of the body

effusion *n.* an escape of liquid into body parts or tissues

EFL early fetal loss

egg *n. see* **ovum**

egg-bar shoe a shoe with a convex bar connecting its heels; provides support to the horse's heel and lifts the fetlock

egg-butt bit a bit which has the ends of the mouthpiece molded around the rings to avoid pinching of the lips; it includes various types of mouthpiece such as jointed or straight-bar, mullen mouth, etc.

egg-butt bit

Ehrlichia risticii a microbe which causes Potomac horse fever

EHV equine herpesvirus

EIA equine infectious anemia

Einsiedler *n.* a Swiss breed used for riding and driving; 15.3–16.2 h.h.

EIPH exercise induced pulmonary hemorrhage

ejaculation *n.* emission of semen from a stallion — **ejaculate** *vt., vi.* — **ejaculatory** *adj.*

elbow *n.* the joint in the foreleg between the humerus and radius

elbow pull a headsetting aid used when lunging the horse; consists of a stiff rope that runs from over the poll, through the bit rings, down between the forelegs, then behind the elbows, and around the barrel

Elburz *n.* a breed that developed in the Elburz Mountains of Persia; used under saddle and as pack horses; about 12 h.h.

electrocardiogram (ECG) *n.* a graph recording electrical impulses of the heart; used to detect abnormalities or disease of the heart

electrocardiograph *n.* an instrument for tracing an electrocardiogram — **electrocardiography** *n.* the process of making an electrocardiogram — **electrocardiographic** *adj.* — **electrocardiographically** *adv.*

electrocardiophonogram *n.* a tape recording of heart sounds recorded by an **electrocardiophonograph**

electrocautery *n.* 1. the process of cutting and or searing tissue for healing purposes by use of an electrical instrument having a heating element 2. an electrical instrument used for this process

electroencephalogram *n.* a recording of the brain waves; used to detect brain disease

electroencephalograph *n.* an instrument used to make an electroencephalogram — **electroencephalography** *n.* the process of making an electroencephalograph

electrogoniometry *n.* an electronic process of determining or measuring angular positions of a leg

electrolyte *n.* any of various simple inorganic compounds or trace minerals that are essential for many of the

chemical processes in the body and for proper metabolism

electromyograph (EMG) a machine used to record and analyze muscle response to nerve stimulation; used to detect tail blocking —**electromyography** *n.* the process of using an electromyograph

electron microscope an instrument that focuses a beam of electrons to produce an enlargement of an object on a fluorescent screen or photographic plate

electrophoresis *n.* a method for study of molecules suspended in fluid by which they can be separated and identified by movement caused by application of an electric field —**electrophoretic** *adj.*

electroretinograph *n.* an instrument that records the electrical responses of the retina of the eye to stimulation by light —**electroretinography** *n.* the process of using this instrument

electrosurgery *n.* surgery which involves the use of an electric current, as in cauterizing

electrotonus *n.* the altered condition of a nerve or muscle when an electric current passes through it —**electrotonic** *adj.*

electuary *n.* a medicinal paste or ball made by mixing medicine with syrup

element *n.* the natural environment, or situation, for a horse

elephantiasis *n. see* **pachydermia**

elimination *n.* the disqualification of a competitor from a particular competition

ELISA enzyme-linked immunosorbent assay

elk lip *see* **parrot mouth**

el pato *see* **pato**

emaciation *n.* a condition of extreme leanness due to starvation or disease —**emaciate** *vt.* to cause to become abnormally lean —**emaciated** *adj.*

emasculate *vt.* to geld; castrate —**emasculation** *n.*

emasculator *n.* an instrument used for gelding

embolic nephritis *see* **pyemic nephritis**

embolism *n.* the obstruction of an artery by an embolus

embolus *n.* foreign matter, such as a blood clot or air bubble, in the bloodstream —**embolic** *adj.*

embrocate *vt.* to rub (an area of the body) with a soothing medicated liquid

embrocation *n.* a medicated liquid used for embrocating

embryo *n.* the earliest or undeveloped stage of the fetus up to 40 days after conception

embryogeny *n.* the formation and development of the embryo —**embryogenic** *adj.*

embryology *n.* the study of the formation and development of embryos

embryonal *adj.* 1. relating to an embryo 2. at an undeveloped or early stage

embryonated *adj.* fertilized and developing

embryonic *adj.* embryonal

embryotomy *n.* the dissection of a fetus in the uterus so as to permit its removal through the pelvis

embryo transfer the transfer of a fertilized ovum from the uterus of one mare to the uterus of another for gestation

EMG electromyograph

emollient *n.* a preparation that has a softening and soothing effect

emphysema *n. see* **heaves**

emphysematous fetus a decaying, gas-filled fetus

empyema *n.* the presence of pus in a body cavity, such as the chest (*see* **guttural pouch**); can happen in foals as a result of bacteria

emulsion *n.* particles of one fluid distributed throughout another fluid, as oil in water

enamel *n.* the hard, white coating of the exposed part of a tooth

enamel spot the enamel floor of the tooth's cup left visible after the cup's cement has worn away; these spots first become visible at age 8 and gradually fade (decreasing in size and moving towards the back of the tooth) until they disappear by age 15 or 16

encephalitis *n.* inflammation of the brain

encephalomyelitis *n.* a usually fatal viral disease affecting the brain and occurring in any of three forms: Eastern, Western, and Venezuelan (VEE); all are carried by mosquitoes and other bloodsucking insects and arachnids, including ticks. The Eastern and Western forms are only transmitted individually by carrier insects, whereas VEE is contagious to humans as well as to horses. Manifested by fever, impaired vision, salivation, lack of coordination, irregular gait, drowsiness, and incontinence of bladder followed by difficulty in swallowing and finally paralysis, coma and death. Vaccinations for all forms are available.

encephalon *n.* the brain

encephalopathy *n.* any degenerative brain disease

encyst *vt., vi.* to enclose or become enclosed in a cyst or sac — **encystment, encystation** *n*

endarteritis *n.* inflammation of the lining of an artery

endobiotic *adj.* parasitic; living within the tissues of the host, as e.g. worms

endocarditis *n.* inflammation of the endocardial valves or lining of the heart

endocardium *n.* the membrane lining the inner cavities of the heart — **endocardial** *adj.*

endocrine *adj.* relating to any gland that produces secretions that are taken by the bloodstream to other parts of the body whose functions they control — *n.* such a gland or its secretions — *see also* **thyroid, adrenal, pituitary glands**

endocrine glands a group of glands, including the pituitary, thyroid, and adrenal glands, that release hormones into the bloodstream

endocrinology *n.* the study of the endocrine glands and internal body secretions

endoderm *n.* the inner layer of embryonic cells which develops the lining of the digestive tract, of other organs, and of certain glands — **endodermal, endodermic** *adj.*

endogeny *n.* a growth originating inside the body — **endogenous** *adj.*

endolymph *n.* the fluid in the membranous part of the ear

endometrial cups areas in the placenta that secrete a hormone called pregnant mare serum gonadotrophin (PMSG); develop about the 35th day of pregnancy

endometritis *n.* inflammation of the endometrium caused by infection

endometrium *n.* the mucous lining of the uterine cavity — **endometrial** *adj.*

endomorphic *adj.* relating to a heavy, round-shaped body, conducive to fatness

endomysium *n.* the internal wrapping of a muscle fiber

endoparasite *n.* a parasite that lives in the internal tissues or organs of the body

endoplasm *n.* the interior part of the cytoplasm of a cell — **endoplasmic** *adj.*

end organ the end of nerve fibers where they enter the skin, muscle or other structure

endorphins *n.* morphine-like proteins produced by nerve tissue to suppress pain and regulate emotional state

endoscope *n.* an instrument inserted through a body passage to reveal its interior. Older instruments consisted of metal tubes with magnifying lenses, an eye-piece, and a light bulb; newer ones consist of a flexible tube containing light-conducting fibers that reflect an image onto the eyepiece.

endoscopy *n.* visual inspection of a body cavity using an endoscope

endosteum *n.* the fine membrane lining the inner surface of the bones

endothelium *n.* the cell layer which forms the inner lining of blood vessels, lymph vessels, and various other cavities —**endothelial** *adj.*

endotoxemia *n.* the existence of endotoxins in the bloodstream; may induce shock

endotoxic laminitis laminitis caused by poisonous bacterial substances

endotoxin *n.* a bacterial pyrogen or poisonous substance produced within certain disease-producing bacterial cells and released when those cells are destroyed —**endotoxic** *adj.*

endotracheal *adj.* of the trachea

endotracheal tube a flexible tube which is inserted into the trachea to draw out liquids and mucus or to administer a gas anesthetic; may also be used to relieve a choke in the esophagus

endurance riding a competition that involves riding over long distances and all types of terrain, in various types of climatic conditions; participants are judged not only on their time of arrival at the destination but also on the condition of their horses; although popular worldwide, the U.S. leads in this sport and the Arabian is the favorite mount

enema *n.* an injection of liquid through the anus as a purgative; used very rarely on adult horses but often on newborn foals to facilitate passage of meconium

energy *n.* strong capacity for work —**energetic** *adj.* —**energetically** *adv.*

enervate *vt.* to deprive of physical strength —**enervated** *adj.*

engaged *adj.* in racing, entered in a particular race

English hackamore a variation of the basic hackamore; all leather, with slightly rounded nosepiece and low-placed side rings; headstall splits into a V about three inches above the noseband, attaching to it in two places; jumping hackamore

English hackamore

English hunt seat *see* seat

English saddle a somewhat flat saddle with a very low pommel and cantle; stirrups are of metal and often referred to as irons; average weight is 18 lbs.; variations accommodate different requirements, such as dressage, jumping, etc.

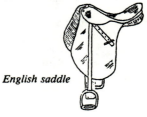

English saddle

enkephalins *n.pl.* chemicals produced in the brain and spinal cord that prevent feeling pain by insulating nerve endings

enteric, enteral *adj.* intestinal

enteritis *n.* inflammation of the intestines from any of various causes, including fungus, bacteria, etc.; can be acute or chronic; when acute, it is characterized initially by trembling, appetite loss, rapid pulse, and frequent defecation; colic sets in and congestion of mucous membranes; in mild forms, colic is either absent or slight

but diarrhea is present and feces are coated with mucus; **ulcerative enteritis** involves ulcers caused by parasitic infestation

enterobacterial *adj.* of or relating to bacteria that live in the intestines

enterobiasis *n.* infestation with pinworms

enterolith *n.* a solidified intestinal growth or stone usually formed of mineral salts; usually gray or green in color with a surface that can be smooth or rough and porous, and rounded or tetrahedral in shape. Can weigh from a few ounces to as much as 6 pounds, although most range between 7 ounces and 3 pounds. An affected horse may have only one or as many as 1,000 small ones. Usually form in the right dorsal colon and can cause intestinal blockage, which, if not relieved by surgery, is fatal; characterized by colic-like symptoms such as kicking and stretching, looking back at the right flank, decreased production of feces (or complete cessation), and a depressed attitude. The average age of horses having this condition ranges from 4 to 14 years.

enteron *n.* the alimentary canal; intestine

enteropathy *n.* any disease of the intestinal wall

enterotomy *n.* surgery of the intestine (enteron) by making an artificial opening into it, as for drainage

enterotoxemia *n.* the presence of intestinally produced toxins in the blood

entire *n.* a stallion

entropion *n.* a condition wherein the eyelid turns in and causes the eyelashes to rub on the surface of the cornea, thus irritating it

entry fee the fee paid by a contestant in order to compete in an event

enucleate *vt.* to surgically remove an organ, such as an eye

enuresis *n.* lack of urinary control; old mares are susceptible, more so than old geldings

enzootic *adj.* relating to diseases that affect animals in a certain area, climate, or season *n.* an enzootic disease

enzootic catarrh a viral infection common in male foals from age 2 months upwards, symptoms are a thick nasal discharge and usually a cough.

enzyme *n.* a chemical or ferment produced by living cells within the body; present in the salivary, gastric, and pancreatic juices; acts as an aid in digestion; for example, when a horse eats, different enzymes in turn immediately come into action, the first being ptyalin (in saliva), followed by pepsin (in the stomach), etc.

enzyme-linked immunosorbent assay (ELISA) a test for antibodies in body fluid and or tissue

Eohippus *n.* the most ancient ancestor of the modern horse; appeared during the Eocene Epoch or dawn period about 55 million years ago (hence the term, which means "dawn horse"); was about 11 inches tall; Hyracotherium

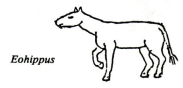

Eohippus

eosin, eosine *n.* a dye used to stain tissues for examination — **eosinic** *adj.*

eosinophil *n.* a type of white blood cell that multiplies during infections, allergies and infestation of parasites — **eosinophilic** *adj.*

eosinophilia *n.* the presence of an abnormally large number of eosinophils

EPE equine protozoal encephalomyelitis

epicardium *n.* the layer of the pericardium on the heart's outer surface — **epicardial** *adj.*

epichloe *n.* a fungus

epicondyle *n.* a projection of bone in the region of a condyle which does not articulate with another bone; e.g., epicondyle of the femur

epidemic *n.* the rapid spreading of a disease among many horses in a particular region —*adj.*

epidemiological *adj.* pertaining to the factors that cause or prevent disease in a particular group of horses

epidemiology *n.* the study of the causes and control of epidemics —**epidemiologic, epidemiological** *adj.* —**epidemiologist** *n.*

epidermis *n.* the outer layer of the skin —**epidermal, epidermic** *adj.*

epididymis *n.* in the stallion, that part of the seminal tube attached to the rear upper portion of each of the testes —**epididymal** *adj.*

epiglottis *n.* the triangular cartilage in the throat that folds over the entrance to the trachea (windpipe) when swallowing, preventing food or liquid from entering the lungs

epimysium *n.* the sheath of tissue encasing a muscle

epinephrine *n.* a hormone secreted by the adrenal gland; it constricts blood vessels and acts as a stimulant; synthetic epinephrine is used to treat the heaves and increase heart rate; adrenalin

epineurium *n.* the connective tissue surrounding a nerve fiber

epiphyseal cartilage *see* **epiphyseal plates**

epiphyseal line the separation, in an immature horse, between the epiphysis and the diaphysis

epiphyseal plates cartilage near the ends of the long bones of the leg; the place where the bone lengthens; growth plates; growth cartilage; physeal plates

epiphysis *n.* one of two ends of a long bone; in immaturity it is separated from the diaphysis or shaft (the main part of the bone) by the open epiphyseal lines —**epipheseal, epiphesial** *adj.*

epiphysitis *n.* stress to the epiphyses due to working an immature horse, resulting in fractures, splints, chronic lameness, and poor development

epiploon *n.* the layer of fat that covers the intestines

episcleritis *n.* inflammation of the sclera (white of the eye)

epistaxis *n.* nosebleed; can be induced by physical strain

epithelioma *n.* a tumor of the epithelium

epithelium *n.* cellular tissue composing the skin and lining internal and external parts of the body —**epithelial** *adj.*

epithelize *vt.* to cover (a raw surface, as a wound or ulcer) with epithelium, which grows in from the periphery —**epitheliazation** *n.*

epizoon *n.* a parasite that lives on the external surface of an animal's body

epizootic *adj.* rapid and widely spreading (as a disease or epidemic)

epizootic cellulitis *see* **arteritis**

epizootic cough *see* **infectious equine bronchitis**

epizootic lymphangitis a contagious chronic disease involving inflammation of glands and lymphatic vessels which develop nodules that rupture and ooze pus; there may also be inflamed eyes and nostrils and pneumonia; similar to glanders; caused by a fungus; recovery can occur after 3–12 months; pseudoglanders, mycotic lymphangitis, equine blastomycosis

epizootiology *n.* the study of epizootic diseases

equestrian *n.* a horseback rider —*adj.* relating to horses, horseback riders, horseback riding, or horsemanship

equestrienne *n.* a female horseback rider

Equidae *n.* a family of mammals that includes the horse, ass and zebra

equid herpesvirus *see* **equine herpesvirus**

equihose *n.* a support bandage for a horse's legs

equilenin *n.* an estrogen hormone

equilin *n.* an estrogen hormone produced by the fetus; excreted in the mare's urine when pregnant from about 4 months to full term; used medicinally for humans and in cosmetics

equine *adj.* of or relating to the horse — *n.*

equine biliary fever *see* **piroplasmosis**

equine blastomycosis *see* **epizootic lymphangitis**

equine chorionic gonadotrophin (ECG) a hormone produced in the pregnant mare from about the 38th to the 120th day of gestation

equine cutaneous papillomatosis *see* **milk warts**

equine degenerative myelopathy (EDM) a disease of the spinal cord in which there is deterioration of myelin resulting in wobbles

equine encephalomyelitis *see* **encephalomyelitis**

equine herpesvirus (EHV) a virus that causes rhinopneumonitis and possibly other diseases

equine infectious anemia (EIA) a communicable viral disease which can be mild or severe and fatal; can be contracted from a carrier through insect bites or by unsterilized hypodermic needles; characterized in acute cases by fever, sweating, and severe depression, and in chronic cases by fluctuating low fever, anemia, loss of appetite and weight, jaundice, staggering or paralyses, hemorrhage of the mucous membranes and frequent urination; swamp fever; river bottom disease —

see also **Coggins test**

equine infectious arteritis *see* **arteritis**

equine malaria *see* **piroplasmosis**

equine metritis *see* **metritis**

equine piroplasmosis *see* **piroplasmosis**

equine protozoal encephalomyelitis (EPE) inflammation of the brain and spinal cord caused by protozoal infection and resulting in wobbles; curable with antibiotic therapy if diagnosed early

equine syphilis *see* **dourine**

equine viral arteritis a serious viral disease manifested by high fever, severe pink eye, weakness, leg swelling, colic, diarrhea, coughing, and wheezing; can cause abortion in mares

equine virus abortion *see* **rhinopneumonitis**

equipage *n.* the horses, carriage, and liveried servants of a person of rank

equisetum *n.* a plant that grows on damp ground; horsetails; if eaten, causes thiamine deficiency; symptoms are similar to those of bracken fern poisoning

equitation *n.* the art of riding; horseback riding

equorum medicus an ancient Roman term for a veterinary surgeon

Equus *n.* the mammalian genus to which the horse belongs

Equus caballus the scientific Latin name of the modern horse; the first true horse, which evolved about 2 million years ago in North America and emigrated to Asia, Europe, Africa, and South America

ergot[1] *n.* the horny growth at the back of the fetlock, hidden by a tuft of hair; thought to be a vestigial toe

ergot[2] *n.* 1. a dark purple or black fungal mass that displaces grass seed, particularly rye 2. the dried part of

the rye fungus from which medicinal alkaloids are extracted and used

Eriskay *n.* a Scottish pony breed

ermine mark *see* **ermine spot**

ermine spot a leg marking which forms an intrusion of the coat color into a stocking or coronet mark, usually at the coronet band

Ermland *n.* a Polish draft breed; about 15.3 h.h.

erythemia *n.* a disease involving an overproduction of red blood cells

Erythrocin *n.* trade name for erythromycin

erythrocyte *n.* a red blood cell

erythrocyte sedimentation rate *see* **ESR**

erythromycin *n.* an antibiotic given to foals with bacterial infections such as joint-ill etc.; trade names Erythrocin, Ilotycin

Escherichia coli rod-shaped bacteria normally present in the intestinal tract; sometimes cause severe infection

escutcheon *n.* the hair pattern made on the horse's coat from below the point of the hip downward on the flank

eserine *n. see* **physostiamine salicylate**

esophagus *n.* gullet; the alimentary tube that extends from the larynx to the stomach — **esophageal** *adj.*

ESR erythrocyte sedimentation rate; a measurement which determines the presence or absence of an infection

essential fever *see* **primary fever**

estrogen *n.* the mare's sex hormone manufactured by the ovaries; influences outward sexual behavior and changes in the estrous cycle

estrogenic *adj.* 1. relating to estrogen 2. producing estrus

estrous *adj.* of or relating to estrus

estrous cycle the mare's reproductive cycle, which includes a period of heat followed by ovulation

estrus, estrum oestrus *n.* a mare's heat or season; the reproductive period in a mare when the ovum (egg) is released into the fallopian tubes and when the mare will accept mating with a stallion; it lasts for five to six days

ethmoid *adj.* like a strainer; relating to the sieve-like bones of the nasal cavity — *n.* an ethmoid bone

ethmoid cells sinus cells

ethmoid hematoma a tissue pocket in the upper area of the nasal passage that swells with blood, bursts and drains, and repeats the process

ethmoiditis *n.* inflammation of the ethmoid sinuses

ethmoid sinus a cavity, or sinus, in the bones of the nasal cavity

ethology *n.* the study of animal behavior

ethyl chloride a chemical used to freeze skin in local anesthesia

etiology *n.* the study of the causes of disease — **etiological, etiologic** *adj.*

eugenics *n.* the science of improving a breed by selective breeding

eustachian tube the auditory tube between the middle ear and the pharynx, which equalizes pressure on both sides of the eardrum

euthanasia *n.* the putting to death of an animal by a human being to end suffering

EVA equine viral arteritis

evens *n.pl.* in racing, the betting odds given on a horse when a person who places the bet stands to win the same amount as wagered; even money

event *n.* a particular contest in a program of competitions — *vi.* to take part in an event

eventer *n.* a competitor

event horse a horse that competes or is capable or competing in a combined training competition

evolution *n.* the developmental change of a species through ongoing genetic adaptation from one form to a successive form. The evolution of the horse (with approximate estimates of periods) is as follows: 1. Eohippus (Hyracotherium), Eocene period (50–38 million years ago); 2. Mesohippus, Oligocene period (38–26 million years ago); 3. Miohippus, Miocene period (27–7 million years ago); 4. Merychippus, latter part of Miocene period; 5. Pliohippus, Pliocene period (7–2 million years ago); 6. Equus, Pleisto-cene period (2 million–10,500 years ago to present day).

ewe neck a neck the crest of which is concavely curved like a U, sometimes called an **upside-down neck**; a conformation fault that often interferes with performance; the head is held so high that the horse is difficult to control —*see also* **swan neck**

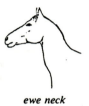

ewe neck

exacta *n.* in racing, a type of wagering in which the bettor must select the first and second place finishers in exact order

examination *n.* an inspection, which may be carried out visually as well as manually; a clinical examination is a detailed and professional inspection of an animal to determine any abnormalities, often conducted with the aid of instruments; a laboratory examination involves tests on body fluids and or solids for analysis; radiographic examination involves the use of X-ray equipment for inspection of internal body parts

exanthem, -thema *n.* an eruptive skin disease

exchange transfusion the process of withdrawing and replacing, with donor blood, most of the body's own blood

excipient *n.* an inert substance added to a drug to facilitate its administration

excise *vt.* to remove surgically, as a tumor —**excision** *n.*

excoriation *n.* a chafing due to movement of a saddle, particularly on perspiring skin —**excoriate** *vt.*

excrement *n.* waste matter; feces

excrete *vt.* to eliminate (waste matter) from the body, as through the kidneys or sweat glands —**excretion** *n.* —**excretory** *adj.*

exercise bandage a bandage wrapping a horse's legs to support tendons and ligaments while exercising

exercise induced pulmonary hemorrhage (EIPH) *see* **nosebleed**

exfoliate *vt., vi.* to shed or peel, as in the superficial layers of the skin —**exfoliation** *n.* —**exfoliative** *adj.*

exhaust *vt.* to tire out to the point of extreme fatigue; horses have been known to run until they drop dead from fatigue

Exmoor *n.* an ancient British pony breed indigenous to the moors of Devon and Somerset; there are records of wild Exmoors that date back to 1085; herds still run wild but are privately owned; unusual physical characteristics include a mealy coloration around the muzzle, eyes and underside between the thighs, unusual "toad" eyes, and a thick "ice" tail with a fan-like appearance at the root; very strong and hardy, intelligent but willful; 12.2–12.3 h.h.

exocrine *adj.* relating to any gland, as the salivary or sweat glands, that secretes onto a surface rather than into the blood; opposite of endocrine

exogenous *adj.* relating to outside causes that affect an organism as food, light, etc.

exostosis *n.* an osteophyte or bony growth that bulges out from a bone —*see also* **ringbone**

expectorant *n.* a medication that induces coughing up of mucus from lungs and bronchial tubes

expiration *n.* 1. exhalation or breathing out 2. breathing final breath; dying —**expiratory** *adj.* —**expire** *vi.*

expression *n.* facial appearance that shows what a horse is feeling

exsanguination *n.* the loss of very large quantities of blood

extended trot *see* **extend stride**

extender-preservative a preservative mixture used to increase the volume of collected semen

extend stride to lengthen the stride without appearing hurried; at horse shows, for example, one can hear the command, "Extend your trot!"; the horses are then asked by their riders to extend their stride and they almost appear to float; extension also applies to the walk or canter

extensor carpi obliquus/radialis muscles the muscles which extend the knee joint

extensor muscles muscles which straighten or extend a limb (as opposed to flexor muscles)

extirpation *n.* the surgical removal of an organ or body part; excision

extracellular *adj.* outside of a cell; e.g., a fluid

extract *vt.* to remove or pull out, as a tooth

extrahepatic *adj.* closely outside the liver

extrasystole *n.* an irregular rhythm of the heart

extrauterine *adj.* outside the uterus

extravasation *n.* the escape of blood, urine, or other body fluid from its normal channel into the tissues, as when a blood vessel ruptures

extremity *n.* a part outermost from the center of the body; e.g., a hoof

extrophy *n.* deformity of an organ

exudate *n.* a substance, such as pus, that is produced from an injured or diseased part of the body; matter exuded from the body; sweat

exudation *n.* something exuded

exude *vt., vi.* to sweat; ooze; discharge from the body

eye *n.* the organ of sight; the color of a horse's eyes is mostly dark brown but may be amber (often in duns), grey, or blue —*see also* **pupil**

eyeball *n.* the part of the eye shaped like a ball, which is enclosed by the socket and eyelids

eyebrow *n.* 1. the bony arch over each eye 2. the long hairs growing from this arch

eyelash *n.* one of the hairs forming a fringe on the upper eyelid

eyelid *n.* either of the two fleshy folds that cover and uncover the eye

eye to hounds in hunting, the experienced rider's ability to know what the fox has done and how the hounds will respond by watching their actions

— F —

facelessness *n.* a freakish congenital abnormality wherein eyes, nostrils, and mouth are absent, usually causing death immediately after birth; aprosopia

facet *n.* a smooth surface, as on a bone

facial marking a mark on the face made by white hairs contrasting with overall coat color; includes blaze, stripe, star, snip (often pink), star-strip-snip, bordering intrusion, bald, race, spot

facial paralysis loss of muscle function in the face; may occur on only one side, in which case the upper lip pulls to the unaffected side

fadge *n.* a half jog or swinging walk

faeces *n.pl.* feces — **faecal** *adj.*

failure of passive transfer (FPT) failure of a newborn foal to receive adequate protective antidotes from its dam's colostrum during the first few hours of life

faint *vi.* to lose consciousness temporarily

fair catch in rodeo team roping, a roping of a steer around the horns, head, or neck; legal catch

Falabella *n.* a miniature horse breed named after the family which developed the breed in Argentina; originated in the 19th century when an Irishman called Newton (Señor Falabella's maternal grandfather) bred a dwarf stallion to small Shetlands and, with the genes for small size proving dominant, thus started a breed of successively smaller miniatures, with the average today at the Falabella ranch being less than 34 inches tall; unlike other breeds, the gestation period is nearly 13 months; since these little horses are too small to ride, they are bred for showing and as pets only — *see also* **Miniature Horse**

Falapen *n.* trade name for benzylpenicillin

fall *vi.* 1. to touch the ground with the shoulders and quarters on the same side (said of horses) 2. to become completely separated from one's horse (said of riders) — *n.*

falling horse a horse trained for Western movies to fall down without injuring itself

fallopian tube either of two uterine tubes through which an ovum travels from the ovary to the uterus

false canter *see* **counter canter**

false cyst a cyst that develops in solid organs where softening or degeneration has occurred; spurious cyst

false nostril a blind pouch in the lateral wall of the nostril, the function of which is unknown

false quarter a condition wherein the inside quarter of the hoof is thin and weak; usually affects the forefeet, although sometimes the hind feet can be involved

false ribs those ribs to the rear of the true ribs which are not attached directly to the breastbone

false sandcrack a superficial defect of the hoof wall that looks like sandcrack but is not deep enough to weaken the hoof wall

false sole *see* **sole**

fan a horse in rodeo, to agitate a bucking bronco by waving one's hat and slapping the horse with it, thereby increasing the bucking and gaining an opportunity to demonstrate skill; reef; dust

fancied *adj.* in racing, favored to win; favorite

fan tail a docked tail that is shortened at the sides near the root to effect the overall appearance of a fan

fantasia *n.* a spectacular riding display which is part of a religious festival in Morocco and is performed in commemoration of ancient wars; a group of handsome horses with highly ornamented tack suddenly gallop into view, their riders carrying weapons which are fired at a given signal in mock attack

Faradism *n.* electrotherapy on muscles to produce rhythmic contractions or for other purposes; named for English physicist Michael Faraday

farcy *n.* a mild, very contagious form of glanders involving ulcerations of the lymphatics of the skin that discharge pus and tend not to heal; lymphangitis

farrier *n.* a horse-shoer; a blacksmith

farriery *n.* the work or the shop of a farrier

far side the right side of a horse if viewed from the rear; off side

fartlek *n.* a Swedish term meaning speed play; varied exercises involving short sprints, hill work, jogging, cantering and skill drills, the purpose of which is to give the horse a series of stresses and recoveries that relax it

fascia *n.* a connective tissue in any of various areas of the body — **fascial** *adj.* — **fascitis** *n.* inflammation of fascia

fastigium *n.* the point of highest severity of a fever or illness

fast-twitch fibers (FT, type IIb) thick muscle fibers that provide energetic, explosive exercise and do not utilize oxygen for contracting the muscles

fast-twitch high-oxidative fibers (FTH, type IIa) muscle fibers that use both oxygen and glycogen to provide either vigorous or sustained exercise, or both

fat *n.* solid or semi-solid, yellow or white, greasy material in animal tissue; adipose — *adj.* having an excess of fat — **fatness** *n.* — **fatten** *vt.*

fatigue *n.* weariness, exhaustion — *vt.* to tire through exertion — **fatigued** *adj.*

fat-soluble vitamins vitamins A, D, E and K

fatty acid an acid that originates from hydrocarbons, such as oleic, stearic, or palmitic acid

fatty degeneration degeneration of an organ when an abnormal presence of fat replaces its normal structure

fauces *n.* the rear area of the mouth leading into the throat — **faucial** *adj.*

fault *n.* 1. in show-jumping, an error or imperfect action recorded on a competitor's score, such as a refusal or knocking down a rail 2. in hunting, a break in the line of scent 3. an imperfection; something that mars a horse's conformation or way of going

favor *vt.* to avoid placing weight on (a leg); to limp

favorite *adj.* in racing, considered likely to win a particular race; having the lowest odds offered — *n.* **fancied**

favus *n.* a parasitic skin disease that is contagious through contact; honeycomb ringworm

feathering *n.* in hunting, the tendency of hounds to show they are uncertain about a scent by moving their rears from side to side while following the line — **feather** *vi.*

feathers *n.pl.* long, shaggy hair below the knee and hock, as typical of Shires and Clydesdales

feathers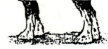

febrifuge *n.* any agent for reducing fever

febrile *adj.* feverish; relating to above-normal body temperature

fecalith *n.* a hard ball of feces within the bowel — **fecaloid** *adj.*

feces *n.pl.* excrement; solid waste — **fecal** *adj.* — *see also* **coprophagy**

fecundate *vt.* to impregnate or make fertile

fecundity *n.* the ability to produce offspring; fertility — **fecund** *adj.*

feed *n.* grain used for nourishment — *vt.* to give grain (or hay) for nourishment

feed bag a bag which is fastened over the muzzle and used for holding feed; nose bag

feed bag

feeler *n.* any of the long hairs around the eyes, as distinguished from the eyelashes

FEI Fédération Equestre Internationale (International Equestrian Federation), the agency that sets rules for international equestrian sports

Fell *n.* a British pony breed of ancient heritage; a registry was formed in 1912; hardy, strong and sure-footed; used for riding and driving; 13–14 h.h.

female *n.* a filly or mare —*adj.*

femur *n.* the thighbone —**femoral** *adj.*

fenbendazole *n.* a dewormer for internal parasites, except bots and tapeworms

fence 1. *n.* in competition, any obstacle to be jumped —*vi., vt.* to jump over an obstacle 2. *n.* a barrier for confinement or as a boundary made of wooden or man-made boards and posts, or wooden or metal posts connected with wire (which, for the safety of horses, should not be barbed) in single strands or mesh —*vt.* to enclose within a fence —**fenced** *adj.*

fenders *n.pl.* the wide flaps on a Western saddle that support the stirrups in front and join the stirrup leathers behind; sudaderos

fenestra *n.* a small window-like opening in a membrane or other body part, as in the middle ear —**fenestral** *adj.*

fentanyl *n.* generic name for a drug with narcotic and painkilling properties which acts as a stimulant

feral *adj.* wild

ferine *adj.* feral

fermentation *n.* the breakdown of complex molecules by the action of enzymes —**ferment** *vi., vt.*

ferric *adj.* containing iron; ferrous

ferrin *n.* a ferric substance found in bile pigment

fertile *adj.* able to produce offspring —**fertility** *n.*

fescue *n.* a genus of tufted, perennial grasses sometimes used for grazing horses; it adapts to shade but not to very high temperatures; ingestion of alkaloids in the grass, as well as the presence of fungus, can result in a thickened placenta in a pregnant mare, causing neonatal death of the foal; another problem may be agalactia (lack of milk production)

fetal dystocia *see* **dystocia**

fetation *n.* fetal development

feticide *n.* abortion induced by a stallion forcibly copulating with a pregnant mare

fetlock *n.* the joint of the leg between the cannon bone and the pastern

fetoscope *n.* an instrument for detection of the heartbeat of a fetus

fetter *vt.* to restrain —*see also* **hobble** —*n.* any device which is used to restrain a horse

fetus *n.* an unborn offspring from the 41st day after conception to birth —**fetal** *adj.*

fever *n.* elevated body temperature —**fevered, feverish** *adj.*

fiador *n.* the part of a hackamore that fastens the back of the bosal to the headstall by a knot; sometimes called theadore

fiber *n.* a threadlike structure that together with others forms tissues in the body

fiber optics the use of flexible plastic fibers to conduct light to internal spaces of the respiratory and intestinal

tracts for viewing purposes — **fiber-optic** *adj.*

fiberscope *n.* an instrument used for fiber-optic examination

fibril *n.* a fine fiber in the body — **fibrillar, fibrillary** *adj.*

fibrillation *n.* an irregular heartbeat

fibrin *n.* a body protein which forms the basis of a blood clot — **fibrinous** *adj.*

fibrinogen *n.* a protein in blood plasma which converts to fibrin during blood clotting by the action of the enzyme thrombin — **fibrinogenic** *adj.*

fibrinolysin *n.* an enzyme, such as plasmin, that can digest fibrin

fibrinolysis *n.* the process by which a blood clot is broken down and fibrin dissolved — **fibrinolytic** *adj.*

fibroblast *n.* a cell in connective tissue of the body that causes the formation of fibers — **fibroblastic** *adj.*

fibroid *adj.* relating to fibrous tissue — *n.* a fibrous tumor

fibroma *n.* a benign, fibrous tumor or neoplasm

fibrosarcoma *n.* a malignant fibrous tumor or neoplasm

fibrosis *n.* the replacement of normal tissue by fibrous tissue — **fibrotic** *adj.*

fibrositis *n.* the accumulation of fibrous tissue due to an injury or inflammation; can be a very painful interference to normal motion

fibrotic myopathy a tearing of the semitendinosus muscle, followed by fibrosis; may occur when a horse fights a side-line (rear foot tied by a rope to a loop around the neck) or catches a rear foot in a loose halter; may also occur in working stock and rodeo horses; characterized by the foot jerking back slightly just before contacting the ground

fibrous tissue gristle; an arrangement of fibroblasts

fibula *n.* a narrow bone behind the tibia of the rear leg

fidding *n.* the cruel application of pepper or ginger to a mare's vagina to make her carry an elevated tail; figging

fiddle-head *n.* a large, ugly head

fiddleneck *n.* a poisonous weed which affects the intestines; amsinckia

field¹ *n.* 1. an open stretch of land 2. an area of cleared land enclosed for pasturing stock

field² *n.* 1. in hunting, the mounted followers of a hunt 2. in racing, (a) all the horses taking part in a race; (b) all the horses not individually favored in the betting

field hunter a horse of any breeding or cross that regularly hunts with a recognized pack of hounds

field master in hunting, the person in charge of the field

fifth leg an advantage a horse is said to have when it smartly avoids a bad result from an error at a jump

figging *n.* *see* **fidding**

figure-eights *n.pl.* a training exercise in which the horse is ridden in two circles, going from one to the other, as in the number 8

filament *n.* a threadlike piece of tissue

filaria *n.* a threadlike parasite that may inhabit the eye and subcutaneous tissue — **filarial, filarian** *adj.*

filled legs swollen legs

filly *n.* a female horse under the age of four years, unless she is bred earlier, at which time she becomes a mare

finish *vi.* in racing, to pass the winning post mounted, provided the horse and rider have jumped all obstacles, if any, as in steeplechase and hurdle racing — *vt.* to complete a competition — *n.* the end of a competition

Finnhorse *n.* an all-purpose cold-blood breed of Finland, strongly built

with a good temperament; there are three types, the draft, trotter, and riding horse; usually about 15.2 h.h. but can vary from 14.2 to 17.3 h.h.

fire brand *see* **brand**

firing *n.* a controversial treatment of a leg injury by burning the skin over the injured area with a hot iron in order that scar tissue may be formed; cauterization —*see also* **acid firing, pin firing, superficial line firing**

first aid any initial help given to an injured horse before professional attention is available

first dung *see* **meconium**

first intention healing the healing of an open wound produced by closing together its edges with sutures and or supportive bandaging; this hastens the healing process with a minimum of granulation tissue and scarring; primary healing

first jockey the principal person engaged by a horse's owner or trainer to ride for him or her

first milk *see* **colostrum**

fissure *n.* 1. a normal groove between parts of an organ 2. an abnormal break in the skin 3. a breaking into parts, as in bone cracks —*vt., vi.* —**fissured** *adj.*

fistula *n.* an abnormal canal that connects an abscess or hollow organ to the skin or to another abscess or hollow organ —**fistulous** *adj.*

fistulous withers a condition affecting the withers wherein fistulas appear as non-infected swelling or as an extensive, weeping infection that starts at the withers; often caused by a badly fitting saddle or harness —*see also* **brucellosis**

fitness *n.* the state of being adapted to a particular level of exercise

fitting *n.* the initial phase of physical conditioning which involves developing the body's system to its existing capacity for work, as opposed to subsequent conditioning that involves building new tissue and extending the body's capacity for work; conditioning —*see also* **condition**

fittings *n.pl.* the parts of an English saddle that can be separated from the saddle, such as stirrup leathers, stirrups, girth

Fitzwygram shoe an iron shoe with a turned-up toe used for stumbling

fixation *n.* the fastening or immobilizing of a body part, such as a broken bone

Fjord *n.* a dun pony breed that originated in Norway but can now be found in Sweden, Denmark, and West Germany; strong and sure-footed and popular for farm work in mountain areas but also used for riding and in harness; 13–14.2 h.h.

flag[1] *vi., vt.* in the mare, to rhythmically lift the tail and expose the clitoris when in estrus

flag[2] *vi.* 1. to tire and slow down 2. dock

flagman *n.* in racing, the person who signals the winning horse; in rodeo, the person who signals the end of time elapsed in timed events

flag racing in playday competition, an event wherein the rider must carry a flag and exchange it at each barrel in a cloverleaf pattern

flake *n.* 1. a section of a square bale of hay; hay is baled into rectangular bales (referred to as square) in such a way as to enable them to separate easily into flakes 2. a small version of the facial marking called a star —**spot**; 3. a tiny piece of something such as skin or dandruff

flame *n.* a marking consisting of a few white hairs in the center of the forehead

Flanders *n.* an ancestor of the various

heavy breeds, such as the Clydesdale, Shire, etc., and said to have been a war horse in medieval times; Flemish

flank *n.* the fleshy area on the side of the hindquarter between the last rib and the hip and extending downward

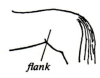

flank

flap *n.* on an English saddle, the large leather piece that forms the side of the saddle under the stirrup leather

flapper *n.* a horse that runs in an unauthorized race

flapping meeting an unofficial, unauthorized race meeting

flare foot a hoof that flares outward due to uneven weight distribution; dished foot, wry foot; flare hoof

flat-catcher *n.* a seemingly all-round attractive horse that is discovered to have undesirable defects

flat foot 1. a foot that has an angle noticeably less than 45 degrees 2. a foot whose sole lacks the usual concavity

flat race a speed contest ridden on a course where there are no obstacles to jump

flat *n.* 1. a race course without obstacles 2. level ground; e.g., "racing on the flat," as opposed to "racing over obstacles"

flat saddle a saddle with a low or cut-back pommel and no knee rolls, used for saddle-seat riding

flat-sided *adj.* slab-sided

flatus *n.* gas in the intestinal tract; flatulence

flatworm *n.* a platyhelminth (e.g., a tapeworm or fluke)

flaxen *adj.* 1. pale yellow or straw-colored 2. describes a chestnut with either white or flaxen mane and tail

flea-bitten *adj.* describes the color pattern of a gray horse that is speckled with small black or brown spots

fleam *n.* a pointed surgical knife used in the 16th century to bleed horses

flecked *adj.* having small areas of white hairs distributed irregularly on the body; the coat may be heavily flecked or lightly flecked

flehmen face an expression made by the horse by stretching the head up and forward, curling up the top lip and showing the upper teeth and gums; a stallion often does this when he smells a mare's urine, but both male and female horses make the flehmen face for no reason apparent to the human

Flemish *see* **Flanders**

flesh fly a fly that deposits its eggs on open wounds; blowfly; the eggs develop into tiny white maggots that eat into the wounds and tear up the tissues

flex *vt.* to bend (a joint or limb) by contracting flexor muscles; usually refers to the neck but can also be applied to the knees and hocks in high action —**flexion** *n.*

flexibility *n.* the physical ability to bend, to be supple and limber; the opposite of stiffness; a poor rider can hinder a horse's flexibility when his or her motion in the saddle opposes that of the horse; to increase flexibility, there are various exercises that may be used, such as to improve lateral flexibility by bending the neck by gently pulling the head to either side with one rein

flexion test a test for inflammation and for degeneration in or around a joint; the joint is forcibly flexed for 30–60 seconds, after which the horse is jogged; appearance or increase of lameness suggests an affirmative diagnosis

flexor *n.* a muscle that bends (flexes) a limb or other body part —**flexural** *adj.*

flexor tendon a tendon that runs from

the knee to the fetlock and can be seen lying behind the cannon bone

float *n.* 1. a trailer for transporting horses 2. a dental rasp —*vt.* to file down irregular molars for a better chewing surface

flora *n.* normal bacteria and protozoa in the digestive tract

fluke *n.* a parasitic flatworm, of which there are several classes (e.g., Trematoda, which lives in the liver and causes anemia and diarrhea; Schistosomatidae, which live in blood vessels)

fluorine poisoning harmful ingestion of fluorine, as from misuse of certain wormers or from consumption of plants covered with dust from industrial works using the chemical

flushing *n.* a widely condemned method of inducing conception whereby a mare is put on a weight-reducing diet, followed, shortly before she is bred, by a high-protein, weight-gaining diet so that the body is building up at conception time —**flush** *vt.*

fly[1] *n.* a flying insect, of which there are many different kinds, that can infect the horse with disease as well as cause extreme annoyance

fly[2] *n.* in hunting, any obstacle that can be cleared in a single jump, as opposed to being jumped on and off

fly a jump to jump an obstacle taking off and landing well away from it while maintaining stride

fly bonnet a fly covering for the upper part of the horse's face; fly mask

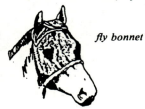

fly bonnet

fly fringe a browband with a fringe of strips to shake away flies; fly guard

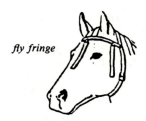

fly fringe

fly guard *see* **fly fringe**

flying lead change a smooth change of lead during a canter or gallop without reducing speed

flying W in playday competition, a timed event involving five poles placed to form a W; the rider weaves through the poles without knocking them down

fly mask *see* **fly bonnet**

fly-shaker muscle a specialized muscle layer which contracts to twitch the skin to shake off flies or other irritants

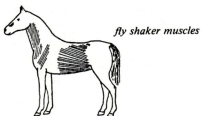

fly shaker muscles

fly sheet a sheet with ties used on a horse for protection against flies

foal *n.* a newborn horse of either sex and up to age 6 months —*vi., vt.* to give birth (to)

foal heat the estrus period of a mare which occurs between 7 and 10 days after parturition

foaling alarm an alarm system used to signal a mare's keeper to the beginning of her parturition

foal jaundice *see* **neonatal isoerythrolysis**

foam *n.* heavy sweat or frothy saliva

fodder *n.* a coarse food, like hay —*vt.* to feed with fodder

foil *vi.* in hunting, to retrace existing

tracks (said of quarry); stain — *see also* **stained line**

follicle *n.* a small gland or cavity from which secretions are generated, such as that in which an ovum develops or in which a hair develops — **follicular** *adj.*

follicle stimulating hormone (FSH) a hormone secreted by the pituitary gland of both mare and stallion; stimulates the development of ova-producing follicles in the mare and growth of sperm in the stallion

foot *n.* the pedal structure from the coronary band to the bottom of the hoof

footfall *n.* the order in which a horse steps in a particular gait

foot warmers cold-weather covers for a rider's feet that fit over English stirrups

foot weights weighted rings placed on the forefeet, especially of Saddlebreds, to cause high action for the show ring

forage acre a measure of the grass available for grazing on a pasture, equal to the total area multiplied by the percentage of land surface covered by usable grass (ex: 10 acres × 30% density = 3 forage acres)

forearm *n.* that part of the front leg that extends from elbow to knee; radius

forefoot[1] *n.* either of the front feet

forefoot[2] *vt.* to break (a horse) by roping around both forefeet while the horse is running so that the horse is brought down with such violence as to often cause injury (knocking out front teeth, etc.)

forehand *n.* the forequarters, including head, neck, shoulders and forefeet

forehead *n.* the front part of the face between eyes and roots of forelock

forelock *n.* the part of the mane that hangs down over the forehead between the ears

forequarters *n.* forehand

forfeit list in racing, a published list of people in debt on entry fees, etc. and the corresponding horses

Forgastrin *n.* trade name for bismuth

forge *vi.* to move in such a way that a hind foot strikes the sole of a forefoot on the same side, causing a clacking sound; a faulty way of going caused by being uncollected or by being in need of a shoeing; over-reach

fork *n.* the part of the Western saddle in front that swells under the horn

form *n.* in racing, any source of information about horses that will run, such as past performances, odds, etc.

fornix *n.* a vault-like structure of the anatomy, as of the pharynx

Forssell's operation the surgical removal of muscles from the neck between the jawbone and breastbone to stop cribbing and or windsucking

forward seat 1. a saddle in which the rider sits just behind the horse's withers, feet back in rather short stirrups with toes in line with knees 2. a rider's position of sitting forward in the saddle; a balanced seat; in jumping, the rider maintains a forward seat with seat bones off the saddle and leaning forward

fossa *n.* a shallow depression on the surface of a body structure

foster *vt.* to nourish and care for (a foal other than the mare's own offspring); possible when the foal's dam has died, has not enough milk, or rejects her foal; depending on the foster mare, this can be either relatively easy or very difficult

founder *n.* an advanced and severe form of laminitis wherein the laminae break down, causing the sole to separate from the hoof wall and drop

down; founder rings develop on the hoof; the pain makes the horse refuse to eat and to sweat and tremble; the horse may be reluctant to move and may change its weight constantly from one foot to another; in extreme cases, the hooves may fall off; condition may be chronic or acute; causes are over-feeding of grain, overwork on hard surfaces, or drinking large amounts of water while still hot after exercise

founder rings very marked rings that develop on foundered hooves clustering around the coronet and pointing down towards the heel

founder stance the typical stance of a horse affected by founder wherein the horse tries to take as much weight as possible off the affected feet. When the forefeet are affected the horse brings them forward in front of its body, moving the hind feet up under its body.

Four-H Club a U.S. government sponsored youth program that encourages horse care and horsemanship among other chiefly agricultural activities

Four Horsemen of the Apocalypse *see* **Apocalypse, Four Horsemen of the**

four-in-hand *n.* a driving team of four horses: two wheelers and two leaders

fox trot a 4-beat gait: left hind, right fore, pause, right hind, left fore; varies from 5 to 10 m.p.h.; head and tail are carried somewhat elevated and head nods; the horse seems to be walking with its forelegs and trotting with its hind legs —*see also* **Missouri Fox Trotter**

fracture *n.* a break in a bone; there are many kinds, including compound, compound-comminuted, comminuted, greenstick or incomplete, simple, fissured, spontaneous, impacted, and riding fracture —*see also* **compression plating** — *vt.*

Franches-Montagnes *n.* a small Swiss draft breed, heavy built with short legs, developed in the Swiss Jura mountain area for agricultural purposes; 15. h.h.

Frederiksborg *n.* a Danish breed whose stud was founded in 1562 by King Frederick with the purpose of developing high-class dressage horses; the breed became famous, but by the 19th century the stud was closed due to deterioration of stock, and today only a few purebreds remain; used for light draft work as well as riding; 15.3–16 h.h.

free fatty acids a group of organic chemicals that form the building blocks of fat and give energy for endurance exercise; triglycerides are their stored forms; together they provide up to a third of a horse's total aerobic metabolism

free rein guidance by a loose rein, with the horse relaxing rather than being collected or even being in light contact with the rider

freeze brand or **-mark** a fairly painless method of branding by freezing hair roots with a copper iron chilled to –320 degrees F.; the hair lost from the branded area grows back white; in the case of gray horses, new hair growth is stopped by longer application of the iron so as to kill the hair roots; developed in 1954

Freiberger *n.* a Swiss breed used by the Swiss army and by farmers in the high mountains of Switzerland where mechanized transport and tractors are impractical; highly regarded and valued, this breed is supported by the government; also used for crossbreeding with Thoroughbreds to produce hunters and sports horses; 15–17 h.h.

fremitus *n.* a vibration that can be felt, as by palpating the chest

French Saddle Horse *see* **Selle Français**

French Trotting Horse a French breed

used in harness and for racing; also called Norman Trotter; up to 16.2 h.h.

frenum *n.* a fold of skin or mucous membrane that limits the movement of an organ or part; e.g., the fold under the tongue; **frenulum** is a small frenum

fresh *adj.* in high spirits, especially at the beginning of a ride, due to lack of exercise, cold weather, or exuberance over getting out for a jaunt

fret *n.* colic — *vi.* to act in a disturbed way

Friesian *n.* an old European breed at one time heavy and used for agricultural work; now lighter, though strong; a good, all-round, attractive riding horse with great presence, high knee action and a very fast trot; has a gentle and willing nature; always completely black; around 15 h.h.

frog *n.* the triangular-shaped, horny structure in the rear half of the sole of the foot which is a partial weight-bearing area of the hoof and serves to absorb concussion

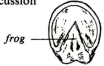

frog

frog-pressure theory the theory that the frog should come in contact with the ground for the foot to function naturally and should not be pared down by the farrier

frontal boss the bony protrusion in the forehead above and between the eyes

frostbite *n.* necrotic damage to body tissues by exposure to severe cold, particularly affecting the legs when a horse is forced to stand in mud and water in very cold conditions or when in similar conditions the legs are washed, especially without immediate and thorough drying

frost nail a shoe nail with a large

pointed or wedge-shaped head used to prevent slipping. There are two basic kinds: (a) those that have flat bases under the heads and (b) those with conical necks which require special holes adapted to insertion into the shoe only and not the hoof

frosty *adj.* having white hairs at the base of the tail, in the mane, down the back, and over bony prominences; skunk tail

fructose *n.* sugar or carbohydrate in the bloodstream of the fetus and newborn foal, which is used up by the body within two days after birth

FSH follicle stimulating hormone

Fulani *n.* a West African all-purpose breed; about 14 h.h.

full *adj.* ungelded

full cheek snaffle bit a plain broken snaffle with full cheeks which prevent the rings from sliding through the mouth

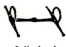

full cheek snaffle bit

fullering *n.* *see* **swaging**

full mouth the mouth of a mature horse having all of the permanent teeth

full stocking *see* **stocking**

full-thickness skin wound a wound that cuts completely through the skin

Fulmer snaffle bit *see* **full cheek snaffle bit**

fundus *n.* the base of an organ

fungal abortion abortion caused by a fungus that grows on the placenta and impedes the nourishment of the fetus; the fungus can also enter the fetal bloodstream, causing lesions in the liver and lungs

fungate *vi.* to grow quickly, like a fungus, as do some tumors

fungicide *n.* an anti-fungal substance

fungus *n.pl.* **fungi** a thallophyte

organism that can cause infection
—**fungous, fungal** *adj.*

Furioso *n.* a Hungarian all-purpose
cross-breed developed in the mid–19th
century from a Thoroughbred stallion
called Furioso bred onto local Nonius-
type mares; later the Thoroughbred
called North Star contributed further
to the breed; excels in competition
such as dressage, show-jumping, and
eventing; 16 h.h.

furniture *n.* any item of harness or
saddlery put on a horse

furosemide *n. see* **Lasix**

furuncle *n.* a boil or abscess; a small
pimple-like skin lump

fusarium *n.* a fungus that produces a
poison called aflatoxin and affects
grain, especially corn. The early
presence of infestation in the horse's
grain is usually invisible and can be
sporadic, with the result that testing
one sample may not be a true indication of contamination, and by the time
visible symptoms appear, it is too late
to treat a horse that has eaten it in
significant quantities.

fuse *vt., vi.* to join together, in reference to parts of the body —**fused** *adj.*
(a fused joint, as in advanced arthritis)

futurity *n.* a contest involving young
horses

futurity race a race in which the contestants are selected long beforehand

fuzztail running the act of herding
and catching wild horses

F waves abnormal pattern on an electrocardiogram that results from excessive electric signals originating in
the base of the heart

– G –

GABA gamma-aminobutyric acid, a
chemical that inhibits the transmission
of nerve impulses

gadfly *n.* horse fly

gag *n. see* **speculum**

gag bridle a severe form of corrective
bridle; cheek pieces of rounded leather
or rope pass through holes at the top
and bottom of round bit rings before
attaching to the reins; should be used
only by experts and with a second pair
of reins thereby restricting its use to
correction only, chiefly to raise the head

gait *n.* the sequence in which a horse
moves its feet in forward motion—
walk, trot, canter, and gallop being
the basic gaits — *vi.* to move in a manner other than a basic gait, either naturally or through training, such as the
natural 4-beat single-foot of the Paso
Fino or a pace, rack, running walk,
fox trot, amble, or tolt —**in gait** *adv.*

gait analysis an analytical, computerized tracing of a horse in motion. One
method is to use sensor to record information about its gait particularly in
regard to leg pressure. Another method
is done by using a high speed movie
camera to determine angular changes
in joints, stride lengths and frequen-
cies, and relative leg positions during
each phase of the stride. In jumping,
characteristics of the approach and recovery strides, jump clearance and arc
of hoof motion can be analyzed.

gaited *adj.* 1. having a particular gait
other than the walk, trot, canter, or
gallop 2. referring to the horse's general way of running, i.e. heavy-gaited,
smooth-gaited, etc.

gaiting strap a trotting harness strap
that prevents a trotter from moving
sideways in gait; sidestrap

galactagogue *n.* a substance that promotes the flow of milk

Galiceno *n.* a pony breed, native to Mexico but found throughout the U.S.A.; used in harness and for riding; has the gait of a fast running walk and is hardy and intelligent; 12–13.2 h.h.

gall *n.* a raised circular skin sore, usually caused by rubbing or chafing of the saddle or by the girth or harness — *vi.* to get sore from rubbing or chafing — *vt.* to make sore by rubbing or chafing

gallop *n.* 1. the fastest gait a horse is capable of, a full 3-beat run of leaping strides with all four feet leaving the ground at one time; may be led from either side (*see* **lead**); on a right lead the sequence is LH, RH and LF together, RF, suspension; on left lead RH, LH and RF together, LF — *vi.* 2. an area of ground surface used for riding or training

galloping boots *see* **brushing boots**

galloping sheet *see* **quarter sheet**

Galloway *n.* an Australian showring category based on a horse's height; measurement is from 14 to 15 h.h.

Galvayne's groove a brown-colored, furrowed streak on the upper corner incisor tooth; it appears just below the gum at the age of 10; it lengthens down the tooth with advancing age, reaching mid-tooth at around age 15 and the bottom of the tooth at age 20; at this time it will also begin to recede from the gum line and by around age 25 it will have disappeared as far down as mid-tooth; by about age 30 the groove may have disappeared completely

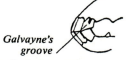

Galvayne's groove

Galvayne's strap a strap, or rope, that extends between the headstall and tail sometimes used for breaking a horse since under this restraint the horse is limited to moving in a circle which soon wears it out

gamete *n.* a reproductive cell

gamma-aminobutyric acid *see* **GABA**

ganglion *n.* any mass of nerve cells outside the spinal cord

gang plow a plow with several blades arranged in a series

gangrene *n.* necrosis, usually from loss of blood supply; putrefied external or internal body tissue. There are two forms, dry and moist, the latter being the commonest form. Gangrene is rare in horses but can occur. — **gangrenous** *adj.* — *see also* **gas gangrene**

ganted up looking starved

garde *n.* a knobby head on the outside splintbone of the hock, sometimes mistaken for a curb. Unlike the curb, which is directly on the back of the leg, the garde is slightly toward the side; also, while the curb yields slightly to pressure, the garde is hard bone.

Garrano *n.* a pony breed of Portugal, used for light agricultural work and riding; 10–12 h.h.; also called Minho

Garron *n.* a native pony of Scotland or Ireland; has a thick, fine-haired mane and tail and usually a dorsal stripe; also called Highland Pony; 13.2–14 h.h.

Garvolin *n.* a Polish draft breed; 14.3–16.2 h.h.

gas *n.* vapor in the stomach or intestines; flatus — **gaseous** *adj.*

gas bacillus a species of the clostridium bacteria that infects wounds, causing gas formation in them

gas chromatograph an instrument used to separate certain organic compounds by means of vaporization to determine their amounts

gas gangrene a usually fatal condition that results when wounds infected by clostridium bacteria cause tissues to fill with gas and pus

gaskin *n.* the area of the hind leg between the stifle and the hock; the second thigh

gastric *adj.* of or relating to the stomach

gastric dilation a permanent distension of the stomach caused by regular ingestion of indigestible foods or sand, or by windsucking

gastric juice the acid digestive secretion of the stomach lining

gastric ulcer an ulcer of the mucous membrane lining of the stomach, usually caused by an invasion of bots or hebronema

gastritis *n.* an inflammation of the stomach caused by defective food or chemical irritants; mild attacks may be characterized by fatigue and unwarranted sweating, a sour mouth odor and furred tongue and hard, mucus coated feces; severe attacks bring colic

gastrocnemius *n.* a muscle which controls the hock and flexes the stifle joints

gastroenteritis *n.* inflammation of the stomach and intestines

gastrointestinal *adj.* of the stomach and intestines

gastrointestinal tract *see* **alimentary tract**

gastrophilidae *n.pl.* equine parasites, or bots, that are the larvae of gadflies — *see also* **bots**

Gastrophilus equi a species of gadfly that produces the most common form of bots; it is ½ to ⅔ inches long and brownish-yellow in color, with bands across its underside; its wings are cream-colored with dark bands and spots; the bots are reddish; also called gadfly, common horse botfly, *G. intestinalis*

Gastrophilus hemorrhoidalis a small species of botfly with a yellowish band across its underside that ends in an orange tip; usually lays its eggs on the horse's facial hair, muzzle, lips and cheeks; the larvae, after traveling through the stomach and duodenum, reach the rectum and anus; they are reddish, turning greenish later; also called nose botfly, red-tailed botfly

Gastrophilus intestinalis see **bot** or **gadfly**

Gastrophilus nasalis a species of botfly having orange and and gray hairs (no spots), that lays eggs in the region of the throat; also called *G. veterinus,* throat horse botfly

Gastrophilus pecorum a species of botfly that produces red bots, similar to those of the *Gastrophilus hemorrhoidalis*; common in eastern Europe

Gastrophilus veterinus see Gastrophilus nasalis

gastrula *n.* the stage of the embryo after blastula

gate *n.* 1. a movable barrier for controlling the start of a horse in a race 2. an upright obstacle in show-jumping competitions

gauze *n.* a fine, loosely woven material used for dressings

GCMS gas chromatography and mass spectrometry; a type of dope test

Gelderland *n.* a breed, native to the Netherlands, used in harness and for riding; 15.2 h.h.

gelding *n.* a castrated male horse — **gelded** *adj.* — **geld** *vt.*

Gelineau's syndrome *see* **narcolepsy**

gemellus *n.* a thigh muscle which rotates the femur outward

gene *n.* a chromosomal unit that generates hereditary characteristics; each carries the DNA and protein code necessary for the development of a specific characteristic in offspring cells; genes are present in the sperm cells of the stallion and the egg cells of the mare; a **dominant gene** is one that breeds true to character even if only one parent possesses it; a **recessive gene** only breeds true to character if both parents possess it; a **lethal gene** is one that kills the individual

generalized *adj.* spread throughout the body, as opposed to localized

generate *vt.* to produce (offspring)

generic *adj.* in pharmacology, named by the chemical ingredient (of a drug), as opposed to the commercial trade name; for example, ivermectin (generic name) is sold under the trade name of Zimecterin

generous *adj.* willingly performing at maximum of ability in competition; such a horse may also be described as having "lots of heart"

genio-hyoideus a muscle that draws the hyoid bone and tongue forward

genitals, genitalia *n.pl.* the external sex organs — **genital** *adj.*

genome *n.* the complete set of chromosomes responsible for the offspring's characteristics — **genomic** *adj.*

genotype *n.* the horse's total genetic makeup

gentamycin *n.* an antibiotic efficacious in treating infestations of pseudomonas and a broad spectrum of other bacteria; may have toxic effects on kidneys

gentian *n.* a substance taken from the root of a plant (*Gentiana litea*) and given to improve appetite; **gentian violet** is an antiseptic dye used for wounds and proud flesh

gentle *adj.* tame and easily handled — *vt.* to make tame with patience and kindness

genus *n.* in biological classification, the main subdivision of a family or subfamily, usually including two or more species; organisms are often referred to by their genus and species

geophagy *n.* the eating of dirt

germ *n.* a microorganism, especially one that can cause disease

German Olympic martingale a martingale that passes through the ring of the bit and snaps onto a dee on each rein

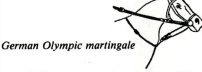
German Olympic martingale

germicide *n.* an antiseptic for killing germs

germinal skin layer the deepest layer of skin, from which outer layers grow

gestation *n.* the period in which the mare is in foal or pregnant, averaging 340 days (12½ months for a jenny)

gestational age length of gestation at the time the fetus is born or aborted

Gestyl *n.* see **serum gonadotropin**

get *n.* the progeny of a stallion

getting down behind a fault wherein a horse, when cantering or galloping, grazes the back of the hind fetlock; horses with long, sloping pasterns are prone to this

get under in jumping, to be too near (the obstacle) when taking off

gharry, gharri *n.* in India, a horse-drawn taxi

giant cell tumor a malignant growth comprising very large cells; may arise from a foreign substance in the tissues or may occur in the bones

gibbing *n.* see **jibbing**

Gidran Arabian a Hungarian breed of mixed Arab descent that encompasses two distinct types: the Middle European, the heavier of the two, about 17. h.h., and the Southern and Eastern European, a lighter, all-purpose competition horse about 16.1 h.h.

gig *n.* a two-wheeled open carriage drawn by one horse

gingering *n.* the act of putting something that burns (such as ginger or pepper) into a horse's rectum to force a high tail carriage

gingiva *n.* see **gum** — **gingival** *adj.*

gingivitis *n.* inflammation of the gums

girth *n.* 1. a band that encircles a horse's belly to hold a saddle or pack on his back 2. the circumference of the deepest part of the body measured behind the withers — *vt.* to fasten with a girth

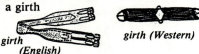

girth (English)   *girth (Western)*

girth buckle safe a safe that protects the saddle flaps on an English saddle from the buckles

girth cover a sleeve of sheepskin or rubber through which a girth may be slipped to prevent galling; girth sleeve

girth gal a sore from excessive pressure and or friction rub from the girth

girth sleeve *see* **girth cover**

girth strap *see* **billet strap**

girth tightener a leverage device for tightening girths on English saddles; should be used with care so as not to tighten too much; useful for young or short riders with tall horses

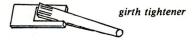

girth tightener

give tongue in hunting, to bark (said of hounds) continuously when after a quarry

gland *n.* an organ or special group of cells that manufactures certain elements and secretes them in a form suitable for the body to use or throw off; if the secretions go into the bloodstream, the gland is of the endocrine system (e.g., pituitary gland); if through a duct to surrounding tissues, it is an exocrine gland (e.g., salivary gland) — **glandular** *adj.*

glanders *n.* a severe and contagious but rare lymphatic disease of the respiratory passages; characterized by a pussy nasal discharge, fever, weight loss, sores in the lining of the nose and lymph nodes, and sometimes a cough and pneumonia; death may occur within a few weeks. Subcutaneous nodules that discharge pus, when the lymphatics of the skin are affected, are a milder form of glanders called *farcy,* and horses having this form may live for years. The chief cause of infection is ingestion of the germ glanders bacillus in water, contaminated food, or contaminated drinking and food containers; may also, however, be contracted through inhalation, particularly in stables.

glans *n.* 1. the head of the penis 2. the corresponding part of the clitoris

glass eye a figurative term for an eye that has a lightly pigmented iris rather than a dark one; also called *blue eye* or *wall eye* or *watch eye*

glaucoma *n.* an eye disease caused by increased pressure within the eye; can result in blindness — **glaucomatous** *adj.*

gleet *n.* a pus-like discharge from a part of the body, as from the nose

globin *n.* a protein component of hemoglobin

globulin *n.* a protein found in body tissues that is soluble only in saline

globulinuria *n.* a condition wherein globulin is abnormally present in urine

glomerulonephritis *n.* a form of nephritis in which capillary loops in glomeruli are affected

glomerulus *n., pl.* **-li** a small round cluster of the kidney having capillary loops that act as filters to separate waste matter from the blood and pass it out as urine

glossitis *n.* inflammation of the tongue; caused by sharp edges on the lower molar teeth, irritating foreign substances or careless handling during rasping of the teeth, etc.; severe bits badly used may also be a cause; compounding the problem, when the tongue is swollen, the horse may bite it while feeding

glottis *n.* the vocal chords and the opening between them

gluck *n.* an abnormal clucking sound made by a soft palate

glucocorticoid *n.* any of a group of steroid hormones secreted by the cortex of the adrenal gland; they help in the synthesis and storage of glucose, control inflammation and regulate metabolism

glucose *n.* a form of sugar which, in its natural form is found in fruit, honey, etc., but is also produced commercially

glucose tolerance the ability of the body to metabolize, use, and store sugar; a test to determine same

glutamate dehydrogenase an enzyme in the liver and kidneys

glutathione peroxidase an enzyme in red blood cells

gluteus muscles the three muscles of the rump which act to extend, retract, and rotate the thigh: gluteus medius, -superficialis, -profundus — **gluteal** *adj.*

glycemia *n.* sugar in the blood; a certain amount is normal but too much is called **hyperglycemia** and too little is called **hypoglycemia**

glycerin *n.* commercial name for **glycerol**, a syrupy liquid derived from the breakdown of fats and used as a base for local skin or throat medications

glycogen *n.* animal starch stored chiefly in the liver and muscles and released as sugar when needed by the body — **glycogenic** *adj.*

glyconeogenesis, gluco- *n.* the accumulation of glycogen and blood sugar

glycoprotein *n.* a compound combining protein with a carbohydrate

glycoside *n.* a sugar derivative in plants — **glycosidic** *adj.*

glycosuria *n.* the abnormal presence of sugar in the urine (rare in horses)

gnat *n.* a tiny, parasitic flying insect that can infect a horse with disease carried from another infected horse; particularly bothersome in the area of the horse's eyes

gnat

gnathic *adj.* relating to the jaw

goal post in polo, the usually collapsible pair of posts at either end of the field through which a goal is scored when a high ball passes between them

goat ribbon pull in rodeo, a contest in which the rider goes after a goat, dismounts, pulls a small amount of hair, and runs back to the starting point

goblet cell a cell lining the intestinal tract, name derived from its shape

going *n.* 1. the forward motion of the horse 2. the condition of ground over which a horse may be traveling

going amiss in racing, said of a mare coming into estrus at the time of her race

goiter *n.* an enlarged thyroid gland in the neck just behind the jaw

gomphrena poisoning a poisoning from eating large quantities of the gomphrena plant that grows in Australia on the Central Queensland coast and inland; symptoms are lack of coordination, dullness, appetite loss and swaying of the body; also called coastal ataxia

gonad *n.* a sex gland; the ovary of the mare or testicle of the stallion — **gonadal** *adj.* — **gonadectomy** *n.* the removal of a testis or ovary

gonadotropin *n.* a hormone that stimulates the sex glands or gonads

gonadotropin test a test which determines the presence of gonad secretions and or tumors via an injection of gonadotropin to stimulate the release of

testosterone by the sex organs or tumor cells; blood samples are taken before and after the injection and results are then based on change in hormone level

gone away in hunting, a cry that announces a fox is out, hounds are away after it, and the field should get ready to ride in pursuit

gone in the wind having diminished lung capacity or other lung deficiencies

gone to the ground in hunting, said of a fox that has hidden underground or in a drain

goniometer *n.* instrument for angular measurements, as of the hoof's angle

goniometry *n.* the measurement of angular changes in joints during a stride as part of gait analysis

gonitis *n.* inflammation of the stifle joint which may be acute and very painful or chronic with slowly developing lameness; among various causes are strain and infection in the stifle after a wound

good bone refers to cannon bones that are well constructed; i.e., fairly short, quite wide looking from the side and, of course, straight; also applied to a desirable measurement of the circumference of bone just below the knee or hock

good hands the tendency to hold the reins and control a horse with a light touch

good mouth a soft, responsive mouth, sensitive to the rider's hands

goose-rumped *adj.* having a croup that slopes down excessively

gordian worm *see* **hairworm**

goose-rumped

go-round *n.* in rodeo, that part of an event in which every contestant has competed on one head of stock

go short to take unusually short steps, indicating lameness or bad shoeing

Gotland *n.* an ancient pony breed of Sweden originally on Gotland Island; used there for light farm work and in trotting races. Strong and intelligent with a good disposition. After the breed nearly became extinct in the U.S.A., efforts began to restore the breed in Kentucky; 12–14 h.h.; also called Skogsruss.

Graafian follicle an ovarian follicle

grab the apple to pull leather

gracilis muscle the muscle which adducts the leg

grade horse a horse whose ancestry is unregistered or uncertain

graft *vt.* to transplant (a piece of skin or other living tissue) from one part of the body to another — *n.* the skin or tissue so used *see* **transplant**

grain *n.* the seed or seedlike fruit of cereal grasses, such as oats, corn, or barley; used as feed

gram *n.* a unit of metric weight amounting to 1 c.c. or about 15 drops of water

gram negative bacteria bacteria that do not retain a special blue stain in laboratory examination; **gram positive bacteria** are those that do

Grande Breton *see* **Breton**

grand entry in rodeo, the opening event during which the colors are carried on horseback into the arena, followed by mounted entries and participants in a mounted drill

Grand National Steeplechase the most difficult of all steeplechases, run annually at Aintree, near Liverpool, England, and dating back to 1837; course is just over 4 miles, with 30 jumps

granulation *n.* newly formed tissue at the base of a wound when healing

granule *n.* a small particle

granulocyte *n.* a white blood cell having granules or grains — **granulocytic** *adj.*

granulomatous enteritis intestinal inflammation resulting in fibrous thickening of the intestinal wall as well as the presence of necrotic tissue and large infection-fighting cells; characteristic of severe parasitic infestation

granulose cell tumor a particular type of ovarian tumor that may cause abnormal changes in the horse's personality

grass *n.* 1. plants on which horses graze having narrow leaves called blades and jointed stems 2. pasture; ground covered with grass — *vt.* 1. to put (a horse) out to pasture 2. to cover with grass — *vi.* to become covered with grass

grass founder *see* **grass laminitis**

grass laminitis a condition caused by overconsumption of lush spring grass especially when exposed to it suddenly and it is eaten greedily without periodic cessation; grass founder — *see also* **laminitis**

grass sickness a fatal disease that can attack horses in Scotland, England, and sometimes Ireland and France; there are four types varying from 24 hours to over 21 days in time taken for the sickness to take its toll; cause is unknown but is not related to grass; symptoms include absence of gut activity, colonic impaction, fetid green regurgitation through the nostrils, tremors

grass staggers *see* **stomach staggers**

grass tetany a rare spastic or convulsive condition caused by a sudden drop in blood magnesium

gravel *n.* a condition characterized by the spread of infection up through the white line of the hoof, which may reach the coronary band where it breaks out; causes acute lameness

gravida *n.* a mare in foal; **primigravida** is a mare in foal for the first time; **multigravida** is a mare in foal for the second or successive time

gray, grey *adj.* describes a dark-skinned horse with a coat of black and white hairs mixed; gray horses may be a very dark gray or almost totally white, except for gray areas on their legs — *vi.* to become gray

gray-ticked *adj.* having a sparse sprinkling of white hairs on a contrasting coat on any part of the body

graze *vi.* to feed on growing grass or herbage — *vt.* 1. to eat growing grass or herbage, as to graze a pasture 2. to provide growing grass or herbage for, as to graze horses on a pasture

grease *n.* a skin inflammation of the back of the fetlock and pasterns, especially of the hind legs; the skin feels hot, becomes inflamed and covered with a gray, foul-smelling greasy exudation; as it worsens, the swollen skin thickens and wrinkles; now rare; also called seborrhea; scratches; chorioptic mange

greasy heel *see* **mud fever; rain scald**

Great Horse a very large horse used in medieval times to carry heavily armored riders who could weigh up to 340 lbs.; thought to be the ancestor of the Shire

greedy *adj.* describes a horse which, having finished its own grain or hay, may aggressively take another horse's rations — **greed** *n.*

green *adj.* 1. describes a horse, usually a young one, which is broken but not fully trained; green broke 2. describes an untimed trotter or pacer 3. inexperienced

green broke (*colloq.*) partially tamed and trained

green osselet inflammation of the joint capsule at the front of the fetlock

green ribbon in hunting, a ribbon

sometimes worn on the tail of a young, unreliable horse — *see also* **red ribbon**

green splint an acute splint

green-stick fracture a fracture in which one side of the bone is broken while the other side is only bent; an incomplete fracture

Gretna Green race a game in which a pony and rider gallop to a designated point to pick up a second rider and gallop back to the starting point

grief *n.* sorrow; sadness; while many people scoff at the possibility of horses grieving, it is now acknowledged that they are indeed capable of feeling this emotion, as has been observed by many horsemen — *vi.* grieve

Griffin *n.* A Mongolian pony imported to China for use in racing and polo; 12.2–13 h.h.

gripes *n.* colic

groan *vi.* to utter a deep sound, as from pain — *n.*

Groningen *n.* a Dutch breed which nearly became extinct in the 1970s but was preserved by the Dutch government; although formerly used on farms, it is now used for riding and in harness; 15.3–16 h.h.

groom *n.* a person who looks after horses — *vt.* to clean and brush (a horse)

groomer *n.* a tool with teeth to clean and massage — *see also* **currycomb**

groomer

grooming kit a collection of brushes and other items to groom a horse

grooming mitt a flexible rubber mitt with many rubber tips to wipe away loose hair and dust   *grooming mitt*

ground money in rodeo, the entry fee and purse money split equally among all contestants in an event when there is no outright winner

ground poles *see* **cavalletti**

groundsel *n.* a plant which usually has small yellow clusters; probably poisonous if ingested; ragwort

ground tie to drop the reins to the ground after dismounting as a command to a Western trained horse to remain standing without being tied to anything

grow *vi.* to develop or increase in size

growth *n.* 1. the process of developing toward adulthood 2. the amount of development or size increase 3. an abnormal body tissue mass, such as a tumor

growth cartilage *see* **growth plates**

growth hormone protein secreted by the pituitary glands to stimulate growth; somatotrophin

growth plates the cartilage at the end of a long bone, where growth of the bone occurs; this growth or lengthening involves production of cartilage cells which then change into bone; a failure of this orderly transfer of cartilage to bone may cause pain and or collapse of the plate; also called *growth cartilage, epiphyseal cartilage, epiphyseal plates, physeal plates*

grub *n.* 1. a fly larva sometimes found in small abscesses beneath a horse's skin 2. a bot in the stomach

grub line rider a cowboy who goes from job to job, staying in one place only long enough to earn some food (grub)

grullo, gruella *adj.* having a type of dun coloration with a bluish, slate-colored coat with black points and dark head and usually primitive stripes. In England the terms "mouse dun" and "blue dun" are used to describe this color. Silver grullo is a cream color with slate-blue points and head and blue eyes. The term is from a Spanish word for the similarly colored sandhill crane. — *n.*

grunt *vi.* to make a short, forced audible expiration; a probable precursor to roaring or whistling, but a horse in severe pain may grunt —*n.*

grunter *n.* a horse that grunts habitually

grunting *n.* the act of testing a horse to see if its reactions are that of a grunter; the horse is placed against a wall and threatened with some object, such as a stick; bulling

Guajira *n.* a Colombian Criollo breed

Gudbrandsdal *n. see* **Dole Gudbrandsdal**

gullet *n.* 1. esophagus; the alimentary tube which connects the mouth with the stomach   2. in a Western saddle, the open space under the horn between the swells

gulp *vt.* to swallow quickly or in large quantities —*vi.* to catch the breath in swallowing a large amount —*n.* 1. the act of gulping   2. the quantity swallowed at once

gum *n.* the flesh in the mouth that covers the jaws and base of the teeth

gurgling *n. see* **tongue swallowing**

gustatory *adj.* relating to the sense of taste —**gustative**, —**gustatorial**

gut *n.* the intestine

guttural *adj.* pertaining to the throat

guttural pouches two sacs formed by a naturally distended section of the Eustachian tube which extends from the middle ear to the throat; can sometimes become infected or distended (*see* **empyema**), causing swelling below the ear, resulting in discomfort and difficult breathing

gymkhana *n.* a riding meet consisting of informal contests, such as egg-and-spoon and other races on horseback

gymnastics *n.pl.* acrobatic mounted exercises such as vaulting on and off a galloping horse, standing on two galloping horses, etc.; monkey drill

gyrus *n.* a convoluted ridge of the brain

— H —

habit *n.* 1. a characteristic action done often, which may be good or bad   2. the costume worn by a rider

habronema *n. pl.* a parasite which inhabits the stomach and is transmitted by flies; larvae can be ingested or can infect an open wound causing summer sores

habronemiases *see* **summer sores**

hack, hackney *n.* 1. a horse for hire   2. a horse for all sorts of work   3. a saddle horse; a **covert hack** is a horse used to carry a person across country to a hunt while the hunters are ridden by road to the meet; a **park hack** is a perfectly turned out horse ridden by ladies and gentlemen of leisure in a park   4. an old, worn-out horse   5. a horse-drawn carriage for hire

hackamore *n.* (from Spanish *jaquima*) a type of simple bridle with no mouthpiece; the basic hackamore, attached to a headstall, consists of a noseband (bosal) which comes together at the chin with a rawhide knot or heel knot (fiador); the reins (mecate), consist of one rope long enough to be looped with enough left over to be used as a lead rope which may be tied to the saddle; there are four variations of the basic hackamore: bosal, Lindell sidepull, English or jumping hackamore, and mechanical hackamore

Hackney *n.* a British breed descended from Arab-Thoroughbred crosses, having a very high-stepping trot, great presence, and a spirited character, making a very attractive carriage horse for the show ring; 14–15.3 h.h.

Hackney Pony a pony version of the Hackney horse; spirited and popularly used in harness but rarely ridden; the breed's outstanding feature is its extraordinary high action; the knee is raised as high as possible and the foot thrown forward in a round movement; the hock bends well under the body and lifts so high that it nearly touches the body; under 14 h.h.

Haflinger *n.* an Austrian mountain pony breed; thickset, sure-footed and always chestnut colored with flaxen mane, and tail; a very tractable temperament makes horses of this breed good beginners' mounts; 13.1–14.2 h.h.

Hailar *n. see* **Mongolian**

hair *n.* one or the overall mass of thread-like growths from the skin that covers the horse's body; most is very fine, but that which comprises the mane and tail is coarser —*see also* **horsehair**

haircloth *n.* cloth woven from horsehair or the hair from another animal

hair follicle a saclike cavity in the skin from which a hair shaft grows

hair polish a liquid spray applied to a horse's coat, mane, and tail to make the hair shinier, softer, and more manageable; also helps repel dust

hairworm *n.* an uncommon intestinal and stomach parasite not usually harmful except in association with other parasites; gordian worm

half-blood *n.* a horse with only one purebred parent —**half-blooded** *adj.*

half-breed *n.* half-blood —*adj.*

half-halt *n.* an interruption of forward motion wherein a rider asks the horse to halt but cues it to continue before it has come to a complete stop; this is a training exercise which improves collection and, by momentarily shifting the horse's weight to the hindquarters, enables the horse to change gait correctly

half hitch a knot in which the end of a rope is passed around the rope and then through the loop thus made

half-pass *n.* a movement in which a horse travels simultaneously forward and laterally with a crossover step; traversal; lateral march

half-round *n.* a horseshoe the bottom of which is convex or rounded; used chiefly on Standardbreds to ease breakover

half stocking *see* **stocking**

halt *vi., vt.* to stop; in riding, the rider bears down with the seat while using leg pressure and pulling in the reins to order the horse to halt

halter *n.* a headpiece of rope, leather, or nylon, with or without a lead; called a **head-collar** in some countries — *vt.* to put a halter on (a horse)

halter class *see* **in hand class**

halter

Hambletonian *n.* a breed of trotters descended from a stallion of the same name foaled in 1849 in Virginia; the Hambletonian Association, formed in 1923, represents the world's fastest trotters; today's Standardbred's heritage comes from this famous sire

hame *n.* in a harness, either of two rigid pieces along the sides of the collar attaching it to the traces; a **hame strap** secures the hames and keeps them in place on the collar

hamstring *n.* the large tendon at the back of the hind leg above the hock; Achilles tendon

hand *n.* a standard of equine height measurement equalling 4 inches, with fractions expressed in inches (e.g., 15.2 hands = 15 hands, 2 inches); term derives from the width of a human hand

hand breeding a breeding technique involving both mare and stallion being under direct human control

hand gallop a fast canter

hand horse the offside horse of a pair ridden by a postilion

handicap *n.* 1. in racing, the weight imposed on a superior contesting horse so as to distribute the chances of winning among other contestants more evenly 2. a race in which these weights are used 3. in polo, points given to players according to ability

handle *n.* 1. in rodeo, a rawhide grip attached to the rigging in bareback bronc riding 2. in racing, the monetary amount of a bet — *vt.* to touch, lead or manually control a horse

Hanoverian *n.* a German warm-blood so named after members of the House of Hanover promoted the breed long ago; the modern Hanoverian is popular in dressage and show-jumping; 16–17 h.h.

hansom *n.* a one horse, two-wheeled covered carriage for two people; the driver sits above and behind the cab

haploid *n.* a cell having a single set of chromosomes; e.g., a sex cell

hard and fast a cowboy team referring to the double half-hitching of the rope around the saddle horn

hard mouth a mouth in which the nerves on the main bone of the bar of the jaw have been deadened by harsh bits and mishandling; a mouth that is hard to rein

harness *n.* the leather straps and metal pieces by which a horse is fastened to a vehicle, plow, or load

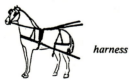

harness

harness horse a driving horse trained to pull a vehicle or farm equipment

harvest mite chigger; a parasite that attacks the head and legs while a horse

grazes, causing much irritation to the skin

haunches *n.pl.* the hips and buttocks

haute école classical equitation

haw *n.* a command made by a driver of a team of horses to direct them to the left — *vt., vi.* to turn to the left

hay *n.* a variety of different regional grasses and legumes that have been cured, dried, and baled to serve as the bulk of a horse's diet

hay feeder *see* **hay rack**

hay fork a 3- or 4-tined fork used for handling hay

hayloft *n.* an upper area in a barn for storing hay

haymow *see* **mow**

hay net a coarsely woven bag for holding hay at shoulder height

hay rack a wall-mounted metal framework to hold hay; hay feeder

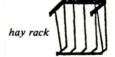

hay rack   *hay net*

haze *vt.* to herd (horses) by frightening with pistol shots, shouts, etc.

hazer *n.* in rodeo, the person who rides on the off side of the calf or steer to keep it running straight for the roper or dogger; in bronc busting the hazer rides next to the bronc, keeping it away from fences or rough ground, and standing ready to pick up the rider from the bronc; a **hazing horse** is the horse ridden by a hazer

Hazule *n.* a hardy mountain pony breed mainly bred in Rumania but also found in Poland, Czechoslovakia, Austria, etc.

head *n.* in racing, the length of a horse's head, used as a measurement of distance by which a horse may have won a race (*by a head*)

head a cow in cutting, to force a cow to change direction

head a fox in hunting, to turn back a fox, an error made by inexperienced hunters; if the fox is then (unfairly) killed, it is **headed to death**

headband *n.* the section of bridle over a horse's forehead, which prevents the bridle from slipping back; browband

head bumper a protective cap for the poll which attaches to the halter

head bumper

head-collar *n see* **halter**

header *n.* in rodeo, one of two riding partners (the other being a healer) in team roping, who must rope a steer by the horns

headlessness *n. see* **acephalia**

head pole a pole used in harness racing that extends from the harness saddle to a ring on the halter and keeps the horse's neck straight

head shy tending to be sensitive about the head and to jerk away when touched there

headstall *n.* the pieces of a bridle not including the bit and reins; i.e., cheek strap, throatlatch, browband, and noseband if used —*see also* **one-eared headstall**

heal *vi.* to become cured, as from a disease or wound

healer *n.* in rodeo, one of two riding partners (the other being a header) in team roping who must rope a steer by the hind legs

heart[1] *n.* the hollow, muscular organ in the chest that pumps blood throughout the body, receiving the blood from the veins and pumping it out through the arteries by alternate dilation and contraction —**heartbeat** *n.* one pulsation of the heart —**heart failure** a breakdown of normal heart function

heart[2] *n.* a quality in a horse that involves a desire to perform as well as possible in response to demand

heart block a disorder involving a defective heartbeat, resulting in independent contractions of the atria and ventricles

heart-rate monitor a device that interprets the heart's electric signal and displays a digital readout of the rate

heart room circumference of the chest

heat *n.* 1. the period of time during which a mare may be bred, occurring at approximately 3-week intervals and lasting from 4 to 6 days; estrus 2. a single race that forms one part of a competition (e.g., *three heats of one mile each*)

heat increment (HI) the value given to feedstuff that corresponds to the internal heat it produces in the horse as it is digested and metabolized; the lower the HI, the less heat the horse must get rid of in hot weather

heat prostration heat exhaustion; characterized by poor heart rate and shock caused by prolonged exposure to high external temperature and poor ventilation

heat stroke a serious, often fatal form of heat prostration in which sweating stops

heave line a muscular ridge developed on the rib cage due to heaves

heaves *n.* a chronic lung ailment (not to be confused with other respiratory ailments which may have similar manifestions) in which the pulmonary alveoli, tiny air sacs in the lungs, lose their elasticity, rupture and break down to form spaces filled with residual air. The first symptom is a cough which persists and worsens with exercise or exposure to dust; wheezing lung sounds may be heard and, while inhalation is normal, expiration is performed with effort and two distinct movements as air is forced out. Over a

long time, the rib cage extends, the diaphragmatic muscles and abdominal muscles enlarge, and a heave line develops. The heart is weakened and the horse is short winded and lacking in stamina; due to flatulence, odorous gas is passed and there may be indigestion and diarrhea. Infection and allergy are believed to cause this disease. Also called pulmonary alveolar emphysema; broken wind.

heavy hands a lack of flexibility and feeling in a rider's hands, combined with excessive forcefulness

heavy in the forehand describes a horse who pulls with its head and neck so that it is putting too much weight toward the front of the body; uncollected

heavyweight hunter a hunting horse capable of carrying a rider weighing over 205 lbs

heel *n.* the bulbs at the back of the hoof; horny in texture but softer than the hoof wall — *vi.* in hunting, to run backward on the line (said of hounds) — *vt.* to impel (a horse) with the heel

heel bug *see* **rain scald; mud fever; grease**

heel crack a vertical crack in the hoof's heel that may affect the laminae

heel nerving a procedure of cutting the nerves of the heel in the presence of navicular disease when it does not respond to any other treatment; often fails to achieve beneficial results

Heilung Chiang *n.* a type of Mongolian breed — *see also* **Mongolian**

hellebore *n.* a plant genus of the lily family, an extract from which is used in medicine as well as insecticide

hell for leather at full speed

helmet *n.* a hard, velvet-covered piece of riding headwear; cap

helmet

helminth *n.* a worm, especially an intestinal parasite — **helminthic** *adj.* 1. relating to helminths 2. expelling or destroying helminths *n.* helminthic medicine

helminthosporium *n.* a fungal disease of grass

hemacytometer *n.* a device used to test the concentration of cells in body fluids, especially the red and white blood cells

hemagglutinate *vt.* to cause clumping of red blood cells, as by the substance hemagglutinin — **hemagglutination** *n.*

hemal *adj.* pertaining to the blood or blood vessels

hemarthrosis *n.* painful bleeding into a joint; may follow an injury

hematinic *n.* any substance that increases the hemoglobin content in the blood

hematocrit *n.* 1. a device used to measure the proportions of cells and fluid in the blood 2. the percentage of cells and fluid in the blood as measured by a hematocrit; also called a **hematocrit reading**

hematogenous *adj.* 1. forming blood 2. spread by the bloodstream

hematology *n.* the study of blood and its diseases — **hematologic, -ical** *adj.* — **hematologist** *n.* a person who specializes in this study

hematoma *n.* a subcutaneous hemorrhage forming a blood clot and swelling; usually caused by an injury or blow that damages the skin and underlying tissues badly enough to rupture local blood vessels

hematophagous *adj.* feeding on blood, as e.g. mosquitoes

hematozoon *n.* a parasitic organism in the blood

hematuria *n.* the passing of blood in the urine, which may or may not be in clots

hemiplegia *n.* paralysis of one side of the body —**hemiplegic** *adj.*

hemisphere *n.* one half of the brain, either right or left

hemlock *n. see* **poison hemlock**

hemoconcentration *n.* a greater than normal proportion of blood cells to plasma; i.e., above 50 percent; occurs normally after exercise or excitement and abnormally in dehydration

hemocyte *n.* a blood cell

hemocytometer *n.* a measuring device that counts the number of cells in a blood sample

hemoglobin *n.* the pigment of red blood cells that carries oxygen to the tissues

hemoglobinometer *n.* a device for measurement of hemoglobin in the blood

hemoglobinuria *n.* the passing of hemoglobin in the urine, making it red or brown

hemogram *n.* red blood cell count

hemolysin *n.* a naturally produced substance that causes destruction of red blood cells, a condition called hemolysis; a mare rarely produces hemolysin against the red blood cells of her fetus, causing the foal to absorb hemolysin from the colostrum and get hemolytic jaundice

hemolysis *n.* the breakdown of red blood cells and escape of hemoglobin into surrounding fluid

hemolytic anemia anemia caused by the destruction of red blood cells by infection or chemicals —*see also* **neonatal isoerythrolysis**

hemolytic jaundice a rare disease of newborn foals caused by the presence of hemolysin in the colostrum which the foal takes; characterized by red urine and increase in heart rate; an affected foal dies within a short time, if not treated —*see also* **isoimmune disease**

hemophilia *n.* a rare inherited disease in which there is a lack of normal blood clotting capabilities; characterized by prolonged bleeding even from minor cuts; can result in fatal hemorrhaging —**hemophilic** *adj.*

Hemopis sanguisuga a water leech

hemopoiesis *n.* formation of red blood cells in tissues such as bone marrow

hemorrhage *n.* excessive bleeding —*vi.* —**hemorrhagic** *adj.*

hemostasis *n.* cessation of bleeding; the clamping and tying off of a blood vessel, as with a hemostat

hemostat *n.* an instrument for clamping a bleeding artery or vein

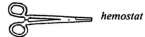
hemostat

hemostatic *n.* an agent that hastens blood clotting —*adj.*

hemotoxin *n.* a substance that destroys erythrocytes, such as snake's venom —**hemotoxic** *adj.*

heparin *n.* an anticoagulant found in the body, especially the liver, which prevents blood clotting; used in surgery and medicine

hepatitis *n.* inflammation of the liver

herb *n.* 1. a seed plant as distinguished from a bush or tree 2. a plant used as a medicine 3. vegetative growth; grass; herbage —**herbaceous, herbal** *adj.*

herbage *n.* grass or green foliage

herbivore *n.* an animal that feeds mainly on herbage —**herbivorous** *adj.*

herd *n.* a group of horses together —*vi.* to move together in a group —*vt.* to drive together in a group

herd bound 1. refusing to leave a herd of horses 2. describes a form of balking; in training, if a horse is ridden too long in a corral, it will become herd-bound and will not ride away from the corral

herd holders in cutting, the two riders on each side of the herd who help the

cutter make a selection (or cut) and keep the herd together while it is being cut

herd instinct the desire or defensive habit of horses to group together

herd's grass redtop or timothy grass

heredity *n.* the passing on of characteristics from parents to offspring — **hereditary** *adj.*

hermaphrodite *n.* a horse with the rare abnormality of having both male and female reproductive organs — **hermaphroditism, hermaphrodism** *n.* — **hermaphroditic** *adj.* — **hermaphroditically** *adv.*

hernia *n.* a rupture; a protrusion of an organ or tissue through its surrounding tissue or muscle or through a natural body opening; occurs especially in the following forms: *diaphragmatic, inguinal, scrotal, umbilical, ventral* — **hernial** *adj.*

herniate *vi.* to protrude and form a hernia — **herniation** *n.*

herpesvirus *n.* a virus that causes rhinopneumonitis, abortion and possibly other diseases; equine herpesvirus

herring gutted having the conformation fault of a barrel that slants sharply upward from the forehand; while unattractive, it does not interfere with function

heterosis *n.* a result of hybridization wherein the offspring has greater vigor, size, etc. than the parents — **heterotic** *adj.*

heterozygote *n.* hybrid; a horse which, as opposed to a homozygote, has two different genes for a particular characteristic; a heterozygote may inherit the dominant characteristics of the parents but transmit recessive characteristics to the offspring; one that does not breed true to type — **heterozygous** *adj.*

hexamine *n.* a drug given to acidify

urine in treatment of urinary infection

h.h. *(abbr.).* hands

HI heat increment

Hibitane *n.* trade name for chlorhexidine hydrochloride

hiccup *n.* a sudden, involuntary contraction of the diaphragm producing a sharp, quick sound; very unusual, but horses are capable of hiccupping — *vi.*

hide *n.* animal skin, either raw or tanned

hidebound *adj.* having hide drawn tightly over the ribs due to loss of subcutaneous fat; caused by nutritional defects or disease

high *adj.* spirited

high blowing *see* **trumpeting**

highbred *adj.* of very good stock or breed

high-goal polo polo in which the total handicap of each competing team in a particular competition is about 19 or more

Highland *n.* a very old pony breed, native to Scotland and the Western Isles, examples from the latter being lighter in weight; docile, strong and sure-footed, these ponies are used on the hills for pack purposes, in harness and for general riding; usually have a dorsal stripe and sometimes zebra markings on the legs; 13–14 h.h. — *see also* **shelt**

high roller in rodeo, a bucking horse that leaps high into the air

high school training *see* **dressage**

hightail *vi.* to gallop across country; derived from the high tails horses often maintain when excited or running

hill topper a rider who participates in a fox hunt by looking from the hilltops to decide where the quarry will be caught; point-to-pointer

hilus *n., pl.* **-li** a small recess or opening in an organ, as where vessels and nerves enter

hind *adj.* rear; referring to the posterior area

hindquarters *n.pl.* the part of the body behind the barrel

hinny *n.* the offspring of a stallion and a female donkey

hip *n.* the joint formed by the meeting of the thighbone and pelvic bone; the fleshy area of the upper thigh

hip dysplasia a faulty development of the hip joint which impairs function

Hipparchikos *n.* the Greek title ("Cavalry Commander") or the first known treatise dealing only with cavalry training, written by Xenophon about 365 B.C.

Hippike *n.* a treatise written by Xenophon in 365 B.C. on horsemanship

hippocampus *n.* *1.* a mythical sea monster with head and forequarters of a horse and tail of a dolphin or fish *2.* a sea horse (small saltwater fish) *3.* a pair of ridges in the front part of the brain —**hippocampal** *adj.*

Hippocrene *n.* in Greek mythology, a fountain and source of poetic inspiration on Mount Helicon said to have begun where Pegasus struck his hoof

hippodrome *n.* 1. in ancient Greece and Rome, an oval racecourse for chariots with spectator seats around it 2. an arena surrounded with seats

hippogriff, -gryff *n.* a mythical creature with the head and wings of a griffin or eagle, the hindquarters of a horse, and the forelegs of a lion

hippolith *n.* a calcification in the intestines

Hippological Hethica the first known writing on horses written on clay tablets in the 14th century B.C. by a chariot-horse trainer

hippology *n.* the acquired knowledge of horses —**hippologist** *n.* a person knowledgeable about horses

hippomane *n.* a rubbery structure of unknown function in the placental fluid of a mare; develops during the first 4 months of gestation and forms a flat, oval or rectangular shape about 4 in. by 2 in. and ½ in. thick

hippopathology *n.* veterinary medicine

hippophagy *n.* the eating of horseflesh

hippophile *n.* a person who loves horses

hippophobia *n.* the fear of horses

hippotherapy *n.* horseback riding as a therapy for the mentally or physically handicapped

Hispano *n.* a Spanish Anglo-Arab breed; intelligent and courageous and very agile; used in the bull ring among other sports; about 16 h.h.

histamine *n.* a breakdown product of histidine (essential amino acid) metabolism in the body; produced by the body in cases of allergy, injury, or infection; its actions include lowering blood pressure, stimulating gastric juices, etc. —**histaminic** *adj.*

histopathology *n.* the study of tissue changes caused by disease —**histopathological** *adj.*

histoplasma farciminosum a fungus responsible for epizootic lymphangitis

hitch *vt.* to fasten (a horse) to something, as by a rope or reins —*vi.* to brush the feet together when moving; forge

hitching post a post, usually having a ring, used to secure a horse

hit the line in hunting, to pick up the scent of the quarry (said of hounds)

hit the wall in endurance riding, to reach the end of energy reserves and fall into complete exhaustion (applies to horses)

hives *n.* *see* **urticaria**

hobble *n.* a strap used on a pair of feet to restrain movement; a fetter —*vt.* to re-

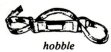

hobble

strain foot movement by means of strapping one foot to another; to fetter — *see also* **hopple**

Hobday operation a surgical procedure performed for the relief of a respiratory disease called roaring; a burr is used to strip mucous membrane from the cups formed by the vocal cords; when healing, the cords are pulled back so that they do not continue to obstruct the air passage but the horse is then mute; this operation is not considered ideal but in most cases it does enable the horse to continue working

hock *n.* the joint between the gaskin and cannon bone; the bony protuberance at the back is called the point of hock

hog *vt.* to clip (the mane) flat to the neck, usually leaving a handhold (a wisp of hair at the withers) and forelock unclipped; roach — **hogged** *adj.*

hogback *n.* a conformation fault that describes a convex back

hog's back in show jumping, a spread fence consisting of three sets of poles; the first is the lowest, set close to the ground; the second is the highest; and the third is slightly lower than the second

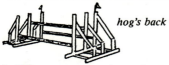

hog's back

hollihan *n.* a type of rope loop used to catch horses

holloa *n.* in hunting, the vocal signal called out to indicate a sighting of a fox

Hollywood bridge a custom-made cover of plastic teeth that can be temporarily affixed to a horse's discolored front teeth for shows

holocrine *n.* a type of gland the secretion of which results from the disintegration of its cells; e.g., sebaceous gland

Holstein *n.* a German breed of med-

ium-heavy build descended from 14th century war horses; infusions of other lighter breeds since then have produced a general-purpose saddle mount well adapted to show-jumping; 15.3–17 h.h.

homeopathy *n.* a method of disease treatment in which very small doses of drugs or other products of the same disease are administered; in a healthy patient large doses of the same medication would produce symptoms of the disease being treated — **homeopathic** *adj.*

homeostasis *n.* stability of body functions at normal levels — **homeostatic** *adj.*

homogeneous, -genous *adj.* similar in conformation because of common ancestry; — **homogeny** *n.*

homograft *n.* a graft of tissue taken from another horse

homologous *adj.* corresponding in structure and position, as a horse's fetlock is homologous to a human's wrist — **homology** *n.*

homozygosis *n.* 1. the state of being a homozygote 2. the production of a homozygote

homozygote *n.* a horse which has two identical genes for a particular characteristic, thus breeding true to type for the particular characteristic involved; purebred; opposite of heterozygote — **homozygous** *adj.*

honda *n.* the small knotted loop at one end of a rope through which the other end is passed to form a large loop; it may be tied in the rope or may be made of brass or aluminum

honeycomb ringworm *see* **favus**

hood *n.* a cloth covering that fits over the horse's head and neck; often used with a blanket

hood

hooded stirrup a Western stirrup, the front of which is

leather covered; it is particularly useful in very cold weather when it helps to keep the feet warm; English stirrup irons can be covered for this purpose with separate foot warmers; also called tapadero

hooey *n.* in calf-roping, a half-hitch by means of which the rope is tied off after taking one or two wraps around the calf's feet

hoof *n.* the horny wall, sole, and frog of the foot

hoof axis the imaginary line passing through the center of the pastern and on through the coffin bone parallel to its front surface

hoof beat the sound of a horse's hoofs striking the ground

hoof bound *adj.* having a dry, contracted hoof, resulting in pain and lameness

hoof brush a brush used to clean off the hoof, inside and outside

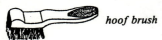 *hoof brush*

hoof knife a knife used by a farrier to pare off dead material from the sole and frog of the hoof

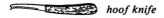 *hoof knife*

hoof nipper an implement used to cut off the lower hoof edges

hoof pick an implement used to clean out the bottom of the hoof

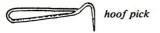 *hoof pick*

hoof rasp a rasp used to file the bottom of the hoof wall and tidy the edges after shoeing

hoof testers pincers used to test the hoof for bruises, or other weaknesses by applying pressure to various parts of it

hook *n.* a sharp projection on a tooth,

usually caused by an uneven bite

hookworm *n.* a parasitic roundworm that infests the small intestine; the name is derived from the hooks present around the worm's mouth

Hoppengarten cough *see* **infectious equine bronchitis**

hopple *n.* a type of hobble used on pacers to prevent breaking gait — *vt.*

hormone *n.* a substance formed by a gland or other organ in the body to stimulate and regulate body functions, such as growth, reproduction, etc. — **hormonal, hormonic** *adj.*

horn *n.* 1. the projection above the pommel of a Western saddle 2. the exterior of the hoof wall 3. a pointed projection in the body, as the uterine horn

Horner's syndrome a condition resulting from sympathetic nerve destruction in the neck, characterized by a drooping of the upper eyelid, protrusion of the third eyelid, abnormal warmth of facial skin and sweating; caused by injury to the neck, surgery in the region of the carotid artery and vagus nerve, tumors, or infected guttural pouch

horn fly a fly which breeds on fresh cow manure and feeds on a host by day or by night

horn tubules multiple spring-like formations that comprise the hoof wall

horn tumor *see* **keratoma**

horse *n.* a member of the order *Ungulata,* the family *Equidae,* the genus *Equus* and the species *caballus*; technically measures 14.2 h.h. or over, with smaller specimens being termed ponies, but ponies generally can still be called horses

horseback *n.* the back of a horse — *adj.* — **on horseback** *adv.* astride

horsebox *n.* an English horse trailer

horsecar *n.* 1. a streetcar drawn by

horses, which was prevalent in cities before electricity was used   2. a vehicle for carrying horses

horse coper *see* **horse dealer**

horse dealer a person who buys and sells horses for a profit; horse coper

horseflesh *n.* 1. the flesh of a horse, usually applied to its use as food   2. a group of horses

horsefly *n.* like the deerfly, a fly that is extremely bothersome to horses, stubbornly clinging on once it alights; the bite is painful and often leaves a blood mark on the animal's coat; the female is known to transmit several diseases, but males are harmless; there are various kinds; also called gadfly

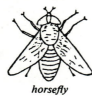

horsefly

horsehair *n.* 1. hair from the mane or tail   2. a fabric made from this hair

horsehide *n.* 1. the hide of a horse   2. leather made from horsehide

horse latitudes regions of the ocean in latitudes 25 degrees N. and 30 degrees S. noted for lack of winds; so named by sailors in the 16th century for when horses were transported over these waters in ships which became becalmed, they died from thirst; doldrums

horse-leech *n.* a leech said to attach itself to the muzzle while a horse is drinking

horse length eight feet; the distance between horses in a column

horseless carriage an automobile

horseman *n.* 1. a skilled male rider   2. a man who trains, breeds, or cares for horses   3. a cavalryman

horse opera a motion picture or play about cowboys, cattle rustlers, and life in the American West, particularly in the 19th century.

horsepower *n.* 1. the power of a horse to pull something   2. a unit for measuring the power of motors or engines, equal to 550 foot-pounds of work per second

horsepox *n.* a mild form of smallpox, variola equina, that affects horses and is characterized by pus-filled eruptions on the skin, particularly on the hollow of the pastern, lips, and nose

horse race a contest of speed between two or more horses that are ridden or driven over a designated course

horse sacrifice an ancient practice of offering a horse to the gods or burying it with its owner when the latter died

horseshoe *n. see* **shoe**

horseshoe nail a thin piece of tapered steel, the thickness of which is half its width; has a wedge-shaped, flat-topped head on one end and bevelled point on the other; used *horseshoe nail* to fasten shoes to the hoof —*see also* **clinch**

horseshoe superstition the notion that it is good luck to find a horseshoe; a shoe may also be worn as a good-luck charm

horse show a public exhibition in which horses compete with one another in executing various maneuvers or in comparing conformation and behavior; they may be ridden, driven, or led by people on foot

horse-tail *n.* 1. the tail of a horse   2. *vt.* to take charge of (a band of horses) for use when herding cattle or sheep over long distances

horsetail *n. see* **equisetum**

horse tick fever *see* **piroplasmosis**

horse trade exchange of horses and the bargaining involved

horsewhip *n.* a whip for driving or managing horses —*vt.* to lash with a whip

horsewoman *n.* 1. a skilled female rider   2. a woman who trains, breeds or cares for horses

horsey, horsy *adj.* pertaining to horses, horsemen or horsewomen, or horse racing, etc. —**horsiness** *n.* —**horsily** *adv.*

hostler *n.* someone who takes care of horses, especially at a livery stable

hotblood *n.* a horse having Mid-Eastern or North African blood in its pedigree; the term refers to type of temperament and has nothing to do with blood temperature; hotbloods tend to be active and high-spirited; Arabians and Thoroughbreds are hotbloods —**hotblooded** *adj.*

hots *n.pl.* in racing jargon, horses after a race, before cooling out

hot shoeing forging a horseshoe and putting it on the hoof while still hot

hot shot a battery-operated electric prod for moving horses, especially at an auction; illegal —*vt.*

hot spot *see* **scintigraphy**

hotting up showing signs of the first stage of labor

hot walker a device for cooling out or exercising a horse; the arms of the walker extend about 16 feet from center; powered by a ½–1 HP electric motor that adjusts for different speeds; will handle 2, 4, or 6 horses at one time —*see also* **walker**

HP horsepower

Hucul *n.* a Polish pony breed; strong, hardy, sure-footed and docile; popular for pack and draft work in hilly areas; 12.1–13.1 h.h.

hull *n.* a saddle

humerus *n.* the main shoulder bone, the equine equivalent of the human upper arm

humor *n.* body fluid, such as blood, bile, etc.; can be a secretion —**humoral** *adj.*

hunt *n.* the pursuit on horseback of game for food or sport, which is done by following hounds chasing a fox or hare or an artificially laid drag line; occasionally deer are hunted —*vi., vt.*

hunt button a button with a symbol or lettering of a particular hunt on it

hunter *n.* 1. a horse bred and trained to be ridden for the sport of hunting 2. a person who hunts and may use a horse doing so

hunter bump a dislocation of the sacroiliac joint —*see also* **luxation**

hunter classes classes in which horses are judged either in the ring over fences or over an outside course with fences resembling obstacles that might be found in the hunt field; horses are judged on their manners, way of going and sometimes conformation

hunter clip the trim over the entire body of the horse, except the legs and a patch under the saddle

hunter pace a timed competition in which riders go out in teams of 2 or 3, leaving a starting point every 2 minutes and riding across a marked course in typical hunting country, usually 7 or more miles long; the top teams must navigate the course over or around many fences in ideal time, usually 360 yards per minute, which requires that a rider be skilled in pacing the horse; there are 2 checkpoints where a 5-minute rest is taken; originated in New York state around 1971 and was sponsored by the fox hunts to raise money

hunter seat a style of riding suited for jumping and hunting, differing from the balanced seat primarily in that there is less ankle flexion in the hunter seat and a slight bend at the rider's hips at the trot, so that the rider is posting; the heel, seat and shoulder should be in line when the rider is seated in the center of the saddle; forward seat

hunter trial a competitive event to be completed within a certain time and held over typical hunting country comprising uneven terrain with

natural obstacles; the course is usually 1 to 2 miles long

hunting cap a protective riding hat covered with velvet

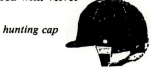

hunting cap

hunting horn a copper horn used to give signals during a hunt; about 9–10 inches long with a nickel or silver mouthpiece

hunting thong a long braided lash that hangs from the hunting crop and used to discipline hounds; the professional hangs the thong along the horse's withers, whereas the amateur holds it coiled in his or her hand

hunting whip *see* **whip**

hunt livery a hunter's coat that is characteristic of a particular hunt

huntress *n.* 1. a mare used for hunting 2. a woman who hunts

hunt secretary a person who performs secretarial work in connection with the hunt and whose duties include keeping contact with farmers and landowners within the hunting area and collecting the cap money at the meet

hunt servant any salaried employee of a hunt

huntsman *n.* 1. a hunter (def. 2) 2. a person in charge of hounds during a hunt

hunt subscription the fee paid by a participant in a hunt

hurdle *n.* one of a number of barriers, made of brush, over which horses jump in hurdle racing; may also be a type of fence used in jumping competition

hurdle race a race over a series of hurdles

husbandry *n.* the management of domestic animals

hyalin *n.* a translucent substance normally present in vertebrate cartilage — **hyaline, hyaloid** *adj.*

hyalogen *n.* an insoluble, slimy substance in animal tissue which produces hyalin

hyaloid membrane a membrane of the eye containing its vitreous humor

hyaloplasm *n.* the clear fluid base of the cellular protoplasm

hyaluronic acid a lubricating substance present in body fluids, such as those of the joints and eyes; a component of synovial fluid

hyaluronidase *n.* an enzyme that breaks down hyaluronic acid; also an enzymatic substance that is used to increase the penetrating diffusion of certain injected medications; found in sperm cells, bacteria, etc.

hybrid *n.* a horse of mixed parentage; opposite of purebred — *see also* **heterozygote** — **hybridize** *vt., vi.* to crossbreed

hybrid vigor *see* **heterosis**

hydration *n.* adequate content of water in the body

hydremia *n.* excessive fluid content of the blood

hydrocele *n.* a collection of fluid in the scrotum

hydrocelectomy *n.* surgical removal of a hydrocele

hydrocephalus *n.* a condition which occurs shortly after birth and involves abnormal amounts of fluid in the cranium, resulting in an enlarged head and brain destruction — **hydrocephalic, hydrocephalous** *adj.*

hydrochloric acid an acid secreted by the cells lining the stomach; helps to digest food

hydrochlorothiazide *n.* a drug that increases excretion of sodium in urine, used to treat edema; trade names Direma, Vetidrex

hydrocortisone *n.* a cortisone medication

hydrogen peroxide solution an antiseptic used on wounds

hydropericardium *n.* fluid accumulation in the pericardium

hydrophobia *n.* fear of water —**hydrophobic** *adj.*

hydrops *n.* accumulation of fluid in an organ or tissue; **hydrops amnii** is an abnormal collection of fluid in membranes around the fetus **hydropic** *adj.*

hydrotherapy *n.* the treatment of inflammation by the use of a force of water or of turbulent water

hydrothorax *n.* abnormal collection of fluid in the pleural cavity (around the lungs)

hydroxyapatite *n.* a bone mineral comprising calcium, magnesium, sodium, phosphates, carbonates and chloride

hygroma *n.* a swelling of the knee or hock, usually caused by bruising but sometimes caused by a foreign body, such as a thorn, buried in the skin; big knee, capped knee, popped knee; a broken carpal bone may also be a cause —*see also* **carpitis**

hymen *n.* the mucous membrane which partially or completely covers the entrance to the vagina **hymenal** *adj.*

hyoid bone the bone to which the tongue muscles are attached

hyoid muscles the muscles of the tongue, including the mylo-hyoideus, stylo-hyoideus, occipito-hyoideus, genio-hyoideus, kerato-hyoideus, hyoideus transversus

hypercalcemia *n.* an excessive amount of calcium in the blood, which may, in severe cases, result in increased bone density and even mental deterioration

hypercapnia *n.* an excessive amount of carbon dioxide in the blood

hyperemia *n.* an increased blood collection in an organ or other part of the body, as may be seen in an inflamed area —*see also* **active hyperemia, venous hyperemia**

hyperextension *n.* the overextension of a leg —**hyperextend** *vt.*

hyperflexion *n.* overbending, as the overflexing of a joint

hyperglycemia *n.* excessive sugar content in the blood

hypericin *n.* a toxin found in certain plants

hyperimmune serum a serum of antibodies taken from a horse vaccinated to produce very high levels of antibody in the blood and then injected into another horse as immunization against infection

hyperkalemia *n.* abnormally high content of potassium in the blood

hyperlipemia *n.* excessive amount of fat or lipids in the blood

hyperorexia *n.* excessive appetite; can be caused by parasite infestation or diabetes mellitus

hyperostosis *n.* excessive growth of bone tissue

hyperparathyroidism *n.* excessive production of parathormone by the parathyroid glands, which causes depletion of calcium from the bones

hyperphosphatemia *n.* excessive phosphate content in the blood

hyperplasia *n.* overgrowth of body tissue or organ due to increase of cells —**hyperplastic** *adj.*

hyperpnea *n.* abnormally fast breathing; panting —**hyperpneic** *adj.*

hyperpyrexia *n.* a very high body temperature, 106–110 degrees F.

hypersensitivity *n.* an abnormal response to a foreign agent —**hypersensitive** *adj.*

hypertension *n.* high blood pressure — **hypertensive** *adj.*

hyperthermia *n.* heat exhaustion with raised body temperature

hypertrophic pulmonary osteoarthropathy an abnormal condition characterized by extreme thickening of leg bones; occurs as a secondary effect of chest or abdominal disorders

hypertrophy *n.* a significant enlargement of an organ or tissue — **hypertrophic** *adj.*

hyperventilation *n.* excessive rapid breathing that upsets the balance of oxygen inhalation and carbon dioxide exhalation — **hyperventilate** *vi., vt.*

hypervitaminosis *n.* the result of excessive vitamin intake

hypnotic *n.* an agent that induces sleep, as used when performing surgery — *adj.*

hypocalcemia *n.* excessively low blood calcium

hypochromia *n.* decreased level of hemoglobin in red blood cells

hypoderma *n. see* **warble fly**

hypodermic *adj.* 1. relating to subcutaneous parts   2. injected under the skin

hypodermic syringe *see* **syringe**

hypoflexion of limbs abnormally limited flexion in muscles and tendons of the legs; sometimes appears in newborn foals and usually affects all 4 legs; characterized by the fetlock being close to or even on the ground

hypoflexion of limbs

hypogammaglobulinemia *n.* insufficiency of gammaglobulin in the blood

hypoglycemia *n.* abnormally low level of sugar in the blood

hypokalemia *n.* deficiency of potassium in the blood

hypoplasia *n.* the underdevelopment of an organ or tissue — **hypoplastic** *adj.*

hypopyon *n.* an accumulation of pus inside the eyeball

hypothalmus *n.* the section of the brain below the cerebrum which regulates many automatic body functions

hypothermia *n.* abnormally low body temperature — **hypothermal** *adj.*

hypothyroidism *n.* decreased function of the thyroid gland and the disorder resulting from this

hypotonia *n.* reduction of muscle tone — **hypotonic** *adj.*

hypoventilation *n.* lower than normal air and oxygen in the lungs from reduced rate of breathing

hypovolemia *n.* abnormal decrease of the body's blood volume due to bleeding, dehydration or shock

hypoxemia *n.* an abnormal decrease of oxygen in the blood due to exhaustive tissue demand or reduced inhalation; may be caused by overexertion

hypoxia *n.* an abnormal decrease of oxygen in body tissues; causes considerable pain; may be caused by overexertion

hypsodonty *n.* the old age condition of having long teeth

Hyracotherium *n.* the remains of an animal resembling the hyrax (small hoofed mammal) were discovered in Kent, England, in 1838 and named Hyracotherium (hyrax-like); this mammal was determined to be the most primitive ancestor of *Equus caballus*; in 1871 similar remains were discovered in North America and named Eohippus; later Eohippus and Hyracotherium were realized to be one and the same; had 4 toes on each foot

— I —

Iberian *n.* the ancestral breed of the Tarbenian

Icelandic *n.* a native pony breed of Iceland. There are two types: one heavier type, used for draft and pack work, and a lighter-weight type used under saddle. A thick mane and tail are typical, but the chief characteristic is a fast, smooth gait called the tôlt; 12–13 h.h.

ice tail a color pattern of the tail wherein it is pale or white from its tip up a certain distance

ichthammol *n.* an ointment made from a coal-tar base and used for treating abscesses and bacterial infections; has a soothing, drawing effect

ichthyosis *n.* a dry, scaly condition of the skin resulting from excessive thickening of the horny layer —**ichthyotic** *adj.*

ICSH interstitial cell stimulating hormone

icterus *n. see* **jaundice** —**icteric** *adj.*

idiopathic spontaneous progressive vitiligo *see* **pinky syndrome**

idiopathy *n.* a disease of unknown cause —**idiopathic** *adj.*

idiosyncrasy *n.* 1. a characteristic peculiarity, as a particular habit 2. an abnormal reaction of an individual to a drug, food, etc. —**idiosyncratic** *adj.* —**idiosyncratically** *adv.*

IgG *see* **immunoglobulin**

ileocecal *adj.* pertaining to the ileum and cecum

ileocecal valve the muscular valve that regulates the flow of food from the ileum to the cecum

ileum *n.* the lowest part of the small intestine, terminating in the cecum —**ileac, ileal** *adj.*

ileus *n.* obstruction of the intestines due to intestinal contents not moving on normally; **meconium ileus** is obstruction in the newborn's intestines by the first dung; **paralytic ileus** is caused by colic

Ili *n. see* **Mongolian**

iliac thrombosis a thrombosis, or blood clot, of the iliac arteries which interferes with the blood supply to the hind legs; may be caused by arterial disease or redworms; characterized by lameness, painful muscle spasms when exercised, abnormal sweating

iliacus *n.* a hip muscle

iliopsoas muscle the tenderloin muscle by which the hip is flexed; **ilio-haunch, psoas-loin**

ilium *n.* the largest pelvic bone forming the point of hip —**iliac** *adj.*

Ilotycin *n.* trade name for erythromycin

imidocarb *n.* generic name for a drug used to treat equine piroplasmosis

immature *adj.* not fully developed or mature; may be applied to the horse's character or body, either in part or whole —**immaturity** *n.*

immune *adj.* having protection or resistance against a particular disease through the presence of corresponding antibodies —**immunity** *n.*

immune body an antibody

immune system the combined parts of the body having the ability to recognize and combat foreign material; includes the lymph system, spleen, bone marrow, thymus, intestinal tissues, wandering tissue cells and other elements

immunization *n.* the process of developing or giving protection against a contagious disease —**immunize** *vt.*

immunodiffusion test a laboratory test to determine the presence of specific antibodies in the bloodstream,

based on the tendency of antibodies and their corresponding antigens to diffuse towards each other when placed in adjacent chambers of a dish or transparent agar gel

immunofluorescence *n.* a laboratory test to determine the presence of specific antibodies in the bloodstream by tagging the antibodies with fluorescent dye, then monitoring the pattern they produce when placed with their corresponding antigens

immunogenetics *n.pl.* (sing. in constr.) the science of immunology which deals with the relationship between immunity and genetics

immunogenic *adj.* producing immunity —**immunogenically** *adv.*

immunoglobulin (IgG) *n.* a globulin protein that forms part of the immune reaction as the antibody for particular antigen

immunohematology *n.* the science that deals with blood cells and the antibodies and antigens in the blood

immunomodulation *n.* a method of supplementing the body's defenses against foreign invaders; used against sarcoid tumors, early stages of respiratory infections, etc.

immunosorbent *n.* an insoluble support for antigens used to take up antibodies from a mixture

immunotherapy *n.* the use of immunization to treat a disease

impacted fracture a bone fracture in which the hard bone of one fragment has penetrated into the softer bone of another fragment; when an impacted fracture is overlapping, it is called a riding fracture

impaction *n.* 1. an obstruction of a body passage caused by an accumulation of deposited material; usually refers to a type of colic caused by partly digested food accumulated in the gut 2. a bit of material tightly wedged or

lodged into another, as a piece of fractured bone lodged into another —**impacted** *adj.*

impalpable *adj.* unable to be palpated or felt with the hands, such as certain tumors

implant *vt.* to embed within the body, as (a) a piece of tissue taken from another part of the body or (b) a slow-releasing medicinal tablet placed under the skin —*n.* the tissue, tablet, etc. so implanted

impotent *adj.* unable to engage in normal sexual intercourse due chiefly to inability to have an erection or ejaculate; **temporary impotence** can be caused by illness or inexperience

impregnate *vt.* to fertilize (an ovum) —**impregnation** *n.*

impression smear a tissue sample obtained by pressing a slide to a lesion for analysis

impulsion *n.* the forward movement of a horse, generating from the hindquarters and hocks

inbreed *vt.* to mate closely related horses, such as a brother and sister, sire and daughter, or son and dam — *vi.* to mate with close relatives —**inbred** *adj.* —**inbreeding** *n.*

incise *vt.* to cut into with a sharp implement, as in surgery —**incision** *n.*

incised wound a clean-cut wound

incisivus inferior a muscle that raises the lower lip

incisivus superior a muscle that depresses the upper lip

incisor *n.* one of the front teeth, of which there are 6 upper incisors and 6 lower incisors

Incitatus *n.* (literally, "swift speeding") a famous racing stallion owned by the deranged Roman emperor, Caligula (Gaius Caesar, A.D. 12–41) who held him in such high esteem that the horse was kept in a marble stable, had an ivory manger and drank from a gold

pail; he was even made a Roman citizen and a senator

inclusion body a foreign material within the protoplasm of a cell which a virus has penetrated

inclusion cyst a cyst composed of one type of tissue enclosing another; sometimes it is the result of a cut when a piece of skin is buried into subcutaneous tissues

incompatible *adj.* describes a horse that does not get along well with another one; it may also be said that the personality of a particular horse is incompatible with that of a person, usually a prospective buyer — **incompatibility** *n.* — **incompatibly** *adv.*

incontinence *n.* inability to contain feces or urine; urinary incontinence is often caused by extreme nervousness but also may be caused by pathological disorders — **incontinent** *adj.* — **incontinently** *adv.*

incoordination *n.* a condition in which the muscles are not in a state of tonus, thereby incurring violent movement and consequent damage under stress in unfit or fatigued horses

incrustation *n.* a scale or scab — **incrust** *vt.* to cover with a crust

incubate *vt.* to put through the process of incubation — **incubational, incubative** *adj.*

incubation *n.* 1. the time taken for a disease to develop from exposure to an infection to the appearance of its symptoms 2. a laboratory procedure in which a virus or bacterium is kept in a suitable temperature and grown or cultivated

incus *n.* one of the three bones in the middle ear

independent seat the holding of a firm, balanced position on a horse's back without relying on reins or stirrups

indeterminate cleavage the division of an egg resulting in the production of twins

Indiana pants a kind of leg harness worn by pacers to hold them to their gait; hopples

indigestion *n.* 1. failure of, or difficulty in, digesting food; causes include insufficient chewing due to defective teeth or bolting, irritating food, parasites, cribbing and windsucking; manifested by irregular appetite, poor condition, dry skin, whole grain or hay strands in the dung 2. the distress caused by digestive failure or difficulty

indigofera poisoning *see* **Birdsville horse disease**

indirect rein a rein used to displace a horse's weight laterally from one side to the other or to make turns and to put the horse into a canter — *see also* **neck rein**

indolent *adj.* slow to heal, such as a wound or ulcer

induce *vt.* 1. to persuade 2. to bring about or cause — **inducement** *n.*

induction *n.* 1. the bringing about or causation of something 2. the initial stages of anesthesia before the patient is completely asleep 3. the influence of one tissue on the development of an adjacent tissue

infanticide *n.* killing of a foal by a stallion

infarct, infarction *n.* an area of degenerated tissue caused by deprivation of blood supply due to a clot within the supplying artery — **infarcted** *adj.*

infection *n.* the presence and growth of disease-causing bacteria, viruses, fungus or parasites within the body

infectious *adj.* relating to that which can cause infection — **infectiousness** *n.*

infectious equine bronchitis a virus-caused, contagious disease marked by a cough which becomes more obvious

when the horse exercises. If an afflicted horse is being ridden, it may suddenly stop in its tracks, lower its head, arch its back and cough loudly; Newmarket cough

inferior check ligament a band of connecting tissue between the deep flexor tendon and the knee which enables the tendon to support the knee without muscular effort; tarsal check ligament

inferior maxilla the lower jaw

infertility inability to produce offspring; sterility —**infertile** *adj.*

inflammation *n.* a reaction of body tissues to an irritant, material, chemical, or bacterial, manifested by pain, heat, swelling, and redness, although not necessarily all of these —**inflame** *vt.* —**inflammatory** *adj.*

influenza *n.* a viral infection of the respiratory system causing inflammation of the respiratory tract and characterized by cough, fever, nasal discharge, and general malaise. Very contagious and transmitted through mucous membranes and direct or indirect contact. Has a very brief incubation period in the host. A vaccination is available.

in foal pregnant

infraorbital region the area below the orbit floor of the eye

infraspinatus *n.* the muscle below the spine of the scapula (shoulder blade)

infundibulum *n.* the dark mark, or cup, that normally appears in the center of a permanent incisor's biting surface and disappears with age

infuse *vt.* to inject (a liquid) into a vein or beneath the skin —**infusion** *n.*

ingest *vt.* to eat or drink —**ingestion** *n.* —**ingestive** *adj.* —**ingesta** *n.pl.* all things that are ingested

inguinal *adj.* relating to the groin

inhalant *n.* a medication that is breathed in

inhalation *n.* the act of breathing in —**inhale** *vt., vi.*

in hand 1. being led rather than ridden; at halter —*see also* **in hand class** 2. prefixed by a number (example: four-in-hand), refers to the number of horses in harness 3. collected (said of a mounted horse)

in-hand class a show class in which the horses are led in a halter with no saddle (draft horses are often shown in their harnesses), and are judged chiefly for conformation and condition; halter class

inherent *adj.* inborn

inherit *vt.* to receive certain characteristics passed on hereditarily by parents —**inheritance** *n.*

inject *vt.* to introduce (a fluid) into a part of the body by needle or syringe —**injection** *n.*

injectable *n.* a medication that is suited to injection rather than oral administration

innate *adj.* existing as part of the horse's nature, as opposed to acquired —**innately** *adj.* —**innateness** *n.*

innervate *vt.* 1. to stimulate a nerve, muscle, etc. to action 2. to supply (a part of the body) with nerves —**innervation** *n.*

inoculant *n. see* **inoculum**

inoculate *vt.* to immunize against a disease by means of injecting a vaccine or other substance —**inoculation** *n.* —**inoculative** *adj.*

inoculum *n.* a substance used in an inoculation, like bacteria; also inoculant

inoperable *adj.* not curable or reversible by surgery

inorganic *adj.* not originating from plant or animal life

insalivate *vt.* to mix food with saliva in chewing

insanity *n.* an abnormality of the brain resulting in irrational behavior; extremely rare in horses —**insane** *adj.*

insecticide *n.* a poisonous substance used to kill insects, such as flies and mosquitoes, etc.; may be applied to a horse's coat in the form of a spray or wiped on as a deterrent to these pests

inseminate *vt.* to inject semen into the vagina either naturally (by the stallion) or artificially (artificial insemination) —**insemination** *n.*

insensitive laminae *see* **laminar horn**

insertion *n.* 1. the introduction of something into something else; e.g. the insertion of a thermometer into the anus to take a horse's temperature —*vt.* **insert** 2. the point at which a muscle is attached to the part it moves

inside *adv.* the inner edge of a circle when working a horse on a circle or in a ring; in racing, the position nearest the rails

inspiration *n.* the intake of air into the lung; inhalation —*vi., vt.* **inspire** to inhale

instinct *n.* an inborn behavioral characteristic; a natural response to stimuli —**instinctive** *adj.*

insufficiency *n.* a deficiency or inadequacy, such as cardiac insufficiency, which is an inadequate pumping of the heart

insulin *n.* a hormone produced in the pancreas and secreted into the bloodstream; it controls blood sugar levels and the metabolism of sugar

insurance *n.* a system of protection against loss (as of a horse)

insurance policy the contract between the owner of a horse and an insurance company which obligates the owner to pay premiums, in return for which the company guarantees to pay a stipulated sum of money in case of loss of the insured horse due to agreed upon circumstances

intelligence *n.* mental ability; according to one train of thought the horse's intelligence is very low and the horse relies only on instinct, habit, or training to function; the other opinion is that horses are indeed very intelligent, some more than others —**intelligent** *adj.* able to learn quickly or showing mental ability beyond mere instinct

interbreed *vt., vi.* crossbreed

intercostal *adj.* between the ribs, such as intercostal spaces or muscle —**intercostally** *adv.*

interdental *adj.* between teeth; **interdental space** the section in the mouth between the incisors and molars, where the bit rests; the bar

interference[1] *n.* a faulty way of going in which one foot strikes against another foot; interfering; forging

interference[2] *n.* in racing, a jockey's act of deliberately or carelessly impeding another competitor, which may incur disqualification

interferon *n.* a cellular substance released to inhibit the growth of viral infection; can be synthetic

intermittent fever a fever which subsides with apparent recovery only to be followed by reoccurence; relapsing fever

internal blistering injection of a counterirritant

international horse shows 1. CSI (Concours de Sauts d'Obstacles Internationale) a horse show open to foreign competitors authorized by their national federation but not officially sent; they are invited by the host federation or personally 2. CSIO (Concours de Sauts d'Obstacles Internationale Officiel) a horse show to which competitors are officially sent by national federations; it is authorized by its national federation and is entered in the FEI (Fédération Equestre Internationale) calendar

interosseous ligament any ligament that lies between bones, as, for example, the thick ligament that attaches the two splint bones to the cannon bone in the leg

interstitial *adj.* of or relating to small spaces (interstices) between tissues —**interstitially** *adv.* —**interstice** *n.*

interstitial cell stimulating hormone (ICSH) a hormone of the stallion that stimulates the cells of the testes to produce testosterone

intertransversalis colli a neck muscle

intertransversalis lumborum a back muscle

interval training a conditioning program involving controlled speed exercise over regulated distances alternating with controlled relief exercise allowing partial recovery of the horse's resting pulse

interventricular *adj.* between the two ventricles of the heart

interventricular septal defect in the fetus, defective development of the heart's septum

intestinal flora bacteria normally present in the intestines

intestinal motility the natural movement the intestines make to pass along food, fluids, and gases

intestinal pacemaker an independent nerve center in the colon which regulates the passage of digested material

intestine *n.* the portion of the digestive system that extends from the exit of the stomach to the anus

in the soup having a problem; originally used in hunting and said of a rider who fell into a ditch of water

intra-arterial *adj.* within an artery

intra-atrial *adj.* within an atrium of the heart

intracapsular *adj.* within a joint capsule

intracardiac *adj.* within the heart

intracutaneous *adj.* within the skin

intradermal *adj.* within the dermal layer (below the outer layer) of the skin —**intradermally** *adv.*

intrahepatic *adj.* within the liver

intramammary *adj.* within the mammary gland; an intramammary injection, used in treating mastitis, introduces a drug through the teat canal into the mammary gland

intramedullary *adj.* within bone marrow

intramural *adj.* within the wall of a body organ

intramuscular *adj.* within a muscle, as an injection —**intramuscularly** *adv.*

intraocular *adj.* within the eye; intraorbital

intraorbital *adj.* intraocular

intraperitoneal *adj.* within the abdominal cavity

intrapleural *adj.* within the chest cavity

intrauterine *adj.* within the cavity of the uterus

intravenous (IV) *adj.* within a vein, as an injection; it is difficult to administer an IV injection to a horse which does not stand still, but there are methods to facilitate this such as attaching the IV apparatus to an overhead swivel system which allows the horse freedom of movement —**intravenously** *adv.*

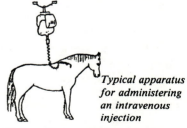

Typical apparatus for administering an intravenous injection

introitus *n.* the mare's vaginal entrance

intromission *n.* the act of penile entry into the vagina

intrusion *n.* in facial coat markings, any dark area within a white mark which contains hairs matching the coat color; occurs often at the whorl in the forehead; when completely surrounded by white, it is sometimes called a night eye or copper penny

intubate *vt.* to administer an anthelcide (deworming agent) by means of a tube which is introduced through one of the nostrils into the stomach —**intubation** *n.*

intumescence *n.* a swelling of a body part —**intumescent** *adj.* —**intumesce** *vi.*

intussusception *n.* the telescoping of a section of the intestine into another, causing colic —**intussuscept** *vt.*

in utero in the uterus; unborn

in vitro in a test tube

in vivo in a live organism

involuntary *adj.* uncontrolled by the will, as an automatic muscle reflex

involution *n.* 1. a body part that curls inward 2. a declining change in the body 3. the return of a body part to its normal size after distension —**involutional** *adj.* —**involutionary** *adj.*

in wear in relation to teeth, the complete contact between a tooth and its opposite member

iodine *(I)* 1. a blue-black element, small quantities of which are normally found in the blood; its metabolism is associated with thyroid function 2. a tincture (solution) of iodine and an iodine ointment can be used as an antiseptic 3. an iodine dye may be introduced internally as a contrast for X-ray examinations

iodoform *n.* a compound of iodine used as an antiseptic in surgical dressings

Iomud (Yomud) *n.* a Russian breed popularly used in long distance races; the outstanding quality of this breed is its endurance of extreme desert temperatures and ability to withstand long periods without water; 14.3–15.1 h.h.

iridocyclitis *n.* a painful infection of the iris and surrounding tissues from any of various irritants such as bacteria or parasites; characterized by inflammation and muscle spasms; also called moon blindness, ophthalmia, uveitis

iris *n.* the colored part of the eye surrounding the pupil and having muscles that dilate and contract the pupil to control the amount of light entering the eye

Irish Draft a light Irish draft breed first registered in 1917; 15–17 h.h.

Irish Horse a sports horse whose registry was started in the 1970s; there are still a variety of types

Irish Hunter usually a cross of seven-eighths Thoroughbred and one-eighth cold-blood (a draft breed such as a Percheron) to produce a rugged mount with a suitable temperament and capable of taking the rough terrain encountered on Irish hunts

iron gray a coat color with an abundance of dark hairs mixed with white; in the Old West such a horse was called a steeldust

iron horse railroad

irons *n.pl.* metal stirrups on an English saddle

isabella 1. *adj.* describes the coal color of a very light Palomino 2. *n.* in Spain, a Palomino (after Queen Isabella, who had a stud of horses of this color, some of which she gave to the Spanish colonies in America)

ischemia *n.* a local anemia of an organ or body part due to blockage of the artery which supplies it

ischium *n., pl.* **ischia** either of the two prominent pelvic bones —**ischial, ischiatic, ischiadic** *adj.*

ischuria *n.* a suppression or retention of urine caused by an obstruction pressurizing the urethra

isoerythrolysis *n. see* **isoimmune disease**

isoimmune disease an uncommon condition of the foal in which there is massive destruction of the red blood cells by antibodies received from the mare's colostrum caused by incompatibility of blood types of mare and foal; characterized by an increasing jaundice with rapid heart and respiratory rates on exertion; signs may appear 12 to 36 hours after the foal's first suckle and include sluggishness, weakness, lack of appetite, and a desire to lie down; results in death within three days of birth, unless treated; also called *hemolytic jaundice, isoerythrolysis, neonatal isoerythrolysis*

isoxsuprine hydrochloride a chemical used to dilate the blood vessels in treatment of laminitis, as well as other vascular problems

Istin *n.* trade name for danthron

Italian Heavy Draft a breed that originated in the mid-19th century with Arab, Thoroughbred, and Hackney blood, though in the 20th century the Breton contributed the most influence; large and strong, docile and fast; due to mechanization on farms, there is now less demand for this draft breed, except for meat, and their numbers are declining; 15–16 h.h.

Italian Saddle Horse a new breed being developed; horses imported from France, Ireland, Germany, the Netherlands and Eastern Europe, have been bred with regional Italian riding horses to create a sports breed; most of the mares have been Anglo-Arabs; it is too early to determine any typical characteristics; 15.3–16.2 h.h.

itch *n.* an irritating feeling of the skin which causes the desire to scratch the part affected; horses can only relieve an itch by scratching with their teeth (if they can reach the spot) or rubbing against something, such as a tree trunk, corner of a stable, etc. — *vt.*

ivermectin *n.* an anthelmintic drug; trade name Zimecterin

ixode *n.* a tick

— J —

jabbing *n.* the act of sharply jerking the horse's mouth

jack[1] *n.* a bony enlargement on the hock

jack[2] *n.* a male donkey; jackass

jackaroo *n.* an Australian cowboy

jackass *n.* a male donkey; jack

jack-knife *vi.* to click the fore and hind legs together while in the air (said of bucking horses)

jackpot *n.* in rodeo or playday events, the total or percentage of the fees charged to entrants; the top winners divide this on a predetermined basis

jack spavin *see* **bone spavin**

jade *n.* a worn-out, valueless horse

Jaf *n.* a breed indigenous to Iran; tough with much stamina; spirited but gentle; has very hard hooves; about 15 h.h.

jaundice *n.* a symptom of a disease or abnormal condition of the body; icterus; characterized by yellowness of the skin, sclera, and tongue; fever may or may not be present; induced by an interference with function of the liver and bile, with the yellow color being due to entrance of the bile into the blood. The most common form in the newborn foal is hemolytic jaundice; there is a clash between the antibodies in the mare's colostrum and the foal's blood cells, which results in death if not arrested; may appear from 12 to 36 hours after the foal's first suckle; the foal seems sluggish and weak, has no desire to suckle and wants to lie down

constantly. —*see also* **isoimmune disease**

jaw *n.* one of two bony parts, upper and lower, that enclose the mouth and contain the teeth

Jennet *n.* a Spanish breed of the Middle Ages descended from Barbs and Oriental stock brought over to Spain by Muslims in the 8th century and bred with native horses; docile and beautiful and known for their 4-beat gait; Jennets were allegedly brought over to America by Columbus and it is from these horses that the Paso breeds of today are descended

jennet *n. see* **jenny**

jenny *n.* a female donkey; jennet

jibbah *n.* the bulge on the face of the Arabian horse between the eyes, up to a point between the ears and down across the first third of the nasal bone; it is a formation of frontal and parietal bones and appears in the form of a shield; it forms the "dish" unique to this breed

jibbing, gibbing *n.* the act of refusing to go forward and instead walking backward, usually in fear of something the horse sees or hears or in objection to a bridle; turning the horse around in a circle and then urging it forward may achieve success but following another calm horse is usually the solution

jig *vi.* to move in a slow, jerky jog-trot —*n.*

jinked back *see* **ricked back**

Jobst boot trade name for an intermittent pressure pump used for therapeutic purposes; it wraps around the horse's leg and, by repeated rhythmic pressure, improves local circulation

jockey[1] *n.* a person who rides a horse in a race

jockey[2] *n.* part of a Western saddle; the **side jockey** is the leather flap, forming part of the seat, that extends over the fender; the **back jockey** is the leather flap behind the cantle that lies over the upper part of the skirt

jockey[3] *vi.* 1. to maneuver for a better position, as in a race 2. to cheat in the horse business —*n.* a horse dealer

jockeys *n.pl.* 1. hunting boots, usually black 2. grease and dirt deposits that may collect on the flaps of a saddle, and should be cleaned off

jockey seat *see* **seat**

jockey's valet someone who attends to the clothes and saddles used by several jockeys

jodhpurs *n.* a style of riding pants that are close-fitting from knee to ankle

jog *n.* a short-paced, slow trot —*vi.*

jogger *n.* a training vehicle for Hackneys

joint *n.* any part of the body where two or more connecting bones capped by cartilage are united; articulation; an **amphiarthrodial joint** involves bones that are directly connected by cartilage and ligaments, with limited movement; a **diarthrodial** joint involves bones connected by a capsule with surfaces in a fluid-filled cavity and having movement; a **synarthrodial joint** involves no movement, as, for example, in the skull; a **joint mouse** is a fragment of broken-off bone in a joint cavity

joint block a test done when there is lameness, wherein an anesthetic is injected into a joint, followed by monitoring of the horse's gait; if the lameness decreases, it is assumed that inflammation or degeneration is present in or around the joint

joint capsule a sac-like membrane that encloses a diarthrodial joint space and secretes synovial fluid

joint ill a serious, often fatal disease that attacks a newborn foal, usually through the navel stump but sometimes in various other ways, as by infection through the dam before birth or through failure of passive transfer. The infection localizes in one or more

joints; symptoms may be swelling and suppuration in the navel area, stiffness and swelling in a joint or joints, and fever, followed by lack of interest in suckling and inability to stand for any length of time. The onset of this disease is usually rapid and, if untreated, the foal may die within 8–10 hours.; also called navel ill

joint-master in hunting, one of two or more people who share the mastership of a pack of hounds, keeping them in order

joint mouse *see* **joint**

jounce *vi.* in riding, to bounce or jolt

joust *n.* a combat between two mounted knights with lances — *vi.*

jowl *n.* the jaw, especially the lower jaw

jugular *adj.* pertaining to the neck or throat

jugular furrows grooves on either side of the neck, the depths of which vary with the horse's condition (deep in an emaciated horse)

jugular vein either of two large veins located on each side of the windpipe in the underside of the neck; carries blood from the head and neck to the chest

jump *vi.* to leap by raising the forelegs and springing from the hind legs — *vt.* to cause to jump, as to jump a horse over an obstacle — *n.* 1. a leap 2. the height jumped 3. that which is jumped over, such as fences, etc.

jump cups the supports for rails in a jumping obstacle which allow the rails to fall when bumped by a horse

jump cups

jumped *adj.* a cowboy's term describing a herd of wild horses when they gallop off at the warning neigh of their stallion leader

jumper *n.* 1. a horse trained to jump 2. a horse who is a natural jumper and therefore not easily confined behind low fences

jumper's bump a protuberance at the top of the croup, inaccurately said to increase a jumper's ability

jumping a wheeler's act of cantering out of fear of the proximity of the coach at the horse's rear

jumping boots protective leather horse boots lined with ridged rubber to protect the tendons; fitted to the backs of the forelegs

jumping boot

jumping hackamore *see* **English hackamore**

jumping lane a narrow fenced-in course with a variety of obstacles used to train a horse to jump

jump jockey a rider who races horses over jumps

jump-off *n.* in show-jumping, an extra round run to decide the final winner when competitors tie for first place

Jutland *n.* a very heavy Danish draft breed of ancient origins; the modern Jutland was lightened in size by crosses with imports from Britain; large-boned, strong, and docile, with generously feathered feet; still used on some Danish farms; 15.1–16.1 h.h.

juvenile *n.* a 2-year-old horse

— K —

Kabardin *n.* a hardy Russian mountainbreed bred by nomadic tribesmen in the Caucasus mountains; 14.2–15 h.h.

kallidin *n.* the product of a group of enzymes that maintain dilation of

blood vessels when inflammation is taking place

kanamycin *n.* a generic name for a powerful antibiotic

kaolin *n.* a fine-particle absorbent pow-

der which may be applied to wounds

Karabair *n.* a Russian breed having great endurance and a spirited but gentle nature; popularly used in mounted games; about 15 h.h.

Karabakh *n.* a spirited Russian breed of ancient heritage that is now becoming rare and is indigenous to the Karabakh Mountains; today is often crossed with small Arabs; used under saddle and as a pack horse; about 14.1 h.h.

Karacabey *n.* a type of horse bred in Turkey from Arabian, Thoroughbred, Haflinger, and Nonius breeds; used for riding, light draft and pack work; 14–16.1 h.h.

Kathiawari *n.* a lightweight, narrowly built Indian breed; a tough, easy keeper but often bad tempered; tends to be sickle-hocked; its unusual feature is its inwardly pointed ears that nearly and sometimes do touch each other; used for riding, racing, packing, and sports, including polo; 14.2–15.2 h.h.

kayack *n.* a leather pack bag

Kazakh *n.* an extremely hardy Russian (Kazakhstan) pony breed, used chiefly for cattle work; subdivided into two types, the Dzhabe and the Adayev; 12.2–13.2 h.h.

keep *n.* a pasture

keeper *n.* a loop to hold straps on tack in place; runner

keg shoe a commercially made horse shoe, as opposed to one made by hand

keloid *n.* an excess of scar tissue that forms like a ridge around a wound — **keloidal** *adj.*

kelp *n.* brown seaweed, high in iodine content and sometimes fed to horses, particularly mares in foal; can cause malfunction of the fetal thyroid and subsequent deficient thyroid hormone production and goiter

kennel *n.* 1. a housing for a dog (as for hunting hounds) 2. a fox's bed

kennel huntsman a person in charge

of hounds in their kennels, sometimes aided by a kennel man; may also be a whipper-in at the hunt

kennel man a person who works in hunt kennels, performing cleaning, feeding, and other tasks, under the supervision of a huntsman or kennel huntsman

Kentucky Derby a 1¼ mile race for 3-year-olds held at Churchill Downs, Kentucky, in May of every year since 1875; one of the United States' three Classics

Kentucky Futurity a top class trotting race for 3-year-olds held annually in Lexington, Kentucky

Kentucky Saddler *see* **Saddlebred**

keratectomy *n.* the surgical removal of the cornea of the eye

keratitis *n.* corneal inflammation; causes may be conjunctivitis, other infections, or external injury; characterized by closed lids, pain, and discharge at first, followed by dryness; ulceration may develop which may finally result in loss of the eye; pannus

kerato-hyoideus *n.* a muscle that raises the hyoid bone and larynx

keratoma *n.* an uncommon wart-like growth on the interior wall of the hoof's horn; can cause inflammation and pain and can be detected by tapping, hoof testers, or X-ray; caused by injury or pressure of foreign intrusions in the hoof

keratosis *n.* a condition characterized by a wart-like growth

keratotomy *n.* the surgical incision of the cornea

Kerry Pony a strong and hardy pony native to Ireland

ketamine hydrochloride an injectable anesthetic of short duration

keyhole race a timed gymkhana competition; the approximate distance from the starting line to center of keyhole is specified; usually overstepping

any part of the keyhole boundary is a disqualification, although sometimes a 5-second penalty is imposed instead

keys *n.pl.* 1. signals that are given to a horse in track training 2. metal pieces on a bit to encourage mouthing of the bit and keeping the mouth moist with the tongue where it should be; players

Khaylan *n.* *see* **Arabian**

kick *vi., vt.* to aggressively strike out with one or both hind legs or strike forward with one hind leg (cow-kick) — *n.*

kidney *n.* either of two glandular organs in the upper abdominal cavity whose function is to separate water and waste matter from blood and excrete them as urine

kidney stone a calculus in the kidney

Kimberly horse disease a disease caused by poisoning from eating the Crotalaria plant, with resultant serious liver damage; characterized by periods of lethargy alternating with periods of walking about aimlessly through or against any obstacles in the way, jaundice, and passing dark-colored urine; walkabout disease; named for the Kimberly area in northwest Australia

Kimberwicke bit a bit that has a low port or snaffle, short cheek pieces, and curb chain

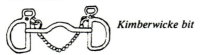

Kimberwicke bit

kinesiology *n.* the study of motion and the gaits

Kirghiz *n.* a Russian mountain breed; due to changes resulting from cross-breeding with Don and Thoroughbred stock, this breed is now known as Novokirghiz; 14.1–15.1 h.h.

Kisber *n.* Hungarian half-bred sports horse; 15.2–16.2 h.h.

Kladruber *n.* a Czechoslovakian breed that originated in Kladruby, Bohemia, in 1572 from Spanish stock;

originally around 18 h.h. but now about 16.2–17 h.h. used in harness; only gray or black in color

klebsiella *n.* a genus of bacteria that may cause a variety of infections in horses, including venereal disease, and is spread by intercourse

Knabstrup *n.* a spotted Danish breed popularly used in circuses and exhibitions but also for riding; 15.1–16 h.h.

knacker *n.* 1. a person who removes carcasses 2. a horse butcher

knee *n.* a joint in the foreleg between the cannon and forearm; carpal joint

knee caps 1. protectors for a horse's knees used for traveling or when training green horses over jumps 2. in polo, protectors for the rider's knees

knee pads 1. the parts of an Australian saddle that protrude behind the pommel 2. knee caps

knee rolls a padding on some English saddle flaps to support the knees

knee spavin *see* **carpitis**

knee sprung having knees set too far forward

knee strap a strap used to restrain a forefoot; the leg is bent at the knee and held by the strap, which may form two loops — one to go around the pastern and the other around the forearm — or just one loop which can be more easily pulled off

knee sprung

knocked-up shoe a shoe having a skate-shaped (rather pointed) inner branch with no nails on the inside, except at the toe; used to counteract brushing

knocker *n.* a derogatory term applied to a sickle-hocked, cow-hocked horse whose hind legs stand far back so that the hocks knock off the balls of excrement

knock-kneed *adj.* having knees set too far inward with the legs angling

from a narrow base at the top out to a splay-footed position of the hooves; splay-footed

knock-kneed

knuckle over 1. to involuntarily flex a leg joint while supporting weight 2. stumble 3. a condition in foals in which the fetlock joint is permanently flexed; caused by a contracted flexor tendon; overshot fetlock; hyperflexion of the fetlock

Konik *n.* a primitive Polish pony breed (name means "small horse") popularly used for farm work, as well as for children to ride; resembles a Tarpan and is dun colored, sometimes with dorsal and zebra stripes; very hardy and long-lived; about 13.1 h.h.

kopar *n.* a Russian mounted game in which a rider carries a goat that competitors try to take from him

Kopoczyk Podlaski the smallest of the Polish draft breeds

Kuhailan *n.* an Arabian subtype bred in Russia

kumiss *n.* a fermented drink made in Mongolia from horses' milk

kunkur *n.* a diseased formation within a bursatti skin tumor

Kurdistan *n.* an all-purpose breed indigenous to the Kurdish region of east Turkey; 14 h.h.

Kushum *n.* a Russian breed developed, chiefly for meat, from crosses of Kazakh mares with Thoroughbred, Orlov Trotter and Don stallions

Kustanair *n.* a Russian breed developed from crosses of Kazakhstan ponies with Don and Thoroughbred stallions and Strelets (Strelets are now extinct); very hardy, with short legs, good bone and much stamina. There are three types: the large Steppe type used in harness and for agriculture; the Saddle or riding type; and the Basic type with characteristics of both the former. About 15 h.h.

Kuznet *n.* the largest breed of Siberia; developed from crosses of local breeds with Thoroughbreds, English heavy draft horses and Orlov Trotters

— L —

labia majora the two major skin folds or lips of the vulva on either side of the vaginal entrance

labia minora the two lesser skin folds or lips within the labia majora

labiate *adj.* having lips

labile *adj.* unstable or apt to change (labile blood pressure is one that fluctuates)

labium *n., pl.* **labia** a lip or lip-like organ

labor *n.* parturition; the process of giving birth

laburnum poisoning poisoning which occurs as a result of eating the laburnum plant

labyrinth *n.* the communicating channels of the inner ear

laceration *n.* a jagged cut or wound —**lacerated** *adj.*

lachrymal, lachrymatory, lacrimal *adj.* relating to tears

lachrymal glands tear sacs beneath the upper eyelids

lacrimal *adj. see* **lachrymal**

lacrimation *n.* excessive shedding of tears

lactalbumin *n.* a protein found in milk

lactase *n.* an enzyme that digests the sugar in milk

lactate *vi.* 1. to secrete milk —**lactation** *n.* 2. —*n.* a salt of lactic acid

lactate dehydrogenase an enzyme in the body

lactation tetany a condition of a newly nursing mare that is stressed by excitement or fatigue, as, for example, when she is being transported over a long distance; characterized by severe distress and muscle spasms, lack of coordination, profuse sweating, rapid breathing, and a temperature rise; a significant drop in blood calcium while milk production rapidly rises causes this pathology

lacteal *adj.* 1. of milk or milky 2. containing chyle in a milky fluid

lacteals *n.pl.* the lymph channels that carry chyle from the intestines to the thoracic duct

lactic *adj.* relating to milk

lactic acid an acid formed in small quantities by sugar metabolism; excessive amounts result from insufficient oxygen supply to cells, especially muscle cells during strenuous exercise

lactic acidosis overproduction of lactic acid present in the bloodstream, often resulting from excessive exercise and causing stiffness

lactiferous *adj.* producing milk

lactobacillus *n.* a species of bacteria in the intestinal tract, helpful in producing lactic acid from carbohydrates in milk

lactoflavin *n.* riboflavin

lactogen *n.* a hormone, produced by the placenta, which induces milk production —**lactogenic** *adj.*

lactoglobulin *n.* protein globulin in milk

lactoprotein *n.* any protein found in milk

lactose *n.* milk sugar

lairage *n.* a resting place for horses traveling

lame *adj.* having an injured leg or foot that manifests pain by making the horse limp or have an irregular gait —*vt.* —**lameness** *n.*

lame hand an inefficient coachman

lamella *n.* a thin plate of bone

laminae *n.pl.* the irreplaceable tissues that bind the hoof horn to the hoof's internal structures —**laminar, laminal** *adj.*

laminar corium the part of the corium by which the upper surface of the coffin bone is attached to the inner surface of the hoof wall; **sensitive laminae; quick**

laminar horn flakes of hoof horn which together with sensitive laminae bind the hoof wall to the underlying bone; insensitive laminae

laminitis *n.* an impairment or inflammation of the soft tissue, or laminae, in the foot; acute laminitis comes on rapidly and lasts briefly, while chronic laminitis is a persistent, long-term disturbance; either, in severe cases, may result in founder

lampas *n.* a swelling of the mucous membrane covering the hard palate behind the upper incisor teeth; may be associated with eruption of the permanent incisor teeth or with feeding

lance *vt.* to cut into (e.g., to lance a boil)

Landais *n.* a French pony breed of very old origins with Arab influence and consequently Arab features; has run wild for centuries on the Landais marshes, which has made the pony tough and wily; although the breed is dwindling, these ponies are used today as childrens' mounts and in harness; up to 13.1 h.h.

landau a four-wheeled, open carriage that has two adjustable leather tops that can be raised or lowered independently; invented in 1757 in Landau, Germany

lane creepers the New Forest ponies that would wander off down lanes and roads to neighboring villages and farms looking for food and being a nuisance before the New Forest in England was fenced

lap and tap in rodeo timed events, an even start between the cattle and contestants, used in small arenas

laparotomy *n.* a surgical operation in which the incision is made through the flank or abdomen

large colon a part of the large intestine which, with the cecum, is where digestion and absorption of cellulose take place; situated between the cecum and small colon; measures 8–18 inches in diameter and 10–12 feet in length

large intestine the lower portion of the digestive system, consisting of the cecum, colon, rectum, and anal canal; the first stage is about 10 feet long with a 70-liter capacity and the second stage is about 10 feet long but with about a 20-liter capacity

large strongyle an intestinal parasite (*see* **strongyles**); also called *bloodworm, palisade worm, sclerostome,* and *redworm*

largo *n.* the fastest speed that the Paso Fino horse performs in gait

lariat *n.* a rope

lark *vi.* in hunting, to jump fences unnecessarily; sometimes indulged in by hunters who are more interested in jumping than following the hounds — *n.*

larva *n., pl.* **-vae** an insect or worm in its immature, wingless stage of development — **larval** *adj.*

larvicide *n.* an agent used to kill larvae — *see also* **ptermalid**

laryngeal *adj.* relating to the larynx

laryngeal hemiplegia a paralysis caused by impaired function of the recurrent nerve supplying the laryngeal muscles; manifested by roaring and whistling

laryngismus *n.* a laryngeal spasm

laryngitis *n.* inflammation of the larynx; characterized by a cough and dysphagia (painful swallowing)

laryngoscope *n.* an endoscopic device for viewing the larynx

laryngotomy *n.* surgery of the larynx — *see also* **Hobday operation**

larynx *n.* the voice box, located just behind the lower jawbones between the throat and windpipe — **laryngeal** *adj.*

laser *n.* an instrument that emits a narrow, intense light beam; used in surgery; acronym for *l*ight *a*mplification by *s*timulated *e*mission of *r*adiation

Lasix *n.* trade name for furosemide, a strong diuretic

lassitude *n.* fatigue, listlessness, weakness

lasso *n.* a lariat or rope, varying in length from 30 to 45 feet and made of rawhide, horsehair, hemp, or nylon; has a running noose and is used for catching wild horses — *vt.* to catch horses with a rope

latent *adj.* hidden or undeveloped — **latency** *n.* — **latently** *adv.*

lateral *adj.* sideways; lying to the side — **laterally** *adv.*

lateral aids the two aids of the hand and rein on one side

lateral cartilage the cartilage which attaches to the upper rear edge of the foot's coffin bone above the coronet and serves as an important aid to the expansion and flexion of the hoof on impact; collateral cartilage

lateral digital extensor muscle the muscle which extends the toe and flexes the hock

lateralis nasi a muscle that dilates the nostrils

lateral lacunae the depressions in the foot on either side of the frog

lateral march *see* **half-pass**

lateral recumbancy lying down all the way on the side with head and neck on the ground

lather *n.* foamy sweat — *vi.* to form lather — **lathery** *adj.* — **lathered** *adj.*

latigo *n.* a strap which secures a girth to a saddle

latissimus dorsi a muscle that flexes the shoulder joint

Latvian *n.* a Russian cold-blood breed with an ancient heritage, native to Latvia; with less demand today for draft horses, this breed has been lightened by crosses with lighter breeds and now there exist a variety of types; now considered a multi-purpose horse; has feathered legs; 15.2–16 h.h.

lavage *n.* the washing out of a body organ with large amounts of water

lawn meet in hunting, a meet held at a private home

laxative *n.* a medicine that promotes evacuation of the bowels — *adj.*

lazy *adj.* deliberately slow and unwilling to work — **laziness** *n.* — **lazily** *adv.*

lead *n.* a metallic chemical element used in various alloys and compounds, such as paint; a horse can be poisoned by chewing painted things such as fences, or by grazing near lead works; symptoms include convulsions, abdominal pain, constipation followed by diarrhea, loss of weight, swelling of the limbs, and paralysis of the hind legs and of the throat

lead[1] *vt.* to hand guide (a horse) on foot by means of a rein or rope 2. to guide by means of going ahead of others, as when a horse leads other horses

lead[2] *n.* 1. the action by the forefoot that takes the first or leading step when entering a canter and while cantering or galloping; when turning a tight circle, a horse must be on its correct lead to be properly balanced (i.e., on its right lead when turning clockwise and on its left lead when turning counterclockwise) 2. a rope or rein used to guide a horse 3. (a) the first or front place, as a horse in the lead; (b) the distance that a horse is ahead, as in a race

leader *n.* in a team of harness horses, either of the two leading horses, referred to as the **near leader** or **off leader** according to position; of tandem driven horses, the one which leads

lead harness the harness used for a leader

lean *adj.* slender

lean-to *n.* an open shelter built onto an adjacent building and open on 2 or 3 sides

lease *vt.* to temporarily take possession of (a horse) for pleasure riding, racing, or use as a stud

leather *n.* hide used for tack, especially cowhide; small amounts of sheepskin, pigskin, doe or buckskin are also used; the flesh side of leather is the inside which is unsealed; the grain side is the outside, which is sealed; rawhide is cowhide that is untanned or only partly tanned; reversed hide is cowhide that has been roughened for better grip

leathers *n.pl.* the straps that hold the stirrups on an English saddle

lecithin *n.* a phosphatide in nerve tissue, semen, bile, blood, etc.

leech *n.* a parasitic worm that has a sucker at each end used primarily for sucking blood. There are two kinds: (a) land leeches that live in wet earth and cling to the legs of horses that traverse their habitats; (b) water leeches, or horse leeches, that live in water and enter a horse's mouth or nostrils when the horse drinks from leech-invested sources, clinging to the mucous membranes therein. Although leeches may reach three inches in length, water leeches are young when they infest the horse and only about one-tenth inch in lenth; as many as 100 may be found in a horse, causing bleeding of the nose, loss of appetite, emaciation and even death from blood loss or suffocation.

left at the post in racing, slow to take off and consequently trailing the rest of the runners

left-hand course a course which is run in a counterclockwise direction

legal catch *see* **fair catch**

leg marking a mark on the leg made by white hairs contrasting with overall coat color. These markings have the following names: stocking, boot, sock, coronet, and ermine spots or marks. Zebra stripes (dark hairs) are also markings.

leg paint a liquid counterirritant

legs out of one hole forelegs that are close together at the top from a narrow chest

leg spray a therapeutic device for spraying a horse's swollen leg with water; consists of a perforated rubber ring joined by T-connection to a hose

legume *n.* any of the leafy grasses characterized by having seed pods, including e.g. clover, lespedeza, and alfalfa; high in protein and vitamins

leg up assistance in mounting a horse; someone on the ground manually hoists the rider with a cupped hand or hands supporting the rider's leg; when one hand is used the assistant bends his or her own left knee and with a cupped hand supports the rider's ankle; he or she then straightens the bent knee and lifts the ankle of the rider, who simultaneously springs up into the saddle; another way is for the assistant to clasp his or her hands together to support the rider's knee and provide a boost

leg up stirrup a single mounting stirrup which hangs lower from a saddle than the regular stirrup to help a rider to mount

leg yielding the desired response of a horse to the pressure of the rider's leg when the rider asks the horse to move sideways away from the pressure

LEM leukoencephalomalacia

length *n.* 1. a distance corresponding to the horizontal measurement of a horse's body by which a horse is said to win a race 2. the measurement from end to end of a part of the body

lens *n.* the portion of the eye lying behind the pupil; focuses entering light rays on the retina, which then transmits them to the brain to form an image

leopard marking a type of marking that features spots of any color on a white or light-colored background; typical of the Appaloosa

leptospirosis *n.* a systemic disease caused by leptospira bacteria; contracted from infected animals or contaminated water; causes red cell destruction, kidney disease, uveitis, and, in pregnant mares, abortion

lesion *n.* damaged tissue due to injury or disease; ulcers, tumors, abscesses, and other disturbances may be called lesions

lespediza *n.* any of a genus of annual or perennial plants of the legume family, cultivated for forage, hay, soil improvement and other purposes

lethal gene a hereditary gene that causes death unless counteracted by medicinal means or special care

lethal white foal syndrome a condition affecting white foals with pink skin and blue eyes (some of which have small color spots) that have defective gut function and die within 3 days of birth; genes that produce an Overo coat pattern are said to be responsible; also called white death

leukemia *n.* a cancerous disease of blood-forming organs causing an excessive number of white blood cells

leukocyte *n.* *see* **white blood cell** — **leukocytic** *adj.*

leukocytosis *n.* an increased number of white blood cells (leukocytes); occurs in the presence of infection or toxemia

leukoderma *n.* an acquired lack of

pigmentation of the skin in hairless areas

leukoencephalomalacia (LEM) *n.* a fatal disease caused by moldy corn; develops within two to several weeks after ingestion of the corn; characterized by loss of appetite followed by an obvious neurological disorder; there may be drowsiness and blindness in one or both eyes, causing the horse to run into obstacles; partial or complete paralyses of the pharynx and muscular twitching may develop, as well as loss of ambulatory control

leukopenia *n.* a decreased number of white blood cells; can be caused by arteritis or excessive radiation

levade *n.* in dressage, an exercise in which a horse balances on its hind legs

levamisole hydrochloride a drug for treating lungworms and gastroenteritis caused by parasites; Nemicide

levatores costarum a muscle that helps breathing (inspiration)

levator labii superioris proprius a muscle that raises the upper lip

levator nasolabialis a muscles that raises the upper lip and nostril

levator palpebrae superioris a muscle that raises the upper eyelid

level mover a horse that maintains a level way of going in all gaits, with all feet pointing straight forward and distance between fore and hind legs correctly paced

LH luteinizing hormone

liberty horse a circus horse that performs without a rider

libido *n.* sexual drive or instinct

lice *n.pl.* *see* **louse**

lick *vt.* 1. to pass the tongue over 2. to whip — *n.* 1. the act of licking 2. short for salt lick or block of salt

Lidzbark *n.* a light Polish draft breed developed from primitive West European cold-blood horses and the North Swedish breed

Lieberkuhn gland an intestinal gland that produces digestive juice

life span the period of existence from birth to death; given good health, the expected life span of the horse may be said to be around 30 years, although certain horses have been recorded to have lived into the forties and fifties and even, in one recorded case, to 62

lift the hounds in hunting, to remove the hounds from a lost line and cast them forward in search of a line farther on

ligament *n.* a tough, fibrous tissue which holds one bone to another or holds organs in place —**ligamentous** *adj.*

ligamentum nuchae a ligament that runs from poll to withers, contributing support to the head

ligation *n.* tying of something, as an artery, with a ligature —**ligate** *vt.*

ligature *n.* a thread or wire used to tie up a bleeding artery — *vt.* to tie with a ligature —**ligate** *vt.*

light bone a smaller than desirable measurement of the circumference of bone just below the knee or hock

light-footed *adj.* stepping lightly and agilely

light horse 1. any horse not of draft ancestry 2. light-armed cavalry

lightness *n.* 1. the art of riding in such a way as only to contribute to rather than counteract or interfere with the horse's movements; the ability to move with the horse 2. a horse's ability to move in a collected or light manner or to respond immediately to the lightest of aids

lightning *n.* an electrical atmospheric discharge, as in a storm; may strike a horse, most often with fatal results and usually when the horse is out at pasture. Signs of this cause of death are a bloody froth at the mouth and dark-colored blood at the anus; the

hair may be singed or there may be a burned line on the coat; sometimes there is grass still clenched in the mouth; the horse's struggle may be evident from dug-up ground around it; sometimes part of the body is torn open. When the electric shock is not so severe, the horse may be dazed or unconscious but alive; the pulse is slow and irregular and respiration labored, the pupils are dilated and convulsions or spasms may be present; paralysis in the limbs may occur and permanent blindness is possible; recovery can take from a few hours to several days.

lightweight hunter a horse that can carry up to 165 lbs.

lilac dun *see* **dun**

limb *n*. a leg

limb bud an embryonic projection which gradually develops into a leg

limber *adj*. supple and able to bend easily — *vt*.

limbic ring, -system a group of subcortical structures (hypothalamus, hippocampus and amygdala) of the brain, which are related to emotion, motivation and various internal organ functions

limbus *n*. a border, often of contrasting color; for example, the limbus of the eye is the area where the colored part of the eye meets the white of the eye

limit class a class at a horse show in which no entrants have won more than 6 blue ribbons at a recognized show

Limousin *n*. a French medieval breed allegedly originating from Barb horses left in France by Muslims in the 8th century; these were crossed through the years with Arabs and Thoroughbreds and today the Limousin is classed as a halfbred; named for the region where it is bred; about 16 h.h.

limp *vi*. to move lamely or with an uneven step — *n*.

Lincolnshire Trotter an extinct English breed once popular in harness

lincomycin *n*. generic name of an antibiotic that is poisonous to horses

Lindell sidepull a variation of the basic hackamore bridle, so named because it has side rings to attach it to the reins

line *n*. in hunting, the scent left by the quarry

lineage *n*. 1. direct descent from an ancestor 2. ancestry

line-back *n*. a horse having a dorsal stripe —**linebacked** *adj*.

linebreed *vi., vt*. to mate horses who are closely related to a single ancestor

lingual *adj*. relating to the tongue

lingulate *adj*. having a tongue-like shape

liniment *n*. a liquid medication for application to the skin to soothe underlying sore or inflamed areas

linoleic acid an unsaturated fatty acid found in linseed oil and other fats and oils; considered essential in animal diets

linseed *n*. the seed of flax generally used in the form of oil, jelly or tea, both as a laxative and to improve the condition of a horse's coat

lip *n*. either of two fleshy edges of the mouth; horses use the lips liberally to pick up grain or gather grass

lip chain *see* **twitch**

Lipican *n*. a Czechoslovakian carriage horse

lipid *n*. any of a group of fats and fat-like substances that form a part of living cells

Lipizzaner, Lipizzan *n*. a breed descended from Spanish Andalusians (9 stallions and 24 mares) imported into Yugoslavia by the Archduke Charles, who founded a stud at the village of Lipizza in 1580. Spanish horses were

imported until the 17th century, then Arab blood was introduced. At the end of World War I the stud was moved to the village of Piber in southern Austria and today this stud supplies the famous Spanish Riding School of Vienna with horses that give spectacular performance shows in many parts of the world. It takes about 7 years to train Lipizzaners to perform the maneuvers for which they are famous. They are intelligent and docile and have compact bodies with strong backs and quarters and strong legs; they mature late, are long-lived and often work into their thirties; although predominantly white, occasionally they are bay or brown; 15–16 h.h.

lipoma *n.* a benign fatty tumor, or neoplasm, usually subcutaneous

lip twitch *see* **twitch**

lithiasis *n.* a condition of stones within the body, as kidney stones

lithotomy *n.* surgery to remove stones

Lithuanian Heavy Draught a Russian draft breed that originated in the late 19th century from Zhmud-Ardennes crosses; heavy though medium-sized, with short feathered legs; 15–15.3 h.h.

liver *n.* the largest glandular organ, located in the upper or anterior part of the abdomen; it secretes bile, metabolizes carbohydrates, fats and proteins, and has a substance essential to the normal production of red blood cells

Liverpool bit a bit, used for driving, which has a straight bar with cheek rings and long, straight shanks with slots for adjustment of severity of the reins

Liverpool bit

Liverpool jump a combination fence having a water jump after it

liver profile a chemical blood test to determine the state of liver function

livery *n.* 1. a place where privately owned horses are kept, exercised and looked after for an agreed fee 2. a place where horses are kept for hire; a **livery stable** 3. distinctive clothing as worn by professional hunt staff

liveryman *n.* a person who owns or works in a livery stable

Llanero *n.* Venezuela's version of the Criollo derived from Iberian stock brought into South America by the Spanish in the 16th century. A fairly light-framed horse. Named after the native plainsmen who ride them

load *vt.* 1. to put (a horse) into something, as a trailer, for transportation 2. —*n.* a burden which a horse is to pull or carry

loaded shoulder a shoulder that has a very thick muscle

loam *n.* rich soil

lobe *n.* a rounded part of an organ or tissue; a small lobe is a **lobule**

lobo dun *see* **dun**

local class a class into which entrance is restricted by management to horses within territory of reasonable size and which is so described in the prize list and catalogue; to be eligible, a horse must be the property of a resident of the prescribed area

lochia *n.* a whitish discharge from the vagina

lock *n.* in a horse-drawn vehicle, the turning capability of the front wheels; a vehicle with "good [or full] lock" can turn within a short space

locked hind leg an inherited condition in which a hind leg locks abnormally, as when a horse is in forward motion. The leg should lock only when the horse wants to stand without muscular effort (as when sleeping while standing up). The kneecap becomes fixed, locking the stifle in such a position that it prevents flexion of the hind limb; the limb can be locked in an extended position for hours or the kneecap may

be released every few steps; this sudden release, with the leg shooting forward, may be mistaken for stringhalt; also referred to as upward fixation of the hind leg

lockjaw *n.* *see* **tetanus**

loco disease a disease caused by ingestion of locoweed, which contains the toxin locoine, and which can affect the horse's brain; the name derives from the wild behavioral symptoms exhibited by the infected horse, which may be so "loco" as to walk off a cliff to its death; other signs include staggering, incoordination, and exaggerated movements of the limbs

loculus, locule *n.* a small cavity in animal tissue

loin *n.* the lower part of the back on either side of the backbone between the hip bones and ribs; the area joining the back to the croup

Lokai *n.* a Russian pony breed used for mountain pack work by the Lokai tribe; popularly used in the game of Kopar; up to 13.1 h.h.

long *n.* a colt, filly, or gelding in the latter part of its second year

longe *vt* *see* **lunge**

long in the tooth old

longissimus capitis et atlantis a muscle which extends or turns the neck

longissiums costarum a muscle that helps breathing (expiration) —*see also* **levatores costarum**

longissimus dorsi the longest of the back muscles, lying parallel and beside the backbone and acting to extend the back or turn to a side

long-reining *n.* a training method, like lunging, using two long reins; teaches response to the bit and does not limit the training to working in a circle

long slow distance (LSD) the first and longest phase of conditioning a horse, involving a 3- to 6-month period of aerobic exercises over increasing distance

longus coli a neck muscle that flexes the head

loose box a large stall in which a horse has ample space to move about

loose rein a rein which hangs loosely, affording no contact between the rider and the horse's mouth; maintained in some classes to show that the horse is not excitable, or as a restful respite for the horse at a walk

loose stifles a defect of the stifle joint wherein the patellar ligament does not move forward over the bulge of the thighbone, thereby manifesting a slight catch in the leg as it strides

lop *vi.* 1. to hang to one side, as the ears (*see* **lop ears**) 2. to move the ears in a hesitant manner

lope *n.* a Western term meaning a type of canter that has a 4-beat rhythm with a pause after the fourth beat —*vi.*

lop ears ears that point outward —**lop-eared** *adj.*

lop neck a very thick neck

lordosis *n.* curvature of the spine producing an excessive hollow of the back or a sway back; can occasionally be congenital and be seen in a newborn foal or can develop as a gradual deterioration and stretching of ligaments in very old horses —**lordotic** *adj.*

loriner *n.* a person who makes the metal parts of tack, such as bits, irons, etc.

louse *n.pl.* **lice** a small parasitic insect that may be found on horses, particularly in the mane and root of the tall —*see also* **nit**

lower school Campagne school

Lowicz *n.* a Polish draft breed derived from Ardennes and Belgian stock; usually chestnut but sometimes bay or roan; 15–16.3 h.h.

low ringbone new bone growth near the coffin joint

low withers withers that are lower than the croup; sometimes seen in trotters

lozenges *n.pl.* small, round pieces of leather or rubber at each side of the mouthpiece of a bit to protect the mouth from chafing; bit guards

LSD long slow distance

lucerne, lucern *n.* alfalfa

lumbar *adj.* relating to the region of the back between the rearmost ribs and the pelvis

lumbosacral *adj.* relating to the area between the last vertebra of the back and the sacrum

lumen *n.* the cavity inside a hollow body organ or structure, as an artery or the bowel

lung *n.* either of two organs of respiration, situated in the thoracic cavity; the horse's lungs are connected; thus if one side of the chest is perforated, both lungs will collapse

lunge *vt.* to train or exercise (a horse) with a lunge line, long whip, and voice by working in a circle. The trainer, on foot, guides the horse in a circle while maintaining contact with the lunge line in one hand and encouraging movement with voice commands and the long whip in the other hand. Horses are usually taught to walk, trot, canter, halt, and reverse on the lunge line before being mounted for the first time; the purposes of lunging are to train an unbroken horse, to retrain a spoiled horse, to relax and supple the schooled horse before riding, and to exercise a horse which for any reason cannot be ridden. —**lunging** *n.* —**longe**

lunge line a rein made of cotton or nylon, about 25 feet long and about 1 inch wide, and attached to the halter with a swivel snap; lunge rein

lunge rein *see* **lunge line**

lunge whip the long whip used as an aid when lunging a horse; does not actually touch the horse but is snapped to reinforce spoken commands; has a small popper on the end that sounds like a cap gun when the whip is snapped

lungworm *n.* a roundworm that spends the final phase of its parasitic life cycle in the lungs, causing inflamed bronchi

Lusitano *n.* a Portuguese breed with an old heritage; attractive, courageous, intelligent, and agile; a valuable horse in the bullring; 15–16 h.h.

lutein *n.* a yellow pigment in certain hormones

luteinization *n.* ovarian changes that occur when a mature egg has just discharged; the cells in that area become enlarged and turn color

luteinizing hormone (LH) a hormone secreted by the pituitary gland, causing ovulation in mares and testosterone production in stallions

luxation *n.* dislocation, as of a vertebra; can refer specifically to dislocation of the sacroiliac joint, which occurs more frequently in hunter-jumper horses; characterized by a bump or protuberance, with pain and reluctance to use the leg; hunter bump —**luxate** *vt.*

lying scent in hunting, a strong scent at ground level

Lyme disease a disease caused by corkscrew-shaped bacteria transmitted by tick bites and characterized by laminitis, fever, skin sensitivity, swollen joints, eye inflammation, heart problems, etc.; these signs are associated with other diseases as well so it is difficult to diagnose the presence of Lyme disease; moreover, blood tests are unreliable, sometimes showing false negative results. False positive results may occur when a horse develops antibodies to bacteria other than that of Lyme disease which cross-react with the latter.

lymph *n.* a clear, yellowish fluid that collects in tissue spaces, drains through lymph channels and lymph nodes, and

helps to combat infection —**lymphatic** *adj.*

lymphadenitis *n.* inflammation of the lymph nodes

lymphangitis *n.* there are two similar types: epizootic (fungal) and ulcerative (bacterial); both affect the lymphatics of the skin through a wound infected by contaminated soil, manure, flies, etc.; may be confused with farcy and glanders but the mallein test confirms a correct diagnosis, giving a reaction in the latter case; often referred to as Monday morning leg, milk leg, big leg

lymphatic *n.* a channel that carries lymph —*adj.*

lymph node any of several small cellular structures, or glands, that lie in groups along the lymph vessels or channels; they collect intercellular fluids and return them to the circulation —**lymphoid** *adj.*

lymphocyte *n.* a type of white blood cell formed in the lymph nodes; important in the production of antibodies —**lymphocytic** *adj.*

lymphoid organ any of several organs which form part of the immune system, including the thymus, lymph nodes, and spleen

lymphoma *n.* a tumor of a lymph node

lymphosarcoma *n.* a malignant cancer of the lymph nodes

lymph system a network of thin-walled vessels which collect cellular fluids and return them to the bloodstream near the heart; important in fighting infections and maintaining the body's fluid balance

lysin *n.* an antibody that can destroy cells

lysine *n.* an amino acid in certain proteins; important to growth and milk production; may also be produced synthetically and added to feed

lysis *n.* 1. the destruction of living cells from the action of certain lysins 2. the receding of disease symptoms

lysosome *n.* any of various tiny particles within a cell that contain digestive enzymes and destroy bacteria

— M —

McClellan saddle a type of saddle named for its designer, "Little Mac," just prior to the Civil War, when it was the standard U.S. Army saddle; it is split down the center; pommel and cantle are lower than those of a Western saddle but higher than those of an English saddle; wooden stirrups are usually leather covered

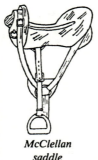

McClellan saddle

macerate *vt.* 1. to soften or break down (food) in the process of digestion 2. to

cause to grow thin —*vi.* to grow thin — **maceration** *n.* —**macerated** *adj.*

macrophage *n.* a white blood cell that devours foreign particles and debris in the body

maggot *n.* the larva of a fly that looks like a fleshy worm; sometimes found in a wound to which the adult fly is attracted and in which it lays eggs

magnesium *n.* a metallic element that forms part of certain compounds given medicinally either as an antacid (**magnesium hydroxide**) or as an absorbent and antacid to treat diarrhea (**magnesium trisilicate**) or as a purgative (**magnesium sulphate**, or epsom salts)

magnetic-field therapy the treatment of a physical disability with electromagnetic energy waves

mahogany bay a seal brown color

maiden *n.* in racing, a horse that has never won a race; in shows, a horse that has not won a first ribbon in a particular division

maiden class a class at a horse show open to entries who have never won a blue ribbon at a recognized show

maiden mare a horse that has never foaled but may be in foal (pregnant)

maiden race a race involving horses that have never won a race

maim *vt.* to disable or cripple —*n.* in injury causing disablement or crippling

maintenance diet a nutritional regimen that is just enough to maintain a horse in good condition without provision for exercise, pregnancy, or nursing a foal

maize *n.* corn

malabsorption syndrome a condition characterized by impaired absorption of nutrients from the gastrointestinal tract

maladjustment *n.* inability to adjust or adapt to a new environment

Malapolski *n.* a Polish breed used mainly for riding; a good jumper; this breed is subdivided into two types according to size: the Sadecki (up to 16.3 h.h.) and the Darbowsko-Tarnowski (about 15.3 h.h.)

malar *adj.* relating to the cheek, cheekbone, or side of the head

malar bone a small bone under the eye

malaris *n.* a muscle that depresses the lower eyelid

mal de caderas a South American term (meaning "sore hips") for an affliction caused by stable flies and characterized by staggering; Spanish American hip disease

male *adj.* describes the sex that fertilizes the female ovum and begets offspring —*n.* a male horse

maleus *n., pl.* **malei** the largest and outermost of the three small bones in the middle ear, shaped slightly like a hammer

malformation *n.* abnormal formation of a body part, usually present at birth

malignant *adj.* dangerous to life; cancerous — **malignancy** *n.*

mallein test one in which mallein (product of glanders bacillus) is injected under the skin for observance of a local swelling reaction, which will occur if glanders has been contracted by the horse

mallender *n.* a callus on the inside of the leg; chestnut[2]

mallenders *n.* a skin condition at the back of the knee wherein dry scabs form and the affected part becomes bald; fissures may form with resultant lameness; sometimes affects draft horses; psoriasis carpi

mallet *n.* a long-handled "hammer" used in playing polo; polo stick

malnutrition *n.* a condition of being undernourished

mallet

malocclusion *n.* faulty meeting of the upper and lower teeth

malposition *n.* abnormal position of a fetus

mamma *n., pl.* **-mae** a milk-secreting gland in the female; **mammary gland**

mammal *n.* a warm-blooded, usually hairy vertebrate belonging to the class Mammalia that feeds its offspring with milk from the female mammary glands; the horse is a mammal — **mammalian** *adj., —n.*

mammary edema a swelling of the udder

mammiferous *adj.* having mammae or udders

mammilla *n., pl.* **-mae** a nipple — **mammillate** *adj.* having mammillae

mandibular artery a blood vessel that supplies the lower jaw and the side of the face

mane *n.* the long hair that grows from the top of the horse's neck

mane banding a Western mane styling, sometimes used in shows, in which over 50 half-inch strands of shortened mane are separated with rubber bands to look somewhat like tassels

manège *n.* 1. the riding and training of horses 2. the exercises of a trained horse 3. a school for the proper training of horses and riders

mane pulling a technique in which long hairs from the underside of the mane are wound around a comb, a few at a time, and pulled to shorten or thin the mane

Manepuri *n.* a pony breed bred in the Asian state of Assama; 11–13 h.h.

mane tamer a wrap to train an untidy mane

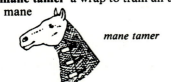

mane tamer

Mangalarga *n.* a Brazilian breed developed in the 19th century by crossing the native Crioulo with imported Alter Real and Andalusian stallions; strong and fast with a comfortable, rocking gait called the marcha; 15 h.h.

mange *n.* *see* **scabies** — **mangy** *adj.*

manger *n.* a feed container of wood or plastic attached to the stall wall

Manipuri *n.* an Indian pony breed (from the state of Manipur) of ancient origins well known for its use in cavalry and in polo; strong and tough; 11–13 h.h.

manners *n.* behavior, particularly in the horse's relation to humans

man on horseback a military man with so much control in his country as to potentially take over as dictator

Man O'War a famous American racehorse, bred in 1917, which won all but one of his 21 races

manta *n.* a horse blanket or cloth

mantee *vt.* to wrap up in tarps, as, for example, feed taken on pack trips that needs protection from moisture or horses

manure *n.* excrement or feces used as soil fertilizer — *vt.*

manure cart a 2-wheeled cart for collecting manure

manure fork a 5- to 10-pronged fork for scooping up manure; apple picker

manure fork

marcha *n.* a comfortable, rocking gait characteristic of the Mangalarga

march fracture a stress-caused bone fracture of the lower extremity

mare *n.* a female horse over the age of 4

Maremmana, Maremma *n.* an Italian breed whose versatility and calm character make it suitable for a variety of uses; e.g., in the mounted police force, light agriculture, herding cattle, etc.; 15 h.h.

Marengo *n.* the horse Napoleon rode in battle in Italy, Austria and Waterloo; its skeleton is kept at the National Army Museum at Sandhurst, England

mare's tail cirrus cloud formations whose long, narrow shape somewhat resembles a horse's tail

mark to ground in hunting, to chase a fox into its lair and then sound the den cry

marrow *n.* the soft tissue inside most bones, consisting of fat and blood cells

marshal *n.* at one time, a groom; in

medieval times, a master of the horse; today, a rider who, before a horse race, leads the competitors past the grandstand

martingale *n*. part of a horse's tack used to control or train a desired head carriage; there are many types: running m., standing m., bib/web m., combination m., chambon m. —*see also* **tie down**

Marwari *n*. a cross-breed in northwest India; about 14 h.h.

mash *n*. a mixture of bran, meal, etc., mixed with warm water and used for feed

mask *n*. 1. in hunting, the head of the killed fox, which is cut off by the huntsman and presented as a trophy to one of the field 2. *see* **fly mask**

mast cells cells in body tissues thought to be related to immunity

Master *n*. a member of a hunt staff who manages and organizes the hunt

Master of the Horse a British title originating in 1377 and held by a person whose responsibilities include being present at all official occasions in which the reigning monarch takes part either mounted or in a horse-drawn carriage and next to whom the Master is privileged to ride; the Master of the Horse has total supervision over all the men and horses on parade

mastitis *n*. an infection of the udder; signs are pain when touched, heat, swelling, hardness, and sometimes lumpiness; it may be difficult to express milk, which may be thick and discolored; in acute cases there may be fever

mastocytosis *n*. an accumulation of mast cells in body tissue; characterized by nodules under the skin

masturbate *vt*. to bounce the erect penis against the belly; often performed by stallions though ejaculation is seldom achieved — *vi*. **masturbation** *n*.

Masuren *n*. a Polish warmblood breed; 16 h.h.

match *n*. 1. a race between two horses owned by different people on terms agreed on by them and to which no money or other prize is added 2. a game played on horseback, such as a polo match

mate *vi*. to join with an individual of the opposite sex in coitus — *vt*. to put (stallion and mare) together for coitus — **mating** *n*. 1. the act of coitus 2. the selection of horses for breeding

maternal *adj*. relating to a mother, particularly in regard to her instincts

maternal dystocia *see* **dystocia**

matrix *n*. 1. intercellular substance embedding living cells, as in bone or cartilage 2. the basis cells from which teeth, etc. are formed

maturate *vt*. 1. to bring to a head, as a boil 2. *vi*. to mature — **maturative** *adj*. — **maturation** *n*.

mature *vi*. to become fully grown — *adj*. generally, having reached 5 years of age, although maturity depends on the breed and may vary between 3 and 6 years — **maturity**

maverick *n*. an unbranded stray horse

maw worm *see* **threadworm**

maxilla *n*. the jaw bone; the upper jaw is called the **superior maxilla** and the lower jaw is called the **inferior maxilla** — **maxillary** *adj*.

maze jumping a competition having a course of jumps laid at odd angles and intervals; one side of each hurdle has a red flag which the rider must keep on the right when jumping; the rider who completes the course in the least time wins regardless of jumping faults

meager, meagre *adj*. thin; emaciated; in poor flesh — **meagerness** *n*.

mealy-mouthed *adj*. having color faded around the mouth, like the color of oatmeal; found especially in bays

and browns but is typical in some breeds such as the Exmoor Pony; sometimes called mulish because many mules are mealy-mouthed

measuring stick a stick marked in inches and hands for measuring the height of a horse; has a sliding, right-angled arm for placement over the withers; some have a spirit level on the arm for accuracy

mebendazole *n.* generic name for a dewormer

mecate *n.* Spanish meaning rope — *see also* **hackamore**

mechanical hackamore a bit consisting of a noseband (made of rope, leather, or rubber-covered chain), a chin strap or chain, and a curb shank, the length of which determines its severity; with a headstall, control is exerted by pressure on the poll, nose, and chin groove

mechanical hackamore

Mecklenburg *n.* an East German breed whose heritage dates back to the 14th century; similar to the Hanoverian; athletic and strong; used for all-purpose riding, including competitions; 15.3–16.2 h.h.

meconium *n.* thick, dark, tarlike waste matter stored in the intestinal tract of the fetus; normally expelled within a few hours after birth

meconium colic colic in a newborn foal caused by alimentary disturbance during passage of the first dung

meconium ileus *see* **ileus**

media *n.* the middle layer of the wall of an artery or vein

medial *adj.* toward the midline of the body

medial patellar ligament the largest of the three ligaments that keep the patella in place

medicine *n.* 1. a remedy for treating a disease or ailment, or pain 2. science of diagnosing and treating disease — **medicinal** *adj.* — **medicinally** *adv.*

medicine hat a rare coloration found on certain mustangs consisting of chestnut or black speckling around the ears, chest, barrel, legs, and rump on an otherwise white coat; considered an extremely lucky marking by American Indian tribes

medium-goal polo polo in which the total handicap of each competing team in a particular competition is about 15–18

medulla *n.* the inner matter of an organ, such as bone marrow, brain matter, etc. — **medullary** *adj.*

medulla oblongata the lowest portion of the brain just above the spinal cord; has nerves that control breathing, circulation, etc.

medullary sheath a sheath or layer of myelin around certain nerve fibers

medullated *adj.* 1. covered by a myelin sheath (as nerves) 2. having a medulla

meet *n.* in hunting, the assembly of hunt staff, followers, and hounds

Megimide *n.* trade name for bemegride sodium

megrims *n.* a disabling condition caused by a parasitic infection of the brain that may affect horses especially while working in harness; symptoms are shaking the head or holding it sideways, rebelliousness, staggering, plunging, falling, then recovering, attacks may reoccur, becoming worse and eventually fatal

meiosis *n.* cell division in which each part of the divided cell (gamete) contains only half the number of chromosomes contained in body (somatic) cells

melanin *n.* a brownish black pigment that occurs in the skin, hair, or retina of the eye

melanism *n.* 1. pigmentation in the skin

or hair 2. darkness of skin, hair, eyes, etc. resulting from high pigmentation — **melanistic** *adj.*

melanize *vt.* to darken as a result of excessive melanin in tissues

melanocyte *n.* a cell containing melanin

melanocyte death the destruction of the pigment-producing cells; characterized by white hair spots often located just behind a riding horse's withers, or along the girth line, or under a harness horse's collar; usually caused by badly fitting tack which destroys the pigment producing cells without destroying the hair's growth

melanoma *n.* a tumor growing from cells containing melanin, or pigment; in its benign form it consists of multiple nodules or a solitary one near body openings; malignant melanomas are found more deeply

melanuria *n.* dark urine caused by the presence of melanin

melch *n. see* **milt**

melena *n.* black stools caused usually from bleeding in the stomach or intestine; dark stools may also appear from eating moldy hay

melioidosis *n.* a bacterial infection contracted chiefly in tropical areas from rats; from the soil the bacteria infect the horse through skin abrasions, inhalation, or insect bites; characterized by high fever, nasal discharge, and slight cough

meloid *n. see* **blister beetle**

melt *n. see* **milt**

membrana tympani the eardrum

membrane *n.* a thin layer of tissue — **membranous** *adj.*

memory *n.* the mental ability to recall things seen, experienced, or learned in the past

Mendel's laws laws of heredity discovered by Gregor Mendel (1822–1884), one of which states that from contrasting characteristics, one is lost in the first generation of offspring but appears in one out of three individuals of the second generation

Meniere's disease a disease affecting the inner ear; characterized by symptoms similar to those of megrims

meninges *n.pl.* membranes that cover the brain and spinal cord and are called the pia mater (innermost and thinnest), the arachnoid (intermediate), and the dura mater (outermost and tough) — **meningeal** *adj.*

meningitis *n.* inflammation of the meninges; usually caused by some disease such as a viral, bacterial, or protozoal infection; characterized by fever, lethargy, or agitation and disorientation

meningo-encephalomyelitis *see* **borna disease**

meperidine hydrochloride generic name for a powerful pain-relieving drug

mercurial blister a strong counterirritant having a mercury compound

mercury *n.* a chemical element used in thermometers and certain medicines, among other things *see* **biniodide of mercury**

Merens *n. see* **Ariegeois**

meridian diagnosis a technique that uses a divining rod to trace the paths of energy flowing through the body; interruption in the flow allegedly indicates the source of a suspected ailment, which is then treated by acupuncture

merocrine *adj.* relating to any gland whose secretions do not obviously harm its cells; e.g., the salivary glands

Merychippus *n.* an ancient (Miocene period) ancestor of the modern horse; had a split hoof with two upper toes well above the roof called dew hooves

mesenteric artery a large blood vessel

which starts from the abdominal aorta and supplies blood to the intestines

mesentery *n.* an abdominal membrane that enfolds the intestines and other organs and connects with the backbone — **mesenteric** *adj.*

mesial *adj.* 1. of, in, toward, or along the midline of the body 2. in dentistry, toward the middle of the face, along the curve of the dental arch — **mesially** *adv.*

mesiodistal *adj.* of the inner part of the tooth

mesocolon *n.* the mesentery of the large intestine

mesoderm *n.* the central germinal or cell layer of an embryo from which develop the muscular, vascular, and other tissues and organs — **mesodermal, mesodermic** *adj.*

mesogastrium *n.* a mesentery of the embryonic stomach — **mesogastric** *adj.*

Mesohippus *n.* an ancient (Miocene period) ancestor in the horse's evolutionary chain; about twice the size of Eohippus, the first horse; appeared about 35 million years ago and had three toes on each foot, the middle one of which had a primitive hoof

Messenger *n.* the well-known Thoroughbred that was the chief founding sire of American trotters

metabolic *adj.* relating to metabolism

metabolic acidosis an abnormal condition of acidity in the body caused by the loss of alkaline substances or retention of acids

metabolic bone disease a condition which involves several interrelated growth disorders in young horses, such osteochondrosis, osteochondritis dissecans, contracted tendons, physitis, synovitis, etc.

metabolism *n.* the chemical and physical processes by which assimilated food is transformed into elements that can be used for growth and energy, and built up (through the process called anabolism) into living tissue, which is then used and broken down (by catabolism) into simpler substances or waste matter — **metabolize** *vi., vt.* — **metabolic** *adj.*

metabolite *n.* any substance in or resulting from metabolism

metacarpal periostitis *see* **bucked shins; mycotic lymphangitis**

metacarpus *n.* the part of the foreleg between the carpus (knee) and the fetlock formed by the three metacarpal bones, which are the cannon bone (third bone) and its two adjacent splint bones (second and fourth bones); these three metacarpal bones are an evolutionary reduction of what once consisted of five — **metacarpal** *adj.*

metamorphosis *n.* a change in the appearance or shape of an organ or part of the body

metaphysis *n.* the wider end of a long bone, next to the epiphysis

metaplasia *n.* an abnormal change or conversion of one type of tissue into another, as of cartilage into bone or scar cells near the hoof into horn — **metaplastic** *adj.*

metaplasm *n.* the part of a cell that consists of lifeless matter

metaprotein *n.* a complex hydrolytic substance resulting from the action of acids or alkalies on proteins

metastasis *n.* the spread of disease (such as cancer) from one part of the body to another not directly connected to it, as by the bloodstream — **metastatically** *adv.* — **metastasize** *vi.*

metatarsus *n.* the part of the hind leg between the tarsus (hock) and fetlock, formed by the three metatarsal bones, which are the cannon bone and its two adjacent splint bones; homologous to the metacarpus in the front leg — **metatarsal** — *adj.*

methionine *n.* an amino acid in proteins containing sulphur and essential for normal growth, especially of the hair and hoof horn; synthetically made methionine can be added to feed to treat weak hooves or founder

methocarbamol *n.* the generic name for a muscle relaxant

methohexitone sodium a short-acting anesthetic which lasts about 3–8 minutes; trade name Brietal sodium

methylphenidate *n.* the generic name for a stimulant to the central nervous system

methylprednisolone acetate a type of cortisone; trade name Depo-Medrone

Metis Trotter a Russian breed originating in the early 1950s from Orlov/American Standardbred crosses; 15.2 h.h.

metriphonate *n.* an insecticide effective against e.g. external parasites

metritis *n.* inflammation of a mare's uterus caused by venereal infection; contagious equine metritis (CEM)

Mezohegyes *n.* Hungarian half-breed used in sports; 15.1–16.2 h.h.

microbe *n.* a disease-causing bacterium; germ — **microbic, microbial, microbian** *adj.*

microbiology *n.* the study of microorganisms

microcotyledon *n.* any of numerous tiny subdivisions of a mare's placenta

microfilariae *n.pl.* minute parasites found in blood and tissues; worm larvae

microfilaricide *n.* worm medicine

microflora *n.* bacteria normally in the body

microhemorrhage *n.* minute leaks of blood into tissue caused by splits in the small blood vessels

micron *n.* a unit of length that measures one thousandth of a millimeter

micronize *vt.* to pulverize into minute particles

microorganism *n.* an organism visible only with the aid of a microscope (e.g., bacteria, viruses, molds, yeasts, protozoa)

microphage *n.* a small cell (phagocyte) which combats and digests germs that may be present in the tissues

microphthalmia *n.* a very rare congenital deformity in which only vestiges of eyeballs exist — *see also* **anophthalmia**

microscope *n.* a device with a number of lenses that enable the viewer to see an enlarged image of minute objects, such as microorganisms — **microscopy** *n.* the use of a microscope

microscopic *adj.* 1. relating to a microscope 2. extremely small or minute

microsphere *n.* a minute globule of various types; can be a radioactive globule that may be injected into a vein and monitored for diagnostic purposes

Microsporum gypseum a fungus from soil that causes skin diseases and ringworm

microsurgery *n.* surgery performed with miniaturized instruments and a microscope upon minute body structures

microtome *n.* a cutting instrument that can cut extremely thin pieces of tissue

micturate *vi.* to urinate — **micturition** *n.*

midden *n.* a heap of dung

middleweight hunter a horse used for hunting and able to carry up to 185 lbs.

midge *n.* a gnatlike fly particularly annoying to horses around the face

Mierzyn *n.* a Polish pony breed

miler *n.* a horse estimated to do well in a flat race of one mile

miliary *adj.* derived from millet, a tiny seed; applied specifically to a disease characterized by similarly small lesions that become widespread in the body

milk *n.* the whitish liquid secreted by the mare's mammary glands through the nipples for suckling her foal — *vt.* to withdraw milk from (a mare's nipples)

milk leg *see* **lymphangitis**

milk pellets white feed pellets containing 23 percent protein and 15 percent oil; they do not heat up horses and are much liked by them; amount given should not exceed 1 lb. per day

milk sugar *see* **lactose**

milk teeth *see* **deciduous teeth**

milk vein a large vein running from the udder forward halfway along the body

milk warts (equine cutaneous papillomatosis) warts that can appear on a foal's muzzle up to 3 years of age; caused by a virus and are infectious to other horses; may ulcerate and bleed; usually disappear within 1–3 months

Miller's disease *see* **big head disease**

milt *n.* a substance resembling a piece of liver which is present in a foal's mouth at birth but is quickly rejected at birth; its purpose is believed to be to prevent water entering through the mouth before and during birth; also called melt or melch

mineral *n.* 1. an inorganic substance found in the earth or water 2. any of certain elements, such as iron, phosphorous, etc., essential to the health of animals and plants

mineralocorticoid *n.* an adrenal hormone that regulates the use of electrolytes

mineral oil a colorless oil from petroleum that may be used as a laxative

Minho *n.* *see* **Garrano**

Miniature Horse a tiny horse whose origins can be traced to the 16th century in Europe where the diminutive size was developed through inbreeding and the horses were used as pets for royalty; then they were worked in coal mines in Europe as early as 1765 and in parts of the U.S. from the late 19th century until the 1950s; today they are increasing in popularity as gentle pets and for shows; the smaller the Miniature, the more valuable it is, 34 inches being the maximum height for registry in the American Miniature Horse Association, and a height of 19 inches is possible — *see also* **Falabella**

Miohippus *n.* an ancient (Oligocene-Miocene period) ancestor in the horse's evolutionary chain, which evolved from Mesohippus and was larger

miosis *n.* 1. abnormal contraction of the pupil of the eye 2. the stage of a disease in which the symptoms decrease — **miotic** *adj.*

miotic drug a drug which causes the pupil of the eye to contract

MIP test mare immunological pregnancy test; used between 45 and 95 days of gestation to detect presence of ECG (equine chorionic gonadotrophin)

misfit *n.* a horse that was bred for a certain requirement (like racing) but that has turned out to be unfit for it

Missouri Fox Trotter an American breed descended from Arab, Morgan, and Southern Plantation horses and developed in Missouri at the beginning of the 19th century; later infusions of Tennessee Walker, Standardbred, and Saddlebred blood were introduced; named because of a special gait in which the forefeet walk quickly while the hind feet trot at a speed of up to 10 m.p.h.; 14–16 h.h.

mitbah *n.* the angle at which the neck of an Arabian horse enters the top of the head; making a slight angle at the top of the crest, it gently curves to the head

mite *n.* a tiny bloodsucking parasite that lays eggs in the furrows of the skin or in the ears, causing irritation, inflammation and itching

mitochondrion *n., pl.* **-dria** a very small structure within most cells, which through enzyme activity breaks down ingested food and produces energy for intracellular processes — **mitochondrial** *adj.*

mitosis *n.* the division of cells — **mitotic** *adj.* — **mitotically** *adv.*

mitral valve the valve between the two left chambers (atrium and ventricle) of the heart; during systole (rhythmic contraction) this valve cuts off a backflow of blood into the atrium

mixed gaits a combination of, or alternation between, gaits. Gaited horses sometimes tend to break from one gait to another, thus mixing their gaits, but if properly trained they hold the desired gait.

mixed meeting in racing, a meeting which involves both flat and steeplechase or hurdle races on the same day

moan *vi.* to utter a low, extended sound, as from pain — *n.*

mob a fox in hunting, to give the fox no chance by surrounding it or overtaking it

mochila *n.* a four-pocketed leather sack once used to carry mail on horseback

model classes conformation show classes

moist rales *see* **rales**

molar tooth any of 12 grinding teeth which are in the back of a horse's mouth and located behind the premolars, 3 on each side on the upper and lower jaws

molassine meal a source of sugar used in feed

mold *n.* 1. a fungal growth on organic surfaces 2. any fungus that produces such a growth — **moldy** *adj.*

molybdenum *n.* a metallic chemical element used in manufacturing various things; can be absorbed by plants from contaminated soil and be poisonous to horses, if ingested, although this rarely occurs; symptoms include diarrhea, abnormal looking coat with loss of color, and loss of weight

Monday morning leg, –disease a condition so named because of its appearance after a weekend of rest with no reduction of the food rations given when working; characterized by a painful swelling of a leg, usually the hind leg, accompanied by fever of 104–105 degrees F., with probable shivering or sweating and severe lameness; these conditions usually last only a few days but tend to reoccur; also called *sporadic lymphangitis*

monensin *n.* generic name for an additive to steer and poultry feed; toxic if fed in large amounts and particularly toxic to horses; it affects the heart muscle and causes necrosis of its cells, usually resulting in heart failure

Mongolian *n.* a pony of ancient origins and native to Mongolia; there are various types according to differences of home territory, climate, and feeding, including the Wuchumutsin, Hailar, Sanho, Sanpeitze, Ili, and Heilung Chiang; raised by Mongol tribes which use them for pack work and some agriculture; mares are milked for making cheese and kumiss; 12.2–14.2 h.h.

monkey drill gymnastics on horseback — *see also* **gymnastics**

monkey mouth a protruding jaw — *see also* **undershot jaw**

monoclonal antibodies antibodies from the descendants of a single or small population of identical white blood cells that are responsive to a single foreign substance

monocyte *n.* a type of white blood cell

monodactyl *n.* one toe; refers to the

hoof, which, now a single "toe," evolved from what originally, in the eohippus stage, consisted of multiple toes

monolayer *n.* a layer having a thickness of one molecule

monorchid *n.* a male horse having only one testicle in the scrotum, the other being either absent or undescended; the condition is considered to be hereditary —**monorchidism** *n.*

monovular *adj.* resulting from one ovum; can be used in reference to twins

moon *n.* a white facial marking in the shape of a moon

moon blindness *see* **iridocyclitis**

Morab *n.* a Morgan-Arabian cross

Morgan *n.* America's oldest domestic breed, named for its foundation sire, Justin Morgan (in turn named after his owner), foaled in 1789 in Vermont; a very attractive, versatile horse with a refined head, sloping, heavy shoulders and wide chest, a short back and well-muscled hindquarters; possesses endurance, a calm disposition, and great presence; an excellent riding horse; 14–15.2 h.h.

morning glory a racehorse that performs excellently in morning workouts but poorly later when run in races; also is bothered by environmental distractions

Morochuco, -guo *n.* a type of Criollo found in mountainous areas of Brazil and Peru

morphine *n.* a strong pain-relieving drug

morphology *n.* the study of the structure of animals

mosquito *n.* a flying, blood-sucking insect, the female of which is responsible for transmitting diseases to the horse, as, for example, equine encephalomyelitis

mosquito

motile *adj.* ability to perform spontaneous motion —**motility** *n.*

motor nerve a nerve that triggers muscles to contract

mottled *adj.* having small white spots on the muzzle, around the eyes, on the genitalia and sometimes on the body

mount *vi.* to get onto a horse —*vt.* 1. (a) to get onto (a horse); (b) to sit on (a horse) 2. to provide with a horse or horses 3. to climb upon (a mare) for copulation —*n.* 1. a riding horse 2. the act or manner of mounting a horse 3. the opportunity for riding a horse, especially in a race —**mounted** *adj.* 1. seated on horseback 2. serving on horseback (mounted police)

mounting *n.* the act of getting onto a horse; it may be done by (a) stepping into a stirrup; (b) using a mounting block; (c) vaulting from the ground up onto the horse's back; or (d) getting a leg up (*see* **leg up**)

mount money in rodeo, money paid to a rider exhibiting but not competing

mouse dun *see* **grullo**

mouth *n.* the opening in the head through which food is taken in and sounds are made; contains the tongue and teeth; horses cannot breathe through their mouths —*see also* **full mouth; good mouth** —*vt.* 1. to take into the mouth or rub with the mouth or lips 2. to accustom (a horse) to the bit

mouth gag *see* **speculum**

mouthing bit a bit having keys on the mouthpiece to encourage salivation

mouthpiece *n.* the part of the bit which goes into the mouth

mow *n.* 1. hay or grain stored in a barn 2. the area in a barn for hay or grain, also called *haymow* or *hayloft*

mucin *n.* a secretion of cells

muck *n.* moist manure —*vt.* to fertilize with muck —**mucky** *adj.*

muck out to remove or clean up horses' manure

muck sweat lathered sweat that is so profuse as to bring out dirt with it

muck worm a worm that grows and lives in manure

mucocele *n.* 1. a cavity having mucous secretion   2. a tumor comprising mucous tissue   3. enlargement of the tear gland of the eye

mucocutaneous junction the meeting area of mucous membrane and skin, as where the lips meet the mucous membrane of the mouth

mucoid *n.* a mucoprotein found in connective tissues, in some types of cysts, etc. *—adj.* like mucus

mucopolysaccharide *n.* a type of carbohydrate containing a small amount of protein, found throughout the body

mucoprotein *n.* a glycoprotein found in animal tissues and fluids

mucopurulent *adj.* having mucus and pus

mucosa *n.* a mucuous membrane *—mucosal adj.*

mucous membrane a covering membrane that secretes mucus and lines the respiratory tract, gastrointestinal tract, or other internal body part

mucus *n.* the thick, slimy secretion of the mucous membranes that keeps them moist *—mucous adj.*

mudder *n.* a racehorse that is not adversely affected by a muddy, wet track

muddy dun *see* **dun**

mud fever inflammation of the heels and or legs that may develop when mud is left on for long periods; there is an exudation from the affected skin which develops scabs; *rain scald; dermatophilosis; mycotic dermatitis; heel bug; greasy heel*

mud tail a style of braiding that consists of a single, thick tail braid that is tucked under and held in place by elastic; used on hunters on muddy days

mug's horse a horse that is gentle to ride but may appear to be the opposite

Mulassier *n.* a French type of horse used to breed mules; some have curly hair at the knees and hocks; 16–16.3 h.h.

mule *n.* the offspring of a donkey and a horse; specifically, that of a jackass and a mare; the offspring of a stallion and female ass is called a *hinny*; usually sterile

mule ears on a horse, ears that are unusually long

mule foot a horse's hoof that looks like that of a mule; i.e., having long straight quarters, contracted heels, and a large frog

mulish *adj. see* **mealy-mouthed**

mullen *n.* the mouthpiece of a snaffle bit which consists of an unjointed bar, either straight or half-mooned in shape; milder than the jointed snaffle

mullen

multifidus cervicis a neck muscle that extends or turns the head and neck

multigravida *n.* a mare in foal for at least the second time

mummification *n.* the shriveling or drying up of a body part, as in dry gangrene

munch *vt., vi.* to chew steadily, often with a crunching sound

Munighi *n.* a subtype of the Arabian bred in the Kirghiz area of Russia

Murakoz *n.* a Hungarian draft breed bred in the Mura River region (also in Poland and Yugoslavia); developed by crossing native mares with Percheron, Belgian Ardennes and Noriker stallions and native stallions; this once populous breed was greatly reduced in numbers in World War II; 16 h.h.

Murghese *n.* an Italian breed named for the Murge area; originated from Barb and Arab stallions; used for riding and farm work as well as for pulling trees in logging; 15–16 h.h.

murmur *n.* an abnormal internal body sound heard with ear or stethescope and having a cardiac (heart) or vascular (blood vessel) origin

muscle *n.* 1. a body organ that consists of cells or fibers and can be contracted and expanded to produce movement —*see also* **skeletal m.; smooth m.; cardiac m.** 2. the tissue making up such an organ 3. muscular strength

muscle belly the thick part of a muscle; a bulge formed by muscle

muscle-bound *adj.* not flexible due to the muscles being enlarged and less elastic, as from too much exercise

muscle fiber typing a technique to assess the type of muscle a particular horse possesses in order to determine performance potential

muscular *adj.* having well developed and prominent muscles —**muscularity** *n.*

musculature *n.* the system of body muscles

musculoskeletal system the system muscles, bones, ligaments, tendons, and joints

musical chairs a gymkhana event in which sacks or tires are used instead of chairs; usually there is one fewer sack than riders, although there may be fewer used in order to speed up the contest when a large number of contestants are involved; while music is played, the riders lope around a circle of sacks; when it stops, each rider dismounts at the nearest sack, taking the reins over his or her horse's head, and steps into the sack; the rider left without a sack is eliminated; when two riders are left, two sacks are placed at one end of the arena; the two riders ride away from them in a parallel line and when the music begins, they race back to the sacks and the first one to reach his or her sack wins

Mustang *n.* an American "wild" breed descended from the horses brought over by the Spanish conquistadores; once largely used by the American Indians, as well as by the early immigrants to cross with their imported horses; tough and wiry and of every color; now reduced in numbers and crossbred almost to extinction but protected in various areas; the American Mustang Association was formed in 1962 and there is also the Spanish Barb Mustang Registry for Mustangs with Barb characteristics; 13.2–15 h.h.

mutation *n.* a change in a hereditary characteristic —**mutate** *vi., vt.* **mutational** *adj.* —**mutationally** *adv.*

mutilate *vt.* to destroy; self-mutilation is sometimes practiced by stallions when they bite themselves on their flanks, often with very injurious results; this behavior is often seasonal and related to the breeding season when it can either worsen or improve

muzzle *n.* 1. that part of the horse's head that includes the nose, nostrils, lips, and chin 2. a covering for a horse's muzzle to prevent cribbing or other undesirable behaviors —*see also* **box muzzle**

myalgia *n.* muscle pain —**myalgic** *adj.*

myasthenia *n.* muscular weakness or fatigue —**myasthenic** *adj.*

myatonia *n.* lack of strength or muscle tone

mycelium *n.* a fungus comprising a network of thread-like growths which can develop on the lining of the guttural pouch and penetrate it with effects on nerves, blood vessels and bone; ulcers can form and bleed; usually one side of the pouch is affected with resultant nasal bleeding on that side, facial paralysis, and difficulty in swal-

lowing; an aneurism may occur on the external artery of the neck and rupture with fatal consequences — **mycelial** *adj.*

mycology *n.* the study of fungi — **mycologic** *adj.*

mycoplasma *n.* minute microorganisms that may cause numerous diseases, especially of joints and lungs

mycosis *n.* 1. the development of parasitic fungi in the body 2. a disease caused by parsitic fungi — **mycotic** *adj.*

Mycostatin *n.* trade name for nystatin

mycotic abortion abortion caused by fungus spreading over the placenta and gradually destroying it, thus robbing the fetus of nourishment; when the fetus is weakened or dies, it is aborted

mycotic dermatitis *see* **mud fever**

mycotic lymphangitis *see* **lymphangitis, epizootic (fungal)**

mycotoxicosis *n.* a poisoning from ingestion of some fungi, among which are molds — **myotoxic** *adj.*

mydriasis *n.* dilation of the pupil of the eye resulting from disease or administration of a drug — **mydriatic** *adj.*

mydriatic *n.* a drug that produces mydriasis

myelin *n.* the fatty sheath surrounding certain nerve fibers, damage to which may cause disease — **myelinic** *adj.*

myelitis *n.* inflammation of the spinal cord or bone marrow; characterized by incoordination; first signs may appear as lameness

myelogram *n.* an X-ray of the spinal canal after injecting a contrast (dye) to show up the spine on the X-ray film; used for diagnosis of spinal injuries **myelography** *n.* the procedure of making myelograms

myeloma *n.* a malignant tumor of the

bone marrow — **myelomatous** *adj.*

myelopathy *n.* disease of the spinal cord — *see also* **encephalomyelitis**

myenteric *adj.* relating to the muscles in the intestinal wall

myiasis *n.* infestation of the body or a body area by fly larvae

mylo-hyoideus *n.* a hyoid muscle that raises the bottom part of the mouth, the tongue, and the hyoid bone

myocardiograph *n.* an instrument for recording the movements of the heart muscle

myocarditis *n.* inflammation of the myocardium

myocardium *n.* the heart muscle

myofascitis *n.* inflammation of a muscle and fibrous coverings of muscle and surrounding ligaments

myofibril *n.* any of the protein strands that comprise a muscle fiber

myogelosis *n.* a hard area within a muscle

myogenic *adj.* coming from a muscle

myoglobin *n.* a protein in muscle that contains iron and stores oxygen and carbon dioxide

myoglobinuria *n.* the presence of myoglobin in the urine — *see also* **azoturia**

myology *n.* the study of the anatomy of muscles — **myological** *adj.*

myoma *n.* a muscle tumor — **myomatous** *adj.*

myometrium *n.* the involuntary muscle of the uterine wall

myopathy *n.* muscle disease

myosin *n.* a protein in muscles which, with actin, enables muscular contractions and relaxation

myositis *n.* inflammation of a muscle

myositis syndrome a term that describes signs of muscle soreness, such as

stiffness, a shortened gait, and a tenderness to pressure on various muscles

myotic *n.* a drug that causes the pupil of the eye to contract

myotome *n.* a part of an embryo which develops into muscle

myotonia *n.* muscle spasm — **myotonic** *adj.*

Myspamol *n.* trade name for proquamezine fumerate

myxoma *n.* a rare subcutaneous tumor composed of connective mucus-like tissue — **myxomatous** *adj.*

— N —

nag *n.* 1. an old, worn-out horse 2. an inferior horse

nagana *n.* a fatal disease transmitted by the tsetse fly; tsetse-fly disease. The first symptom, in acute cases, is fever, which can reach 106 degrees F., with edema of the limbs; after a week or two the horse dies. The more common form is chronic; this also starts with fever, then anemia sets in with accompanying weakness and severe emaciation despite a good appetite; edema is also present on the limbs and under the abdomen; may last from one month to one year.

nagsman *n.* an experienced rider whose aim is to better a horse as a mount or to rid the horse of an existing vice

nail bind *see* **shod too close**

nameplate *n.* a piece of metal or wood having a horse's name inscribed on it; metal ones can be used to personalize bridles or halters; metal or wood ones are used at the entrances of stables

nap¹ *n.* a short sleep; horses take frequent short naps — *vi.*

nap² *vi.* to fail to obey given aids — **nappy** *adj.* —*n.* in racing, a good tip

naproxen, -yn *n.* generic name for an anti-inflammatory pain reliever

narcolepsy *n.* uncontrollable and frequent desire for sleep brought on by inflammation of or damage to the brain; Gelineau's syndrome; paroxysmal sleep; sleep epilepsy

narcosis *n.* a drug-induced condition of unconsciousness — **narcotize** *vt.* to use a narcotic on (a subject) — **narcotization** *n.*

narcotic *n.* a drug that relieves pain and produces sleep or narcosis —*adj.*

Narragansett Pacer a breed developed around the time of the American Revolution in Rhode Island; had a smooth pacing gait which appealed to Southern plantation owners who brought them south where they were among the breeds used to develop the Tennessee Walker; now extinct

narrow behind a narrow appearance of a horse's rear due to lack of muscle in the croup and thighs

nasal *adj.* pertaining to the nose

nasal gleet *see* **ozena**

nasal septum the bone, cartilage, and membranes separating the left and right nasal cavities

nasociliary nerve the nerve connected to the eyeball and nose

nasogastric tube a flexible tube inserted into and through the nostrils to the stomach to introduce or drain fluid

nasolabial *adj.* relating to the nose and lip

nasolacrimal *adj.* relating to the nose, tear glands, and tear ducts

nasolacrimal duct a duct that normally drains the tears from the eye corners

nasopalatine *adj.* relating to the nose and palate

nasopharyngitis *n.* inflammation of the nose and throat

natal *adj.* pertaining to birth

National Federation the governing body of equestrian affairs in any country affiliated with the FEI (Fédération Equestre Internationale)

National Horse Show America's top horse show, held every year since 1883 in November in Madison Square Garden, New York City; it includes all classes; sometimes called "The National" or "The Garden"

National Steeplechase and Hunt Association the ruling body covering steeplechasing and hurdle-racing

Nations' Cup a team competition involving teams from different nations

Native Mexican Horse an agile riding horse indigenous to Mexico and used extensively for ranch work; 15 h.h.

natural aids the aids given with the body, hands, legs, and voice —*see also* **aids**

nature *n.* 1. character or disposition 2. instincts, desires, etc.

navel *n.* the scar in the middle of the abdomen left by the attachment of the umbilical cord; umbilicus

navel ill an infection which is contracted by a newborn foal through a poorly treated umbilical tube —*see also* **joint ill**

navicular apparatus the navicular bone and the navicular bursa, which together regulate the angle at which the deep flexor tendon and coffin bone in the hoof meet

navicular bone a small boat-shaped bone at the back of the foot just above the hoof; shuttle bone, distal sesamoid

navicular bursa the saclike pouch that lies between the navicular bone and the deep flexor tendon

navicular disease a bursitis and ultimately a disintegration of the navicular bone, usually caused by excessive work on hard surfaces or jumping, hoof imbalance, or conformational flaws

near side the left side of the horse as viewed from behind; trained horses are accustomed to being haltered, saddled, led, and mounted from the near side, although Western horses in particular are often trained to be mounted from either side (this is very practical and allows mounting or dismounting on whichever happens to be the safest side in tight situations, particularly on mountainous terrain); the custom of using the near side originated from cavalry officers carrying their swords on the left hip, making it necessary to mount on the near side only; a **nearside horse** is the horse on the left side of a pair

Neats-foot oil an oil obtained by boiling the feet and shinbones of cattle and used as a dressing for leather

neck[1] *n.* 1. the part of the body which joins the head to the body; its formation and its angle with the back is important in judging general conformation as well as assessing the horse's performance capability 2. the narrowest part of an organ

neck[2] *n.* a measurement of distance by which a horse is said to win a race; when horses are said to be running **neck and neck**, they are running evenly

neck cradle a wide wooden or metal collar used to restrain a horse from bending its neck and biting an infected area of his body

neck cradle

neck rein to guide a horse, while mounted, by putting pressure of one rein on the neck, holding both reins in one hand, rather than pulling

on the bit with one rein as in direct reining

neck strap a strap that encircles the base of the neck and through which the martingale is passed to be held in position

neck sweat a covering, usually fastened with Velcro strips, worn on a thick neck to sweat it down; may be wide enough to cover the whole neck or narrow to cover just part of it

neck sweat

necropsy *n.* an autopsy; a dissection and inspection of a dead equine body to search for physical abnormalities

necrosis *n.* the abnormal death of tissue, as caused by infection, burning, etc. —**necrose** *vt., vi.* —**necrotic** *adj.*

needle biopsy the use of a special needle to remove a small piece of tissue for microscopic examination

negative punishment the removal of something pleasant to a horse in response to undesirable behavior

negative reinforcement the removal of something unpleasant to a horse in response to a desired act or behavior

negative result in medical terms, an indication that a test shows normalcy

neigh *vi.* to vocalize loudly —*n.*

nematode *n.* a roundworm

Nembutal *n.* trade name for pentobarbitone sodium

Nemicide *n.* trade name for levamisole hydrochloride

neolithic *adj.* relating to a late Stone Age cultural period, beginning around 10,000 B.C., when humans developed stone and metal tools and began rearing stock and developing agriculture; it was during this time that the horse is first known to have been domesticated

neomycin *n.* an antibiotic

neonatal *adj.* relating to a newborn —**neonate** *n.* newborn

neonatal horn hoof horn in existence when a foal is born

neonatal isoerythrolysis anemia in newborn foals caused by a blood type incompatibility between dam and foal. The foal may inherit from the sire a blood type containing certain antigens that the mare's blood does not have. If some weakness allows blood to penetrate through the placental membrane from fetus to dam, the dam then produces antibodies against the antigens and these are then stored in the colostrum; when the foal ingests these antibodies in its first milk, they will kill the foal's red blood cells. The condition is characterized by weakness and lassitude within 48 hours of birth, followed a day or two later, if the foal is still alive, by jaundiced gums and whites of eyes; also called hemolytic anemia, foal jaundice, isoimmune disease.

neonatal maladjustment syndrome (NMS) a brain disorder in a foal that usually appears within the first day of birth; probably caused by insufficient oxygen or birth trauma; characterized by convulsions, loss of sucking reflex and inability to recognize and follow the dam; the foal produces a "barking" sound when breathing, hence the term barker syndrome; also dummy- or wanderer-foal syndrome

neonatal period the first four days after birth

neoplasm *n.* an abnormal, non-inflammatory and irregular growth of new tissue such as a tumor or wart, although not all tumors are neoplasms; may be benign, as in a lipoma or osteoma, or malignant, as in a sarcoma or carcinoma

Neopolitan noseband a very harsh and

cruel noseband of metal with shanks of considerable leverage; a similar but less severe type is used in Arabia today

neostigmine *n.* a drug used to stimulate and induce smooth muscle control

nephritic *adj.* 1. relating to the kidneys 2. having nephritis

nephritis *n.* an inflammatory kidney disease which may be diagnosed by chemical test of blood and urine; characterized, in acute attacks, by passing large quantities of light-colored urine which later diminish to frequent attempts to urinate with scant results; the horse becomes debilitated, the hind limbs lose flexibility and there is tenderness to any pressure on the loins

nephrogenic *adj.* 1. originating in the kidneys 2. producing kidney tissue

nephrology *n.* the study of kidney diseases

nephron *n.* one of the minute tubes of the kidneys that secrete urine

nephrosis *n.* a kidney disease associated with kidney degeneration

nephrotoxin *n.* anything that is poisonous to the kidney

nerve *n.* any of, or bundles of, the cordlike fibers that transmit impulses from body organs to the brain and spinal cord including e.g., the following types: afferent, autonomic, cerebrospinal, cranial, efferent, motor, parasympathetic, sensory, splanchnic, and sympathetic

nerve block the injection of an anesthetic into or near a nerve to blot out sensation in the area supplied by that nerve

nerve cell *see* **neuron**

nerve center a group of nerve cells that cooperate with each other to control a body function

nerve ending the point at which a nerve enters the area it supplies

nerve fiber one of the threadlike elements, dendrites or axons, that comprise a nerve

nerve impulse an electrical wave transmitted along a stimulated nerve

nerve tract the route of a nerve from its place of origin to its ending

nerve trunk a bundle of nerve fibers covered by a connective tissue sheath outside the brain and spinal cord

nerving *n. see* **neurectomy**

nervous *adj.* 1. of the nerves 2. excitable, agitated, tense 3. fearful —**nervousness** *n.* the state of being nervous

nervous system the entire system of nerves in the body, including the brain, spinal cord, etc.; it controls responses to stimuli and influences behavior

nester *n.* a rancher who seldom leaves his ranch

nettlerash *n. see* **urticaria**

neural *adj.* pertaining to the nerves or a nerve

neural motor response the response activated by certain nerves

neuraminidase *n.* a viral substance that causes disease

neurectomy *n.* the surgical removal of a nerve or part thereof to remove pain from the area it supplies; nerving

neurilemma *n.* the sheath of a nerve fiber

neurilemmoma *n.* a tumor on the neurilemma

neuritis *n.* inflammation of a nerve

neurofibroma *n.* a type of nonmalignant tumor

neurogenic *adj.* relating to a nerve

neurogenic shock the breakdown of vital body systems caused by physical or mental strain to the nervous system

neuroglia *n.* a structure of tissue that supports nerve tissue of the central nervous system —**neuroglial** *adj.*

neurohormones *n.* hormones produced by or acting on nervous tissue

neurohumor *n.* a nerve hormone — **neurohumoral** *adj.*

neurological patterning the superior development of nerve pathways due to conditioning

neurology *n.* the science that deals with diseases of the nervous system

neurolysis *n.* 1. damage to nerve tissue due to over-stimulation 2. the freeing of a nerve from adhesions

neuroma *n.* a nerve tumor

neuromuscular *adj.* relating to both nerves and muscles

neuromuscular junction the junction of a nerve end and a muscle, where an impulse is transmitted by nerve to muscle

neuron *n.* a nerve, including the cell and all its processes

neuropathy *n.* any disease of the nerves

neurotomy *n.* the surgical cutting of a nerve to eliminate pain

neurotoxin *n.* a poison to nerve tissue — **neurotoxic** *adj.*

neurotransmitters *n.* in the nervous system, any of several chemical transmitters of electrical impulses between cells

neutropenia *n.* decrease of neutrophils in the blood

neutrophil, -phile *n.* a white blood cell that constitutes the main antibacterial portion of pus active against bacterial infections

neutrophilia *n.* increase of neutrophils in the blood; indicates infection

New English Road Horse *see* **Norfolk Trotter**

New Forest an English pony breed indigenous to the New Forest area of Hampshire but bred throughout Britian and exported to a number of countries; has a very mixed heritage; possessing a gentle nature, it makes a good family riding pony; 12.2–14.2 h.h.

Newmarket cough *see* **infectious equine bronchitis**

niacin *n.* nicotinic acid, part of the vitamin B complex; it dilates blood vessels and is necessary for energy; present in grains; may be produced in the body by tryptophan

niacinamide *n.* a chemical form of niacin naturally present in the body

nibble *vt.* to gently bite at; horses nibble themselves to relieve an itch or nibble each other as a form of grooming — *n.*

nick *n.* a term used in reference to mating; a "good nick" means a successful mating considered to result in producing a required type — *vt., vi.* 1. to crossbreed to produce improved or certain desired results 2. *see* **cut and set**

nicker *vi.* (of horses) to make a soft sound — *n.*

nicotinic acid *see* **niacin**

nictate *vi. see* **nictitate**

nictitate *vi.* to wink or blink; nictate — **nictitation** *n.*

nictitating membrane a transparent membrane which serves as a third, innermost eyelid to maintain a clean, moist eye

Niedersachsen *n. see* **Rhenish**

Nigerian *n.* a breed indigenous to West Africa and developed from Barb and Arabian stock; about 14.1 h.h.

niggle *vi.* 1. to work the reins in a manner that will induce greater speed, altered gait, etc. 2. to move in a short, jerky trot

night blindness a deficiency of vision in the dark or in dim light due to reduced rhodopsin of the retina; nyctalopia

night eye (*colloq.*) a chestnut on

the leg or an intrusion —*see also* **chestnut²**; **intrusion**

night rider a member of a band of masked riders who performed violent acts, especially the band of such men in the Southern United States after the Civil War

nightshade *n.* a plant whose leaves are toxic to horses, causing gastrointestinal distress

nikethamide *n.* a drug used to increase depth of breathing and regulate the heartbeat; also as a counter-depressant after anesthesia; trade name Coramine

nine-day heat *see* **foal heat**

nip *vt., vi.* to bite —*n.*

nippers *n.pl.* a farrier's instrument for trimming hooves

nippers

nipple *n.* either of two protuberances of the mare's udder through which milk passes to a suckling foal; teat

nit *n.* the egg or young of a louse

nitrate *n.* a salt of nitric acid; **nitrate poisoning** can occur with ingestion of fertilizers and plants that have taken up nitrate resulting in diarrhea, abdominal pain, incoordination, convulsions and, in severe cases, death —*vt.* to treat or combine with nitrate or nitric acid —**nitration** *n.*

nitrate of mercury *see* **citric ointment**

nitric acid a highly corrosive acid that can burn tissues but can be used in dilute solutions to burn warts

nitrofurazone *n.* an antibacterial agent, sold in liquid or ointment form

nitrogen (nonprotein) an element of the blood —*see also* **urea nitrogen**

NMS neonatal maladjustment syndrome

noble *adj.* of a proud bearing, as typical of an Arab

nodder *n.* a horse that moves its head up and down noticeably when in motion; often applied to Tennessee Walkers because they nod their heads in gait more than other breeds because of their fast walk

node *n.* a small, knotty swelling —**nodal** *adj.*

nodule *n.* a small node

Nonius *n.* a Hungarian breed named after the alleged French foundation sire called Nonius (foaled about 1810); he was captured during the Napoleonic wars and taken to Hungary where he was bred with Arabian, Holstein, Lipizzaner, and Anglo-Norman mares. Today the breed is popular under saddle, in competition, and for harness and farm work. A tough, compact horse; quiet and willing with good action. There are two types: one heavier and up to 17 h.h.; the other ranging from 14.2 to 16 h.h. Usually dark bay or black.

nonpyogenic *adj.* not producing pus (describes certain bacteria)

noose *n.* a loop formed in a rope with a slipknot that enables the rope to tighten when pulled

Noram *n.* a French breed chiefly used as a racing trotter; 15.2 h.h.

norepinephrine *n.* a hormone secreted by the adrenal gland; increases heart rate and constricts blood vessels during stress

Norfolk Roadster *see* **Norfolk Trotter**

Norfolk Trotter an English breed of trotters with a very ancient heritage; considered extinct now although a few are still said to exist; originated as a breed in the 18th century by crossing Thoroughbreds with native mares; Bellfounder was famous, was exported to the United States, and was a significant influence in the development of the Standardbred; strong, short-legged but very fast-trotting; also called the New English Road Horse and Norfolk Roadster

Noria *n.* a device for raising water in a series of buckets, or similar containers, attached to a revolving chain on a wheel; there are various kinds, one of which may be pulled by a horse; used in Spain and the Orient

Noriker *n.* an Austrian cold blood draft breed of ancient origins named after the state of Noricum, which was once part of the Roman Empire; the Pinzgauer Norikers (named after the Pinzgau district) are spotted but now rare; good mountain workers, Norikers are used for that purpose and still bred in large numbers; 16–16.2 h.h.

normal *adj.* conforming with an accepted standard; natural

normal horse serum serum taken from healthy horses, which have been immunized against infections, which is prepared for use in treating other horses having antibody deficiencies

Norman *n.* *see* **Selle Français**

Norman Trotter *see* **French Trotting Horse**

Northland *n.* a Norwegian pony breed originated from Tarpan and Mongolian stock; about 13 h.h.

North Swedish a medium sized heavy Swedish breed of ancient origins used in agriculture and in the Swedish army; a breed society was established at the end of the 19th century; has a good temperament, is economical and a healthy keeper, and is long-lived; 15.1–15.3 h.h.

North Swedish Trotter a lighter type of the North Swedish breed; popularly used in harness races; 15.1–15.3 h.h.

Norwegian Trotter *see* **Dole Trotter**

nose *n.* the part of the face between eyes and mouth having two orifices (nostrils) for breathing and smelling — **nasal** *adj.*

nose[1] *n.* the part of the face between eyes and mouth having two orifices (nostrils) for breathing and smelling — **nasal** *adj.*

nose[2] *n.* in racing, the shortest measurement of distance by which a horse can win

nose bag a feed bag hung on a horse's head and over the muzzle; feed bag

noseband *n.* a part of the bridle or halter comprising a strap which goes over the nose; there are many designs for the bridle; a **drop noseband** is so called because it is worn fairly close to the nose to prevent opening of the mouth — *see also* **cavesson**

nosebleed *n.* nasal bleeding, as is sometimes seen in racehorses; epistaxis

nose botfly *see* **Gastrophilus hemorroidalis**

nostril *n.* 1. either of the two orifices of the nose 2. the fleshy part around the orifice

no time in rodeo, a contestant gets "no time" if he or she misses in roping events or if the calf gets free after the tiedown; this result is signalled by the flagman waving the flag from side to side

novice class a show class that is open to entrants that have won not more than three blue ribbons at recognized horse shows

Novokirghiz *n.* a Russian breed, originally the Kirghiz pony of Mongolian stock and native to the Kirghiz and Kazakstan mountain areas; during the 20th century this breed was crossed with Thoroughbreds and Dons to develop a larger horse, which then became known as the Novokirghiz; used for riding, in harness, and for mountain pack work; 14.3–15.2 h.h.

NRA National Reining Horse Association

nucleus *n.* the center of a cell which contains hereditary structures necessary for reproduction, growth, etc.

number cloth a racehorse's saddle cloth worn to clearly show a number corresponding with its number on the race card

Numidian *n.* an ancient breed used by Hannibal (247–183 B.C.) in his 6,000-horse cavalry; an ancestor of the Barb

numnah *n.* a saddle pad cut to the shape of the saddle; may be made of felt, rubber, or sheepskin

nurse *vi.* to be fed milk, as when a foal sucks from the mother's teats — *vt.* to give milk, as when a mare feeds her foal

nursery handicap a handicap race in which only two-year-olds compete

nut *n.* a cube, or other shape, of compound feed; may contain cereal, vitamins, minerals and hay

nut-cracker *n.* a horse that grinds its teeth (rare)

nutcracker twitch *see* **twitch**

nutmeg liver chronic venous liver congestion; usually caused by some heart pathology, lung disease, nephritis, or tumors; occasionally this condition may ensue from lack of exercise; can be alleviated but not cured

nutrient *n.* something, such as food, that is nourishing and promotes growth — *adj.* nourishing; conveying nourishment, as nutrient arteries

nutriment *n.* 1. something that nourishes, as food 2. something that causes growth — **nutrimental** *adj.*

nutrition *n.* 1. that which nourishes; food; nutriment 2. the process by which the body uses food — **nutritional, nutritious, nutritive** *adj.* — **nutritionally** *adv.*

nutritional osteoporosis a mineral bone deficiency which causes deformity and weakness of the bones; results from a deviation in the desired ratio of calcium to phosphorus in the diet

Nuttallia equi a parasite that is said to cause biliary fever

nux vomica 1. the poisonous seed of an Asiatic tree of the same name 2. a medicinal stimulant made from this seed and containing strychnine

nuzzle *vt.* to touch, push, or rub with the muzzle

nyctalopia *n.* night blindness

nystagmus *n.* an involuntary, rapid movement of the eyeball which can be seen in diseases or damage of the brain or under anesthesia — **nystagmic** *adj.*

nystatin *n.* an antifungal antibiotic best used as an ointment as it is poorly absorbed when taken orally; trade name Mycostatin

nyxis *n.* puncturing with a needle to draw out excess fluid

– O –

oakum *n.* hemp fiber often mixed with tar and used as a filler for cracks or space between a hoof pad and the sole

oat *n.* 1. a cereal grass 2. the grain of this grass, which is used as feed

oaten *adj.* made of oats

oat-hair calculus a large intestinal calculus consisting of oat-hairs which are derived of oat husks; removal of husks in preparation of the oats will prevent these calculi

obedient *adj.* willing to obey commands or aids

Oberlander *n.* a draft breed that originated in Germany; 15.1 h.h.

objection *n.* in racing, a disapproval of any of the placed horses which must be heard by the stewards at the race meeting where it is expressed

obliquus abdominis externus and **-internus** abdominal muscles that compress the abdominal cavity to help effect defecation, birth and expiration

obliquus capitis anterior a neck muscle that extends or turns the head

obliquus capitis posterior a neck muscle that rotates the head

obstacle race a race that is run over obstacles, such as the steeplechase and the point-to-point races

obstetrical *adj.* relating to birth —**obstetrically** *adv.*

obstinate *adj.* stubborn; unwilling to comply with commands —**obstinacy** *n.*

obstruction *n.* 1. an obstacle 2. in the body, a condition in which the normal flow of contents through a passageway is blocked

obturate *vt.* to close (an opening in the body) —**obturator** *n.* that which closes, as a disk —**obturation** *n.*

obturator externus a thigh muscle that adducts the thigh

obturator foramen an opening in the pelvis formed by the ischial and pubic bones

obturator internus a thigh muscle that rotates the femur outward

obturator nerve a nerve that originates at the spinal chord and supplies the pelvic cavity; it pierces the membrane that covers the obturator foramen

Obvinski *n. see* **Viatka**

occipital bone the bone which forms the rear of the skull; the poll

occipital puncture the insertion of a needle between the occiput and first neck vertebra to obtain cerebrospinal fluid for analysis

occipito-hyoideus a muscle that moves the hyoid bone during swallowing

occipito mandibularis a lower jaw muscle that opens the mouth

occiput *n., pl.* **occipita** the rear part of the skull —**occipital** *adj.*

occlude *vt. see* **occlusion** —**occludent** *adj.*

occlusion *n.* 1. the fitting together of the upper and lower teeth when the jaws are closed 2. a closing off, as blood flow

occult *adj.* concealed or hard to detect, as in some diseases —**occultness** *n.* —**occultly** *adv.*

occult spavin arthritis of the lower joints of the hock; blind spavin —*see also* **spavin**

OCD osteochondritis dissecans

ocular *adj.* relating to the eye

odds *n.pl.* in racing, the betting quotation on a horse in a particular race

odds-on *adj.* considered to have more than an even chance of winning

odometer *n.* an instrument for measuring distance covered which is attached to the horse's lower foot

odontoma *n.* a very rare tumor that consists of dentine; a **temporal odontoma** is a tumor that relates to the temporal bone

oestrus *n. see* **estrus**

off side the right side of the horse if viewed from behind; far side —**offside horse** the right-hand horse of a pair

ointment *n.* a medicinal substance used externally; salve

old *adj.* 1. having lived a long time; a horse is considered to be old when it reaches the age of about 20 2. having the appearance of being old 3. being a certain age (e.g., *ten years old*)

Oldenburg *n.* a German warmblood breed whose ancestry dates back to the 17th century; an all-purpose saddle horse; a type of Oldenburg called Rottaler in Bavaria is almost always chestnut while the others vary from bay to black; 16.2–17.2 h.h.

olecranon *n.* the elbow point, formed by the ulna

olfaction *n.* 1. the sense of smell 2. the act of smelling —**olfactory** *adj.*

oligenia *n.* lowered blood volume

oligopnoea *n.* abnormal decreased respiration

oliguria *n.* a condition in which urine secretion is greatly decreased

Olympic Games international athletic competitions, including equine events, held every four years at a selected site; the equine events are: 1. a 3-day event which includes dressage, cross-country, and show-jumping; 2. show-jumping; and 3. dressage

omentum *n.* an apron-like extenion of the membrane that covers the stomach and colon; the **great omentum** covers the stomach and intestines; the **lesser omentum** partly covers the stomach and common bile duct — **omental** *adj.*

omo-hyoideus a neck muscle that moves the hyoid bone and root of the tongue

onager *n.* a wild relative of the horse and subspecies of the Asiatic wild ass; small, grayish-white, with long ears and a tufted tail; once ranged all through central Asia and India and westward to Palestine but is now nearly extinct, although there are still a few in zoos in Chicago and Philadelphia, as well as a colony of them at the Catskill Game Farm in New York

onchocerca *n.* a roundworm parasite, carried by flies, found particularly in the skin, eyes, and subcutaneous tissues; **onchocerca microfilariae** are the larvae

onchocerciasis *n.* a skin condition caused by the larvae of the onchocerca worm which is transmitted by flies; manifested by patches of thinned hair, itchy, scaly skin, and sores on the abdominal midline, chest, and face

one day event a variety of competitions completed in one day

one-eared headstall a

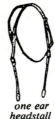

one ear headstall

headstall that has no browband and has a slot for one ear only

on his (her) toes restlessly eager to go

on terms in hunting, steadily pursuing the quarry because of a strong scent (of hounds)

on the bit in a collected state with the neck held correctly according to the pace; contact with the bit is light, and the horse fully accepts the bit without resistance

on the leg having a shallow body and long legs

on the rails in racing, positioned close to the rails

ontogeny, ontogenesis *n.* the biological development of a single organism — **ontogenic, otogenetic,** *adj.*

oocyte *n.* an unfertilized egg cell

oogenesis *n.* the development of an egg cell

ooze *vi., vt.* to slowly exude moisture or fluid — **oozy** *adj.* — **oozily** *adv.* — **ooziness** *n.*

opacity *n.* the state of being opaque

opaque *adj.* resistant to the passage of light, as an opaque area in the eye

open *adj.* in reference to a mare, not bred

open arthritis (*also* **open joint arthritis**) an arthritic condition that arises from wounding or bruising caused by accidents, wounds, or occasionally by a bone splinter from a fracture entering the joint; the wound may discharge synovial (joint) fluid, which suggests open arthritis; swelling may occur when the fetlock and elbow are affected but, if present, is mild; when the hock or stifle is involved, the swelling can be very pronounced; pus may be present; most cases are very painful and in the beginning the horse may be off its feed but drink a lot of water; may develop fever with increased respiration and may lie down frequently

open behind having hocks far apart and feet close together; base narrowed

open class a class open to any horse and rider in a given division

opening meet in hunting, the first meet of the season

open behind

open jumper a horse capable of high jumping in competition; the horse is scored only on faults, not time

open knees a developmental stage in which the end of the forearm bone is still made up of cartilage

open rein in English riding, a training action of holding a rein in each hand and directing a turn by holding one rein down toward the rider's knee on the side of the turn; direct rein; in Western riding, plow rein

open shelter a shelter with one or two sides open; a lean-to is a type of open shelter which is built onto an adjacent building and may be open on three sides; horses like an open shelter (which should always be closed on the side facing the prevailing wind) as it enables them to see about them and gives them a sense of being able to escape if necessary

operable *adj.* capable of being cured or alleviated by surgery

ophidism *n.* poisoning due to a snakebite

ophthalmia *n. see* **iridocyclitis**

ophthalmic *adj.* relating to the eyes

ophthalmology *n.* the science dealing with functions and diseases of the eye

ophthalmoscope *n.* an instrument that reflects light into the eye for examination — **ophthalmoscopic** *adj.* — **ophthalmoscopy** *n.* the use of this instrument

opisthotonos *n.* a spasm of the back muscle causing a pulling back of the head; can be seen in tetanus or an injury to the brain

opsin *n.* a protein constituent of the color- and light-sensitive structures of the eyeball

optic, -cal *adj.* relating to the eye

optic disc a small round spot on the eye where retinal nerve fibers converge and exit the eye toward the brain

optic nerve a nerve which connects the retina with the brain

oral *adj.* of the mouth

orange dun *see* **dun**

orbicularis oculi an eyelid muscle that closes the eyelids

orbicularis oris a cheek and lip muscle that closes the eyelids

orbit *n.* the eye socket

orbital cellulitis inflammation of the tissue surrounding the eyeball

orchidopexy *n.* a surgical procedure in which an undescended testicle is brought into the scrotal sac

orchiectomy *n.* removal of one of both testicles; castration

orchitis *n.* inflammation of a testicle

organ *n.* a part of the body designed for a particular function, as, for example, the organ of hearing — **organic** *adj.*

organism *n.* any individual living thing — **organismic, organismal** *adj.* — **organismically** *adv.*

organography *n.* the study and description of the organs of the body

organophosphate *n.* a type of dewormer; an amount only slightly more than the effective dose is poisonous

Oriental *n.* a horse of the Orient; loosely used for any horse of Eastern origin, such as the Arabian

orifice *n.* any opening leading to or from a body cavity, such as the mouth, nostrils, etc.

Orlov *n.* a Russian trotter breed named for Count Orlov, who founded the Krenov Stud in 1778; used chiefly for trotting races; 15.2–17 h.h.

osmosis *n.* the passage of a fluid through a membrane of the body

osselet *n.* a hard swelling or periostitis, often in both front legs, at the front of and just above or below the fetlock; caused by subjecting immature horses to hard training or the conformation fault of excessively upright pasterns

osseous *adj.* bony

ossicle *n.* a small bone, particularly one of those in the tympanic cavity of the ear

ossify *vt., vi.* to transform from non-bony tissue into bone — **ossification** *n.*

osteal *adj.* bony

osteochondritis *n.* bone and cartilage inflammation

osteochondritis dissecans (OCD) osteochondritis that causes splitting of fragments of cartilage into a joint; causes include trauma to cartilage, malnutrition, and mineral imbalances; initial symptoms are pain and deformity, lameness

osteodystrophia fibrosa *see* **big head disease**

outride *vt.* 1. to ride better or faster than (another rider) 2. to ride ahead of or beside (a horse-drawn vehicle)

outrider *n.* 1. a rider who rides in attendance beside or ahead of a horse-drawn vehicle 2. a rider or cowboy who prevents cattle from straying from a particular range 3. a forerunner on horseback

outside rim shoe a horseshoe having a rim around the outside edge for increased traction; barrel racing special

ovarian follicle any of the cavities in the ovaries in which eggs develop

ovariectomy *n.* a surgical operation to remove an ovary

ovary *n.* either of two reproductive glands in the mare that produce eggs (ova) — **ovarian** *adj.*

over at the knees *see* **knee sprung**

over-bent *adj.* having a neck position with the chin brought in too much by the bridle, so that it rests almost against the neck and the crest is over-arched

overbite *n. see* **parrot mouth**

over-face *vt.* to ask (a horse) to jump too big a fence before the horse is ready

over-mounted *adj.* (of a rider) nervous or inexperienced and tending to overreact to the horse's movements

Overo *n.* a coloration which is mainly a solid color with white patches, especially in the midsection of the body; rarely spreads across the back; often bald-faced; where colors meet, demarcation lines are often blurred; legs frequently dark but usually mixed — *see also* **Pinto**

over-reach *vi.* to hit the foreleg or hoof with a hind toe; can be lessened by corrective shoeing; boots can be used for protection — *see also* **forging**

over-reach boot a round rubber boot fitted to protect the coronet from injury caused by over-reaching

over-reach boot

over-ride *vi.* in hunting, to follow too closely behind the hounds

overshot fetlock *see* **knuckle over**

overshot mouth *see* **parrot mouth**

over the bit having the head raised and the muzzle extended outward in an attempt to shift the bit and avoid bit pressure; a horse that goes over the bit thus becomes what is termed a star gazer

over-tracking an action made visible when the imprint of the hind foot is beyond that of the forefoot on the same side; this should apply to medium, extended, and free walk, as well as medium and extended trot

overweight *adv. see* **underweight**

oviduct *n.* the mare's fallopian tube, connecting the ovary with the uterus and in which fertilization takes place

ovoid *adj.* egg-shaped

ovulation *n.* the process in which an egg (ovum) is released from the ovary; the 24- to 48-hour period in a mare's reproductive cycle when the ovum is discharged from the ovary — **ovulatory** *adj.* — **ovulate** *vi.*

ovum *n.* a mare's egg, which, after fertilization by the stallion, develops into an embryo

owlhead *n.* a horse considered too wild to train

owner *n.* in racing, the person in whose name a racehorse runs, regardless of whether that person is the sole owner or is a member of a syndicate

oxbow stirrup a U-shaped Western stirrup; the term derives from the U-shaped part of an ox yoke

oxbow stirrup

oxer *n.* a jump consisting of two hurdles separated but jumped as one, such as a **bush oxer** (brush between posts and rails or posts and guardrail), **posts and rails oxer** (same as brush oxer without the brush), **posts and planks oxer**, etc.

oxibendazole *n.* one of the benzimidazole group of dewormers

oxidation *n.* the chemical combination of oxygen with another substance, as in burning or rusting — **oxidize** *vt.* — **oxidative** *adj.* — **oxidant** *n.* an agent that oxidizes

oxidative capacity the ability to use oxygen in body metabolism

oxygen *n.* an odorless gas that comprises nearly 20 percent of the earth's atmosphere and is essential to life; the oxygen inhaled is carried to all body tissues by red blood cells; can be administered artificially as an inhalant with other gases during anesthesia, to foals having low blood oxygen, or to resuscitate foals

oxygenase *n.* a chemical enzyme that extracts oxygen from inhaled air for use by body tissues

oxygenation *n.* usage of oxygen as when red blood cells take oxygen during respiration

oxygen debt a depletion of oxygen caused by intense exertion, which must be reversed to normal with subsequent rest

oxyhemoglobin *n.* the red substance of blood, formed in the lungs by the combination of hemoglobin with oxygen

oxyphenbutazone *n.* a chemical excreted in urine when a horse is given phenylbutazone; also produced synthetically

oxytetracycline *n.* generic name of a broad spectrum antibiotic

oxytocin *n.* a hormone produced by the mare's pituitary gland to increase uterine contractions during foaling and to stimulate milk production during lactation; posterior pituitary extract — *see also* **posterior oxytocin principle (POP)**

oxyuriasis *n.* an internal parasitic condition caused by oxyuris equi (pinworms or threadworms) that causes rectal itching with subsequent tail rubbing

ozena *n.* a respiratory disease which is frequently of a catarrhal nature, with discharge from one or both nostrils, and can have a foul odor; nasal gleet

— P —

pace *n.* a two-beat gait wherein the fore and hind legs on one side move in unison; it can be as fast as galloping or as slow as ambling — *vi.*

paced *adj.* in racing, having the pace set by a pacemaker

pacemaker *n.* in racing, a horse that sets the pace for others; a pacesetter

pacer *n.* a horse that paces naturally

pacesetter *n. see* **pacemaker**

pachydermia *n.* an abnormal condition in which areas of the skin become devoid of hair and are thick and hard; often follows repeated attacks of sporadic lymphangitis; because of the skin's similarity to that of an elephant, it is also called elephantiasis

pack *n.* 1. a bundle carried on the back of a horse 2. a number of hounds kept for hunting

packed cell volume (PCV) in a blood sample, that part of the blood that is composed of red and white cells; in a healthy horse at rest, the normal proportion of cells to plasma (fluid) is 40 percent to 60 percent; hematocrit

pack horse a horse used for carrying loads

packsaddle *n.* a saddle used for balancing a load carried by a pack horse

pad[1] *n.* 1. a saddle blanket 2. a soft, stuffed saddle 3. a protective piece used between a horseshoe and the hoof 4. the "saddle" used in harness

pad[2] *n.* a horse with an easy gait (an old term)

paddling *n. see* **dishing** — *vi.* **paddle**

paddock *n.* 1. a small, enclosed piece of land, sometimes near a stable 2. an enclosure at a racetrack where horses are saddled and walked before a race 3. in Australia, a unit of 300 square miles — *vt.* to enclose in a paddock

pad-groom *n.* a person who gently rides a hunter to a hunt meet and returns with the hack the owner has ridden there

Pahlavan *n.* an Iranian cross-breed developed from Thoroughbred, Arab, and Plateau Persian blood

pain *n.* a feeling of hurt transmitted by the nerves and caused by injury or a disorder of the body — *vt.* to cause pain — *vi.* to have pain — **painful** *adj.*

paint *n. see* **Pinto**

palate *n.* the roof of the mouth

Palfrey *n.* an old English name for a small, gentle horse

Palio *n.* an Italian race held twice a year (July and August) in Siena, a city consisting of 17 contradas or neighborhoods represented by their contesting horses. The race dates back to 1310 and is an event of historic pageantry, great excitement and danger; the course is a shell-shaped piazza having two 90-degree downhill turns, and the actual race today lasts only about 71 seconds but is preceded by a three-hour procession; the few existing rules bar the use of saddles and purebreds but the contesting horses are treated with extraordinary care in preparation for the race; jockeys have no restrictions and may even block or unseat other competitors, but a riderless horse is allowed to win; the official prize is the Palio, an ornate flag painted each year by a different artist and carrying great honor; significant sums of money are, nevertheless, exchanged in connection with the competition — *see also* **Sardo**

palisade worm *see* **large strongyle**

palliate *vt.* to relieve (pain) without curing — **palliation, palliator** *n.*

palliative *n.* a medication for relieving pain but not for curing — *adj.*

Palomino *n.* a golden or cream-colored horse with white or ivory mane and tail. Although there are Palomino breed societies, the oldest of which is in America, this horse is judged on color, not conformation, so there are many types. Palominos are found worldwide and have ancient origins; their name may have derived from Count de Palomino of Spain, who

allegedly named some he owned after himself, but quite likely it may have derived from the golden grape of the same name. They are still known in Spain as Isabellas. Palominos sometimes have pink skins, although this is unusual, and often they are dappled; there are many shades of coat color ranging from a very light cream (isabella) to a very dark yellow in which black hairs are mixed in with the yellow (smutty); rarely leopard spots can occur.

palpate *vt.* to examine manually for medical diagnosis — **palpation** *n.* — **palpable** *adj.* able to be palpated

palpebra *n.* the eyelid — **palpebral** *adj.*

palpitate *vi.* (of the heart) to beat rapidly

Pan American Games equine competitions dating to 1951 and modeled after the Olympic equestrian events; they are held in North, South and Central America every four years the year before each Olympiad

pancake *n.* an English saddle

pancreas *n.* a large gland near the stomach which secretes digestive enzymes into the intestines and insulin into the blood — **pancreatic** *adj.*

pancreatitis *n.* inflammation of the pancreas

Pange *n.* a cross-breed of native Baltic mares and trotter stallions

panic snap a snap attached to a lead or rope used when tethering a horse; in case of emergency it is easily released by pulling back the casing

panniculus *n.* a subcutaneous fat layer

panniculus muscles fly-shaker muscles

pannier *n.* a large basket, or either of a pair of baskets, slung across a horse's back for carrying produce

pannus *n.* the growth of tiny blood vessels in the cornea of the eye, which obscures vision; keratitis

panopthalmia *n.* an infection of the eye

pantothenic acid a part of the vitamin B complex which is important for healthy skin, hair, and various internal organs

panus *n.* a swollen and inflamed lymph gland

paper face an all-white head

papilla *n., pl.* -lae a small, nipple-shaped projection of tissue

papilloma *n.* a benign growth of the skin or mucous membranes that comprises a group of enlarged papillae — **papillomatous** *adj.*

papule *n.* a small pimple or inflammatory elevation of the skin — **papular, papulose** *adj.*

parabola *n.* in jumping an obstacle, the arc made by a horse from the take-off point to the landing point

paracentesis *n.* the surgical introduction of a needle into the abdominal cavity to draw off fluid

parade *n.* a public procession for display — *vi., vt.*

parafilaria multipapillosa a parasitic worm that sometimes invades subcutaneous tissue where the skin is raised, usually on shoulders and hindquarters, causing the condition **parafilariasis**

parallel bars in jumping and cross-country competition, a type of fence consisting of two sets of rails paralleling each other

paralysis *n.* a partial or complete loss of muscle function — *see also* **radial nerve paralysis, sweeny, wobbler**

paralytic ileus *see* **ileus**

paralyze *vt.* to cause paralysis in — **paralyzed** *adj.*

parametritis *n.* inflammation of the tissues around the uterus

parametrium *n.* the tissues surrounding the uterus

paranasal sinuses air cavities, lined by mucous membranes, located around the nasal passages

paraphimosis *n.* a constriction of the penis by the shrinkage of its surrounding sheath

paraplegia *n.* paralysis of the hind limbs; equine encephalomylitis —*see also* **encephalomylitis**

parascarisequorum a roundworm

parasite *n.* any of various types of animals that live in or on a host horse and draw sustenance from it, as e.g. intestinal worms, ear mites, ticks, etc.; internal parasites are **endoparasites**; external parasites are **ectoparasites** —**parasitic** *adj.*

parasiticide *n.* an agent that destroys parasites —**parasiticidal** *adj.*

parasitism *n.* the condition of parasite infestation

parasitology *n.* the study of parasites and parasitism —**parasitologist** *n.* a person who specializes in the study of parasites and parasitism

parasympathetic nerves the involuntary nerve system that supplies the eyes, heart, glands, etc., keeping them under control, as opposed to the sympathetic nervous system that stimulates involuntary response, such as increasing the heart rate, dilating the pupils of the eyes, etc.

parathormone *n.* the hormone secreted by the parathyroid glands

parathyroid glands four small endocrine glands located in the neck next to the thyroid gland which secrete a hormone that balances the calcium-phosphorus metabolism of the body

paravertebral *adj.* next to the vertebral column

parenchyma *n.* the tissue of an organ that is responsible for its function, such as glands that line the intestines, air cells in lungs, etc., as opposed to connective tissue —**parenchymal, parenchymatous** *adj.* —**parenchymatously** *adv.*

parenteral *adj.* given by a means other than through the mouth, such as by injection

paresis *n.* partial paralysis

paries *n., pl.* **parietes** a wall in the body —**parietal** *adj.* relating to or forming the walls of a body cavity

parietal bones the major skullbones that form the top of the head

parimutuel *n.* 1. in racing, a system of betting wherein the whole amount bet on the winning horse, less a deduction for tax and operating expenses, is divided among the backers of that winner in proportion to what each one has staked 2. a totalizator or machine for recording such bets

park *vi.* to stand in a stretched position

park hack a perfectly turned out horse ridden in a park by gentlemen and ladies of leisure

park horse a horse with an animated gait; the term originated with horses used for riding or driving in a park

park saddle a flat English saddle with a low or cutback pommel and no knee rolls, used by saddle-seat riders; the center of the seat is close to the cantle

park saddle

park trot a slow, animated, very collected trot with much leg action; called for in the show ring and seen in all harness classes where Hackneys or Saddlebreds perform

parotid *adj.* near the ear

parotid gland the largest of the salivary

glands, located under the ear; produces secretions into the cheek through ducts opening near the upper molars

parotitis *n.* inflammation of the parotid gland

paroxysmal sleep *see* **narcolepsy**

parrot mouth a congenital malformation of the jaw wherein the upper incisors protrude beyond the lower incisors; causes longer than normal front teeth due to lack of contact with opposite teeth. The degree of parrot mouth varies and is classified as quarter-, half-, three-quarter, or full-tooth overbite; with a severe condition, grazing properly is impossible, and the worst cases have to be destroyed. Foals will sometimes outgrow mild cases. Also called brachy gnathia, buck tooth, overbite, elk lip, overshot mouth.

parrot mouth

parturient *adj.* (of a mare) foaling or about to foal — **parturiency**

parturition *n.* foaling; the act of bringing forth a foal

Pasitrotero *n.* a native breed of Costa Rica; small but strong, easy keepers, gentle; their smooth basic 4-beat gait is the pasitrote but they have several 4-beat gaits including the trocha; 13.2–14.1 h.h.

Paso Costaricense a cross-breed developed in Costa Rica from Peruvian Paso stallions, Hackneys, and local trotting horses; used as a parade horse; about 15 h.h.

Paso Fino a gaited breed indigenous to Puerto Rico and Colombia but also bred in other South and Central American countries as well as the United States where it is becoming well known in equine circles and gaining much popularity for shows and pleasure riding. The gait is a 4-beat single-foot in which the footfall is RF-LR-LF-RR and involves three paces: the **paso fino** or **fino fino**, a highly collected, high-action step with little forward speed; the **paso corto**, the same step at medium forward speed; and the **paso largo**, an extension of the same step at a faster speed. At shows, the fino gait is performed on a 48-foot wooden strip to enable this very quick step to be heard and judged. An extremely comfortable horse to ride, and the rider appears motionless in the saddle while in gait. Finely boned, though strong; a maximum height of 15.2 h.h., though usually smaller. —*see also* **trocha**

passade *n.* in dressage, the maneuver in which a horse turns on its haunches

passage *n.* in dressage, an airy, elevated, collected trot in which the horse's feet seem to hover above the ground

passenger *n.* one who rides a horse without control, letting the horse go as it wishes

passive immunity immunity incurred by antibodies transferred from an immune horse to one not previously immune

passive transfer the transfer of antibodies from mare to foal through the colostrum

pastern *n.* the part of the foot between the fetlock and hoof

pasteurellosis *n.* a bacterial disease (caused by pasteurella bacteria) that is uncommon in horses but, if contracted, can cause fever and respiratory tract infection

pasture *n.* a field of grasses used for grazing —*vt.* to put (horses) out to graze in a pasture —*vi.* to graze in a pasture —**put out to pasture** 1. to put out to graze in pasture 2. to retire (a horse)

pat *n.* an affectionate, gentle tap with the hand — *vt.*

patch *n.* an area of hair contrasting with the predominant coat color

patella *n.* the triangular bone situated over the stifle joint; equivalent of the human kneecap — **patellar** *adj.*

patella luxation a slipping or dislocation of the patella caused by arrested growth of part of the femoral trochlia

patella locking an inherited condition, not to be confused with stringhalt, wherein the stifle becomes locked, preventing flexion of the hind limb; the leg is observed to be fully extended with hoof bent backward; when the horse moves, the front of the hoof on the stiff leg drags on the ground; the locked condition may last for hours or may be released suddenly, often with a snapping sound, every few steps, allowing the leg to bend

patent *adj.* open or unobstructed, as in reference to a blood vessel or other body passageway

patent ductus arteriosis a passageway in the fetus that conducts blood from the lungs into the aorta; it normally closes after birth; if it does not, circulation problems cause a murmur and weaken arterial walls

patent urachus a condition in a foal wherein urine drips from the stump of the navel cord; pervious urachus

pathobiologist *n.* a specialist who studies changes in body processes at the microscopic level

pathogen *n.* a bacteria or virus that causes disease

pathogenic *adj.* capable of causing disease

pathognomic *adj.* relating to signs and symptoms that indicate a particular type of disease

pathognomy *n.* the study of signs and symptoms of disease

pathological *adj.* relating to a disease — **pathologically** *adv.*

pathological fracture a bone fracture that is caused by a disease rather than an injury

pathologist *n.* a physician who determines the nature of a disease by studying changes in tissue structure

pathology *n.* 1. the science that attempts to determine the nature of diseases through examination of affected tissues 2. abnormality caused by a disease

pato *n.* (Spanish for duck) an equestrian game originally (1610 or earlier) played in Argentina with a duck which was sewn to a piece of leather, then thrown into the air above a group of riders on horseback, each of whom would try to catch it and then ride to the home of his loved one and throw it on her doorstep; sometimes two teams would take part. This dangerous game lasted for hours and many riders were killed. In 1822 pato was banned; then in 1937 a more humane version was instigated with fixed rules: eight riders (two four-man teams) on a playing field 270 feet by 600 feet, use a heavy ball with leather hand grips which a rider has to pick up at full gallop and throw to a team player or into the opponents' basket which is fixed to the top of a pole; there are six playing periods lasting seven minutes each and separated by five-minute breaks; each rider has to have more than one horse due to the stress involved.

patten shoe a bar shoe with a wide, raised bar used to raise the heel and reduce pain in cases of sprained tendons; also called platten shoe

pattern horse a horse that is proficient in one pattern of trained maneuvers but has not mastered other maneuvers

patulous *adj.* open, as in reference to a body part (e.g., a cervix)

PC phosphocreatine

PCV packed cell volume

peat moss an absorbent plant that grows in wet places such as swamps and bogs and forms partly decayed matter (peat); sometmes spread on ground surfaces used for riding to provide soft, springy footing; sphagnum

Pechora *n.* *see* **Zemaituka**

peck *vi.* 1. to stumble or pitch forward 2. in jumping, to hit a jump lightly with the forefeet or to stumble on landing after the jump

pecking order a social system among a group of horses or even two horses that amounts to a special order of dominance

pectoral *adj.* relating to the chest

pedal *adj.* relating to the foot

pedal bone the end bone in the leg; coffin bone; third phalanx

pedal osteitis inflammation of the pedal bone within the hoof; caused by an inherited conformation that increases the concussion on the pedal bone, by concussion associated with hard work on hard surfaces, or by poor hoof care

pediculi *n.pl.* lice — **pedicular** *adj.* 1. relating to lice   2. infested with lice — **pediculosis** *n.* infestation with lice

pedigree *n.* 1. descent   2. a recorded line of descent

pedometer *n.* an instrument to measure distance covered; strapped to the foot near the fetlock; weighs about 1½ oz.

peel back (of cattle) in rodeo cutting, to return toward the herd from the center of the arena; after some of the cattle are separated and driven to the center of the arena, the rider chooses a cow to cut while the rest of the cattle try to peel back to the herd

Pegasus *n.* the famous winged horse of Greek mythology, whose name meant, literally "from the water"; because horses were often transported by ship and were made to swim ashore, they were associated with the sea and thus named; the wings depicted their speed

pelage *n.* the coat or hair covering the body

pelham *n.* a bit which has rings at the top and bottom ends of the cheekpiece (exclusive of the uppermost ring to which the headstall is attached) and is used with a snaffle (or other types of mouths) and a curb and usually with two sets of reins; if one set is used, a leather couplet links the two rings of the bit

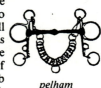

pelham

pellet *n.* a small mass of compressed food; **pellet concentrates** are pellets that can contain concentrated hay, grain, vitamins and minerals, or a combination of these, with high nutrient value; nuts

pelvic flexure a bend of the large colon, around its midpoint, where it folds back upon itself

pelvis *n.* a ring-like group of bones in the hip region — **pelvic** *adj.*

pemoline *n.* generic name of a stimulant for the central nervous system

pemphigus foliaceous an autoimmune skin disease that produces fluid-filled blisters on a horse's body, which burst and form itchy, scabby lesions and skin slough

pen *n.* a small enclosure for confining animals; corral

penalty *n.* in competitions, a disadvantage, such as loss of points, incurred by a competitor for breaking the rules — **penalize** *vt.*

Penavlon *n.* trade name for benzylpenicillin

Peneia *n.* a pony breed indigenous to Greece; used for light farm work and as a pack pony; averages 12.1 h.h.

penicillin *n.* an antibiotic derived from certain molds

penicillin-streptomycin combination a mixture of penicillin G and dihydrostreptomycin marketed under brand names such as Combiotic and Pen-Strep

Penidural *n.* trade name for benzamine pencillin

penis *n.* the male reproductive organ, through which urine is ejected — **penile** *adj.*

Pen-Strep *n.* a brand name for penicillin-streptomycin combination

pentathlete *n.* a contestant who takes part in a pentathlon

pentathlon *n.* 1. an athletic contest comprising five different events 2. an Olympic contest of five events that includes a 5,000 meter cross-country horseback ride

pentazocine *n.* a synthetic drug derived from coal tar and used as a pain killer

pentobarbitone sodium a short-acting barbiturate; trade name, Nembutal

Pentothal *n.* trade name for thiopentone sodium

pepsin *n.* a stomach enzyme that aids in digestion, particularly of protein

pepsinogen *n.* a secretion from the gastric glands of the stomach from which pepsin is produced

peptic *adj.* 1. relating to digestion 2. relating to pepsin

peptone *n.* any of several basic proteins which are converted, through metabolism, into amino acids which pass through the intestinal wall into the bloodstream

peracute *adj.* extremely acute, as in a disease

Percheron *n.* a heavy, cold-blood breed of ancient heritage (one of the oldest) that originated in a part of France called La Perche; infusions of Arab blood made the breed handsome and active; at one time used as a war horse by armored knights, then later used for agricultural work and transport; today this breed is still used for agriculture, as well as for showing and, in France, also for meat; docile and powerful; 15.2–17 h.h.

percussion *n.* the manual tapping of parts of the body in order to diagnose the condition of internal organs from the sound thus produced — **percuss** *vt.*

percutaneous *adj.* through the skin — **percutaneously** *adv.*

percutaneous splitting the separation of tendon fibers by surgical incision

perfecta *n.* in racing, a form of betting which obligates the wagerer to bet on the first and second place horses disregarding the order in which they finish

performance *n.* 1. an exhibition before an audience in a show 2. a particular class in a show

perfusion *n.* the pouring or injecting of a fluid into a part of the body in order to completely permeate it

periarteritis *n.* inflammation along an artery

periarthritis *n.* inflammation of the tissues around a joint

pericarditis *n.* inflammation of the sac (pericardium) around the heart, which stifles circulation by pressure of the swelling; may be caused by a chest wound, pneumonia, pleurisy, streptococcal or viral infection

pericardium *n.* the thin membranous sac encasing the heart — **pericardial, pericardiac** *adj.*

perichondritis *n.* inflammation around the cartilage of a joint

perilymph *n.* fluid in the area that

separates the membranous from the osseous labyrinth of the ear

perimysium *n.* connective tissue which binds together and covers groups of muscle fibers

perinatal *adj.* relating to the time around birth

perineoplasty *n.* surgical repair of the perineum

perinephrium *n.* the connective and fatty tissue enveloping the kidney

perineum *n.* the area between the anus and vulva in the female and between the anus and scrotum in the male — **perineal** *adj.*

perineurium *n.* the sheath surrounding a nerve — **perineureal** *adj.*

periodic iridocyclitis *see* **periodic ophthalmia**

periodic ophthalmia an eye disease involving recurring attacks of inflammation of the pupillary structures; a common cause of blindness; recurrent iridocyclitis; moon blindness

periodontal *adj.* relating to the gums and tissues around the teeth

periodontal cyst an outpouching of the root of a tooth

periople *n.* the exterior, protective covering of the hoof wall; it is a natural varnish that holds in the moisture of the hoof — **perioplic** *adj.*

periosteum *n.* the tough connective membrane that lies between the bones and their surrounding ligaments and tendons, serving as an anchor for ligaments and tendons; it protects, nourishes, and is involved in bone growth — **periosteal** *adj.*

periostitis *n.* inflammation of the periosteum, caused by injury — *see* splints — **periostitic** *adj.*

periotic *adj.* surrounding the inner ear

peripheral 1. away from the center, as peripheral vision, which is the area of vision to the side of the direct line of sight 2. near the surface, as peripheral nerves which supply the legs

peripheral nervous system the system of nerves that connect all body parts to the spine and brain

peripheral vasodilator an agent that widens the arterioles

perirectal *adj.* around the anus

perirenal *adj.* around the kidney

peristalsis *n.* the wavelike contractions of the intestines and various other hollow organs that propel their contents onward — **peristaltic** *adj.* — **peristaltically** *adv.*

peritoneal fluid a clear abdominal lubricating liquid which resists infection

peritoneal tap *see* **paracentesis**

peritoneum *n.* the membranous lining of the abdominal (peritoneal) cavity — **peritoneal** *adj.*

peritonitis *n.* inflammation of the peritoneum, commonly caused by a sharp object, such as a broken fence rail, penetrating the abdominal wall; rupture of the stomach (bots can perforate the stomach wall) or intestines, allowing their contents to spill into the abdominal cavity, usually results in fatal peritonitis; symptoms are abdominal pain, reluctance to lie down, tense abdominal muscles, severe depression, and grunting associated with breathing or when forced to move; also, loss of appetite and weight and debilitation

perlino *adj.* having an off-white coat color similar to cremello with the same blue eyes but slightly red or blue points

permanent teeth the teeth that replace the original temporary or milk teeth by age 5

permeable *adj.* able to be penetrated by fluids — **permeability** *n.* — **permeate** *vt.*

pernicious anemia a type of anemia involving a decrease in red blood cells and gastrointestinal and nervous disorders

peroneal region that which is on the outer side of the leg

peroneus tertius a strong tendon that extends from the front of the stifle to the hock and is part of the apparatus that automatically flexes the hock when the stifle is flexed

Persano *n. see* **Salerno**

persistent root a long narrow sliver of a milk tooth's root left in the gum after the permanent tooth erupts

perspire *vi.* to sweat — **perspiration** *n.*

Peruvian Paso a gaited breed, of gentle disposition, indigenous to Peru but bred in other South American countries as well as the U.S.A. Descended from the Iberian Horse, Barb, Spanish Jennet, and Andalusian. In gait, the forefeet flare out with high knee action called termino, while the hind quarters energetically drive the horse forward in a smooth, ambling, four-beat gait that is very comfortable for the rider; the preferred gait is called the "paso llano," wherein the footfalls are evenly spaced; the faster gait is called the "sobreandando" wherein there is a small time lapse shifting the horse's weight from right to left and then from left to right. Fairly heavy-boned and strong, this horse possesses considerable stamina and is used to travel long distances over the rough, mountainous terrains of Peru while maintaining a relaxed gait of about 11 m.p.h. Has great presence with a proud, arched, elevated head carriage, and long and luxurious mane and tail, presenting a beautiful appearance in its unique gait; 14–15.2 h.h.

pervious *adj.* able to be penetrated or passed through

pervious urachus a condition in a newborn foal in which urine drips constantly from the navel, resulting from failure of the urinary passage within the umbilical cord to close after the cord is cut

pesade *n.* a high-school (haute école) movement in which the horse rears very high

pessary *n.* a device placed in the vagina as a support to maintain the normal position of the uterus or rectum or to prevent conception

pesticide *n.* a chemical used to kill insects and other pests — **pesticidal** *adj.*

petechia *n.* a small, round reddish spot caused by hemorrhage into the skin or mucous membranes

petechial fever *see* **purpura**

pethidine a drug to relieve pain, as in colic (also pethidine hydrochloride)

petrous bone a bone close to the mastoid bone behind the ear

PG prostaglandin

phacofragmentation *n.* a surgical procedure to remove cataracts by using high-energy ultrasound that fragments the clouded lens, the pieces of which are then lifted out with a suction device; this clears up the horse's distance vision although near vision is slightly blurry

phaeton *n.* an open, four-wheeled carriage, drawn by one or two horses, with front and rear seats and usually a folding top

phagocyte *n.* a body cell which can consume foreign matter — **phagocytic** *adj.*

phagocytosis *n.* the destruction by phagocytes of bacteria or foreign matter — **phagocytotic** *adj.*

phalanx, -ange *n.* one of the three bones of the foot: long pastern bone (first phalanx), short pastern bone (second phalanx), or coffin bone (third phalanx)

phallus *n.* the penis — **phallic** *adj.*

phantom *n.* a padded dummy used for a stallion to mount, in place of a mare, when collecting semen for artificial insemination

pharmacodynamics *n.pl.* the study of the effects of drugs on the body, and the body's reactions

pharmacology *n.* 1. the study of drugs and their uses 2. the study of the effect of drugs — **pharmacological, pharmacologic** *adj.* — **pharmacologically** *adv.* — **pharmacologist** *n.* a person trained in pharmacology

pharyngitis *n.* inflammation of the mucous membrane of the pharynx

pharynx *n.* the throat; the cavity behind the nose and mouth and in front of the larynx and esophagus; serves breathing and swallowing

P.H.B.A. Palomino Horse Breeders Association

Phenergan *n.* trade name for promethazine hydrochloride

phenobarbitone *n.* a barbiturate drug

phenol *n. see* **carbolic acid**

phenothiazine *n.* a commercial chemical used in deworming agents and other drugs, including tranquilizers

phenotype *n.* the collective observable characteristics of a horse, including its appearance and its character, which result from both heredity and environment — **phenotypical** *adj.* — **phenotypically** *adv.*

phenylalinine *n.* a necessary amino acid

phenylbutazone *n.* a white anti-inflammatory powder used to treat arthritis, sprains, and wounds; commonly called **bute**

pheromone *n.* an animal scent; specifically, a substance secreted by one animal, the scent of which has an effect on another animal; for example, a pheromone in a mare's urine when she is in estrus excites a stallion

PHF Potomac horse fever

phimosis *n.* an abnormal condition in which the foreskin of the penis is so tight that it cannot be withdrawn, thereby restricting the head within — **phimotic** *adj.*

phlebitis *n.* inflammation of a vein or veins; can be caused by accidentally cutting a vein or by an intravenous injection

phlegm *n.* thick mucus secreted by the respiratory glands — **phlegmy** *adj.*

phlegmatic *adj.* 1. sluggish and slow 2. producing phlegm

phlegmon *n.* infection of connective tissues

phonendoscope *n.* an instrument used for auscultating

phosphatase *n.* an enzyme found in body tissues and fluids

phosphatic calculi gray-colored calculi composed of phosphates (magnesium, calcium, ammonium) developed from food

phosphocreatine (PC) *n.* a chemical which produces immediately available but limited energy for muscle contraction; expended in about 8–10 seconds of an all-out effort; efforts that use this energy are calf roping, dressage capriole, or sprint racing up to 300 yds.

phosphorus *n.* 1. a normal mineral constituent of the body 2. a nonmetallic chemical element present in organophosphorus drugs and poisons, such as rat poisons; these can poison a horse, causing pain, jaundice, and other symptoms, followed by convulsions, coma and death

photo finish the end of a race in which the first horses to come in are so close together that the winner is determined only by a photograph of them

photoperiod *n.* the period of daylight suited to the growth of an organism — **photoperiodic** *adj.*

photophobia *n.* in horses, the action

of avoiding light, by squinting or turning away, when it adversely affects the eyes

photosensitization, -sensitivity *n.* a skin allergy caused by sensitization to sunlight (not to be confused with sunburn); manifested by oozing lesions on white or unpigmented areas of skin; in severe cases the skin dies and sloughs away; caused by certain plants or drugs or liver disease; blue nose disease — **photosensitize** *vt.*

phrenic *adj.* 1. relating to the diaphragm 2. relating to the mind

phycomycete *n.* any of a class of fungi — **phycomycetous** *adj.*

phycomycosis *n.* a common type of internal disease caused by phycomycetes

phylogeny, -genesis 1. the line of descent or evolutionary development of an animal species 2. the origin and evolution of an animal species — **phylogenetic, phylogenic** *adj.* — **phylogenetically** *adv.*

phylum *n.* a broad division of the animal kingdom; horses belong to the phylum *Chordata,* which includes mammals

physeal plates growth plates; epiphyseal plates

physic *n.* a laxative

physical *adj.* 1. natural 2. relating to the body as opposed to the mind

physical therapy *see* **physiotherapy**

physiologic saline solution (PSS) 0.9 percent saline solution used for such purposes as wound cleansing, restoration of blood volume and dilution of drugs

physiology *n.* the science dealing with the processes and functions of living organisms or their parts — **physiologist** *n.* — **physiological, physiologic** *adj.* — **physiologically** *adv.*

physiotherapy *n.* the treatment of

injury or disease by physical means, such as massage, exercise, light (infrared or ultraviolet), heat (electrically heated boots, poultices, etc.) or cold (cold water, packed ice, bandages soaked in cooling lotions, etc.)

physitis *n.* inflammation of growth plates caused by inappropriate amounts and types of feed or excessive exercise; epiphysitis

physostigmine salicylate an alkaloid from the calabar bean used medicinally to stimulate involuntary muscles, such as those of the intestines, and to contract the pupils of the eyes

phytin *n.* an organic form of phosphorus in certain grains, including oats, corn and soybeans, excessive quantities of which may combine with calcium, zinc, copper, and other trace minerals to form insoluble compounds that may reduce the benefits of those foods

piaffe *n.* in dressage, a trot in place — *vi.* to perform the piaffe

pia mater the innermost membrane covering the brain and spinal cord

pica *n.* depraved appetite, such as that for dirt, dung (coprophagy), afterbirth, etc.

picadex *n.* an anthelmintic similar to piperazine salts

picador *n.* in bullfighting, a horseman who pricks the bull's neck with a lance to weaken its muscles

pick-up man in rodeo, a mounted assistant who helps bareback and saddle bronc riders in dismounting from their bucking broncos

Piebald *n.* a horse whose color is black and white; also called Pinto or Paint — **pied** *adj.*

pigeon-toed *adj.* standing with toes pointed inward

pig-eye *n.* a small eye — **pig-eyed** *adj.*

pigging string a soft rope, six feet

long, carried by a calf-roper, usually in his teeth or under his belt, to tie the calf's or steer's legs

pigment *n.* the coloring matter in the cells and tissues

pigmentation *n.* coloration due to pigment in the tissues

pillar *n.* one of two posts to which a horse is tied when learning high school movements

pin bones the bony prominences of the rump

pinched withers withers which are gripped by an ill-fitting saddle

Pindos *n.* a mountain pony breed native to Greece; an ecnomical keeper, strong and hardy; 12–13 h.h.

pineal gland a small gland at the base of the brain; considered to be partly responsible for the body's clock system

pin firing *n.* a treatment for chronic leg injury by means of burning the skin with a hot iron to produce scar tissue and hasten healing; in **point firing,** as opposed to other types of firing, the point of the iron fires deeper, reaching the subcutaneous tissue or tendon and, when indicated, even the bone —see *firing* for other types of firing —**pin fire** *vt.*

pink eye conjunctivitis

pinky syndrome a harmless but unattractive condition wherein the skin loses pigment, showing pink spots, often around the eyes and muzzle but sometimes on the feet near the coronary band; more common among grays and seems to affect chiefly Arabians; cause is unknown but one factor may be genetic; another may be nutritional because many affected horses lose the spots when given special vitamin-mineral supplements; also called idiopathic spontaneous progressive vitiligo

pinna *n.* the cartilaginous part of the ear that sticks up or projects from the head —**pinnal** *adj.*

Pinto *n.* a type of coloration for which horses of various breeds (except purebreds like Arabs and Thoroughbreds) are selectively bred in the U.S.A. Pintos are generally used as all-purpose saddle horses and vary in size and conformation. Pintos may be either piebald (black and white) or skewbald (white with a color other than black); the actual color patterns are termed Overo (basically a dark coat with white patches, the borders often being lacy-edged and jagged) and Tobiano (basically a white coat with large, dark patches with smooth edges). In the U.S.A. Pintos are covered by three different registries: the American Paint Horse Registry registers stock type horses with Quarter Horse and Thoroughbred breeding; the Pinto Registry registers the stock horse type, Hunter type and Saddle type (predominantly Saddlebred); the Moroccan Spotted Horse Cooperative Association registers gaited horses and also those of Hackney, Thoroughbred, Saddlebred, Tennessee Walker, Arabian and Morgan ancestry. Also called Paint.

pinworm *n.* a white, thread-like, parasitic worm up to 10 cm. long, which can be found in the large intestines and is sometimes apparent in the rectum; causes rectal itching with subsequent tail rubbing; seatworm

Pinzgauer *n.* an Austrian breed used chiefly for draft or pack purposes; often spotted; about 15.3 h.h.

piperazine *n.* a chemical used as a dewormer for roundworms and pinworms

piperonyl butoxide an insecticide

Piroplasma caballi see Babesia caballi

piroplasmosis *n.* a contagious viral disease caused by two types of blood parasites —*Babesia equi* or *Nuttallia*

equi — and transmitted by ticks or possibly biting insects such as flies or mosquitoes; it destroys the red blood cells, causing anemia; incubation in the host is 14–21 days; characterized by fever, lack of energy, and loss of appetite; babesiosis, equine biliary fever, horse tick fever, equine malaria

pirouette *n.* in dressage, a turn within the horse's length, including three kinds: a turn on the center, a turn on the forehand, and a turn on the rear

pisiform *n.* a projecting bone at the back of the knee

pit *n.* an indentation or hollow on some part of the body

pitch *vi.* to buck

pith *vt.* to destroy the brain and spinal cord (of a horse) with an instrument in order to kill or make insensible

pit pony a pony used in mining

pitting edema an accumulation of fluid under the skin which will move when pressed, thereby leaving a pit or surface hollow

pituitary gland a small endocrine gland at the base of the brain; produces growth hormones and influences other glands such as the thyroid and the renal glands

pityriasis *n.* a dry skin condition characterized by scaliness like dandruff and sometimes hair loss; may be caused by lack of exercise or grooming or by disease or digestive troubles

pivot *n.* a 90 degree spin in which, with hind feet in place, a horse pushes off with one forefoot and raises its forehand off the ground as it turns on its hindquarters in a full 90 degree angle, either to right or left, without touching the ground with the forefeet — *see also* **spin** — *vi.*

place *vi.* in racing, to finish second

placenta *n.* a membrane that connects an unborn fetus by the umbilical cord to the mother's uterine wall and serves as a means of receiving nourishment from and discharging wastes to the mother's circulatory system; it is expelled after birth; also called afterbirth — **placental** *adj.*

plait *vt.* to braid (the mane or tail) — *n.*

plane *n.* in reference to the body, a natural line between tissues

planks *n.pl.* in show jumping, an obstacle made up of 12-inch boards

plantar *adj.* relating to the sole of the foot

plantar cushion a shock-absorbing pad of fibrous tissue between the navicular and coffin bones and the sole and frog

Plantation Walking Horse *see* **Tennessee Walker**

plaque *n.* 1. an abnormal patch on the skin or other parts of the body 2. a thin film or deposit which forms on the teeth from the interaction of food, water, and saliva; can harden into tartar

plasma *n.* the clear portion of blood that carries the red and white cells

plasma membrane a thin membrane that envelops a body cell

plasma protein protein contained in the plasma portion of the blood

plasma protein concentration (PPC) total protein (TP) or percentage of protein in plasma; in a healthy horse, the PPC should be approximately 7 percent

plasma therapy a method used to treat uterine infections in which some of a mare's blood is taken and separated; the plasma part is then reintroduced into the uterus to try to form a concentrated defense against the infections

plasmin *n.* an enzyme in blood plasma which can dissolve blood clots

plasmolysis *n.* cell shrinkage caused by loss of water —**plasmolyze** *vt., vi.* to cause or go through plasmolysis

plaster cast a mold made from plaster of Paris and used to encase a fractured limb and prevent its movement

plaster of Paris a thick paste which hardens quickly and is used for a plaster cast

plate *n.* 1. a lightweight shoe for a racehorse 2. (a) a prize given to the winner of a race or contest; (b) a race, the prize for which is a plate rather than stakes 3. a thin layer, as of bone

Plateau Persian a light, hardy breed used by tribesmen who roam the area from the Persian Gulf to the Zagros Mountains bordering Iraq

platelet *n.* a tiny disk, smaller than a red blood cell, in circulating blood which contributes to blood clotting

plate luting a bonding process that is incorporated into compression plating; it fills gaps under the plates, making their fit more secure

plater *n.* an inferior race horse

platten shoe *see* **patten shoe**

playday *n.* a competition that includes barrel racing, pole bending, goat tying, and other events without using rough animals, such as wild bulls and broncs

players *n.pl. see* **keys**

pleura *n., pl.* -**rae** the thin serous membrane that lines the chest cavity and covers the lungs —**pleural** *adj.*

pleural space the space around the lungs

pleurisy, pleuritis *n.* inflammation of the lungs and pleura; characterized by fever, pain which worsens with deep breathing or coughing, and fluids in the chest cavity

pleuropneumonia *n.* pneumonia coupled with pleurisy; a serious respiratory disease characterized by fever, cough, runny nose, and chest pain; can be fatal but complete recovery is possible if treated in its early stages; sometimes broadly termed shipping fever because it often follows stressful travel, although this may not necessarily be the cause —**pleuritic** *adj.*

Pleven *n.* a Bulgarian breed used in riding competitions, including jumping; 15.2 h.h.; it is an Anglo-Arab

plexus *n.* a network of blood vessels or nerves

Pliohippus *n.* an ancient ancestor (Pliocene period) of the modern horse that developed from Merychippus; had a split hoof

plod *vi.* to move in a heavy, uncollected way

plow *n.* a farm implement sometimes drawn by a horse or horses and used to break up and prepare the soil for planting; today, in industrial countries, plowing is usually mechanized —*vi., vi.*; **gang plow** a plow that has several blades arranged in a series

plowboy seat an undesirable and unbalanced way of riding bareback in which the rider flaps his or her elbows and legs while hanging on to the reins

plow rein *see* **open rein**

plug *n.* a nondescript, slow, and undesirable horse

PMSG pregnant mare serum gonadotrophin

pneumobacillus *n.* a type of bacterium that causes lung infection

pneumococcemia *n.* septicemia (blood poisoning) caused by pneumococcus bacteria in the blood

pneumonia *n.* inflammation of the lungs caused by pneumococcus bacteria, a virus, or other germs; characterized by increased respiration, loss of appetite, fever, weakness, and probably slight nasal discharge —*see also* **bronchopneumonia** and **pyemic pneumonia**

pneumoperitoneum *n.* the presence of air in the abdominal cavity

pneumothorax *n.* collection of air in the pleural cavity caused by injury to the chest wall; causes the lungs to collapse, resulting in sudden death

pneumovagina *n.* the presence of air in a mare's vagina when the external genital organs fail to seal the entrance; can cause infertility

point¹ *n.* 1. a projection of the body; e.g., point of hip (which is not literally part of the hip but rather part of the pelvis 2. the shape of a tooth when there is a condition of malocclusion; the tooth develops the point by not being worn evenly; older horses in particular are subject to this, which interferes with chewing, and they may be seen dropping their feed while chewing; these points can be removed by floating

point² *vi.* to stand on three feet with one forefoot just touching the ground; indicates unsoundness, particularly founder; not to be confused with a similar frequent way of standing, with either fore or hind foot resting

point award system the system by which rodeo champions are chosen each year; a competitor wins one point for each dollar earned at the PRCA-approved rodeos during the year's rodeo season; at the end of the season the cowboy who has the most points in a particular event is named PRCA world champion and the one who has won the most points in two or more events is a PRCA world all-around champion

point firing *see* **pin firing**

point of hock *see* **hock**

points *n.pl.* 1. in reference to color, the legs, mane, tail and sometimes the tips of ears; a bay, for example, may be described as having black points 2. in judging breeding, the physical characteristics used as a standard

point to points a type of race run in England from February to May with horses used for hunting during the preceding season. Originally this kind of race was run from one designated point to another; later this developed into two kinds of racing. One remained as it had originated; the other became the professional sport of steeplechasing and hurdle racing.

poison *n.* a substance that, when ingested or absorbed, adversely or even fatally affects the health; toxin

poison hemlock a weed, *Conium maculatum,* that contains the alkaloid conine, which, in fresh leaves only, is toxic to horses; ingestion causes incoordination and trembling with paralysis; treatment can produce recovery but in severe cases, when about 4 lbs. have been ingested, death can occur within 6–12 hours after symptoms appear

Poitevin *n.* a French breed of very unattractive qualities, used chiefly to produce mules; 16.2–17 h.h.

pole bending a timed playday event in which horse and rider maneuver in and out of six lined-up poles and return; a missed turn at a pole disqualifies the rider and five seconds are added to the time for each pole knocked down

police *vt.* to throw (a rider)

Polish Arab the Arab breed bred in Poland since the 16th century and reinforced with fresh stock imported from Arabia from time to time; promoted by the Polish government as this breed has become a valuable export

poll *n.* the uppermost part of a horse's head between the ears

poll evil an inflammation of the fluid-filled sac or bursa just above and behind the poll; may be caused by infection or a trauma such as a badly fitting bridle or a blow to the head; characterized by tenderness around the poll, stiffness in head movement, or pus discharge and swelling

pollution ring a ring made of cloth, rubber or metal for fitting around a stallion's sheath to prevent masturbation by causing slight pain if he tries to achieve an erection

polo *n.* a game played on horseback on a field 300 by 170 yards, with goals eight yards wide and 250 yards apart; two opposing teams, of four players each, try to drive a small wooden ball through the opponents' goal with a long handled mallet. The game is divided into 7½ minute periods called chukkas. "Polo" derives from the Tibetan word "pulu," meaning root or ball. This game dates back to at least 600 B.C. when it was played in Persia; in about the 16th century it appeared in India and there in 1863 was first played by Europeans; in 1869 it started in England and in 1876 it spread to the U.S.A. Indoor polo is played with three players to a team and a soft ball.

polocrosse *n.* a mounted game involving two teams of six riders each who use a long, flexible stick with a small net at the end of it to scoop up a soft ball and carry or toss it to a teammate to try to get it through a goal; only one designated player is allowed to score a goal for his or her team, while the opposing team is allowed only one defending player in the goal-scoring area; periods of play, or chukkas, are six minutes; size of the playing area is 160 by 60 yards

polo pony a horse suitable for playing polo. Must have a responsive, even, courageous temperament; stamina; agility; balance; and speed. Must not be too tall, although now these so-called ponies are taller than formerly and are really horses, ranging in height from 14.2 to 15.3 h.h.

polo race a mounted game in which each competitor has a polo mallet and ball and hits the ball while racing to a post, around which he or she must turn and continue to hit the ball back to the starting line

polyarthritis *n.* inflammation of several joints

polycythemia *n.* a condition characterized by excessive red blood cells

polydipsia *n.* a condition wherein a horse drinks water excessively, resulting in diarrhea; may be caused by a physical problem or may be a vice similar to cribbing

polymorphonuclear leucocyte *n.* a white blood cell that has a lobed nucleus

polyp *n.* a fibrous growth, usually benign, that grows from the membranous lining of a body cavity — **polypous** *adj.*

polyphylism *n.* a belief that the modern horse is descended from several wild ancestors

polypnoea *n.* increased respiration, as in fever

polyuria *n.* the passing of excessive amounts of urine; may indicate nephritis and may also be caused by ingestion of defective fodder; associated with diabetes insipidus — **polyuric** *adj.*

pommel *n.* the raised part of the front of a saddle

poncho *n.* a cloak-like rider's garment, especially a waterproof one

pones *n.pl.* (*colloq.*) mounds of fat on a horse

pony[1] *n.* generally speaking, any horse under 14.2 hands; unlike horses, at birth the pony does not have long legs in proportion to the body and proportionately it is stronger; in England, however, a pony is also a child's mount of any size

pony[2] *vt.* to lead (another horse) while riding

pony cunning (*colloq.*) the pony's apparent advantage over the horse in terms of quicker thinking and power of survival

Pony Express a method of transporting and delivering mail on horseback

between the states of Missouri and California from April 1860 to October 1861

pony horse a horse which, while mounted, guides another horse on lead, especially a racehorse at the race-track

Pony of the Americas a breed developed in the 1950s in Iowa from crossing a Shetland stallion with an Appaloosa mare; the pony's conformation resembles both the Quarter Horse and Arab in miniature but has the coloration of the Appaloosa; the hooves are often striped; popular for riding and showing; 11.2–14 h.h.

POP posterior oxytocin principle

popped knee enlargement of the front of the knee due to cartilage damage, often resulting from racing injuries; **big knee; carpitis; capped knee**

pore *n.* a tiny opening in the skin

position *vt.* to place or stand (a horse) in the correct place, as when getting ready to start a race or lining up with other horses in a show *— n.* 1. the place where a horse is put or stood 2. the way a foal is lying during delivery; e.g. **dorsal position** (normal position with back uppermost) or **ventral position** (upside down)

positive punishment physical discipline after an undesirable act or behavior

positive reinforcement a reward given to a horse after a desired performance or behavior; may be physical (as a pat), material (as a treat to eat), or verbal

posology *n.* the science of drug dosages **— posological** *adj.*

post[1] *n.* in racing, a pole indicating the point at which a race begins or ends

post[2] *vi.* in riding, to rise and sit in rhythm with the horse's trot; this term derives from the postilions who rode the near horses of a coach team and

who devised this method of relief from the constant jarring of the trotters

post and rails in show jumping and cross country courses, an obstacle consisting of upright posts between which are horizontally laid rails which in show jumping are just supported by posts but in cross country events are fixed to the post

post and rails

post bet a bet placed on a racehorse after the numbers of the competitors are posted

posterior *n.* the rear area of the horse's body *— adj.*

posterior digital nerves two nerves located at the back of the pastern which serve the sole and back half of the foot

posterior oxytocin principle (POP) an extract from the pituitary gland that served as an impure source of oxytocin; no longer available because oxytocin is now produced synthetically in pure form

posterior pituitary extract *see* **oxytocin**

post horse a horse used for carrying mail for the Pony Express

Postier *n. see* **Breton**

postilion *n.* 1. a person who rides the left-hand leader of a four-horse carriage 2. a person who rides the left-hand horse of a two-horse carriage when there is no driver

posting *n.* 1. when horses provided the chief mode of overland travel, posting was the term given to traveling in hired post carriages, which gave more privacy than stagecoaches; after 10 miles, horses were changed and the original ones were usually ridden back by an attendant called a **postboy** 2. *see* **post**[2]

post-mortem *n.* (literally, "after

death") autopsy or examination of a dead body to discover cause of death and disease damage; necropsy

postnatal *adj.* of the period immediately after the birth of a foal

postpartum *adj.* of the period following the birth of a foal

postparturient toxemia a toxic reaction in the entire body of a mare caused by uterine infection from causes such as a retained placenta

post rider a rider who carried mail for the Pony Express

post time in racing, the starting time

posture *n.* 1. the way a horse stands 2. the alignment of a foal's legs and neck in utero or presentation during delivery

potato picking scramble a mounted team game or gymkhana event in which a heap of potatoes is piled in the center of an arena, a bucket is placed for each team and, during a set time limit, two members of each team race back and forth, putting as many potatoes as they can in their buckets; the horse rounds the bucket in much the same way as a Western barrel racer rounds a barrel

Potomac horse fever a disease of the bloodstream caused by rickettsia microorganisms; so named because it was first recognized as a seasonal disease in 1979 in the Potomac Valley; may cause fever, laminitis, and diarrhea

Pottock *n.* see **Basque**

poultice *n.* a soft substance applied to an area of the body to reduce inflammation or change temperature — *vt.*

povidone iodine an iodine solution which does not burn on application; tamed iodine

pox *n.* see **horsepox**

PPC plasma protein concentration

ppm parts per million (a measurement, as of ammonia gas)

prairie schooner see **Conestoga wagon**

prance *vi.* to move in a very lively way, with high action — *n.* such a movement

PRCA Professional Rodeo Cowboys Association; sets the rules for members who compete in professional rodeos

predispose *vt.* make susceptible, as overeating grain predisposes a horse to colic — **predisposition** *n.*

prednisolone *n.* a synthetic steriod used to reduce inflammation

prednisone *n.* a synthetic steriod used to reduce inflammation

preferred associates horses who share a preference for each other

prefix *n.* a name added before a horse's name when registered to denote the breeder's ranch — *see also* **suffix**

pregnancy toxemia an acute condition in undernourished and stressed mares in their last few weeks of pregnancy, characterized by an abnormal nervous function, coma, and finally death

pregnant *adj.* in foal; having a developing fetus in the uterus — **pregnancy** *n.*

pregnant mare serum gonadotrophin (PMSG) a follicle-stimulating hormone in a pregnant mare from about days 40–90; can be obtained from the mare's blood and administered to male and female recipients to stimulate the sex organs, although this procedure is not very successful and is not generally used any more — *see also* **serum gonadotrophin**

prehensile *adj.* able to grasp, especially by wrapping around the object being grasped, as in the case of the horse's lips when grazing — **prehensility** *n.*

premature *adj.* occurring before the normal time, as in the birth of a foal — **prematurity** *n.*

premolar *n.* any of 12 grinding teeth behind the bar and in front of the molars

prenatal *adj.* before birth — **prenatally** *adv.*

prepartum *n.* before parturition

prepotency *n.* the ability to pass on certain characteristics to offspring — **prepotent** *adj.*

prepuce *n.* the foreskin of the penis — **preputial** *adj.*

presence *n.* a proud bearing or personality; a quality possessed by a horse whose beauty of character, as well as body, commands the attention of the beholder

presentation *n.* the position in which a foal emerges at birth; **anterior presentation:** head first (normal); **posterior presentation:** hindquarters first; **transverse presentation:** crosswise

President's Cup a trophy awarded annually to the country that in one year won the highest number of points in Nation's Cup show-jumping; first awarded by Prince Philip of England in 1965

pressure bandage an elasticized bandage used to apply pressure to a wound or injury to stop bleeding and control swelling

prevesical *adj.* in front of the urinary bladder

priapism *n.* in the male, a prolonged penile erection

prick *n.* a puncture of the bottom of the hoof made either when the horse steps on a nail, wire, etc., or when a farrier hammers in a nail too close to the white line; a spot of blood and lameness may be observed and, if not treated immediately, pus formation and intense pain may develop — *vt.*

prick the ears to hold the ears erect and attentively

primagravida *n.* a mare in foal for the first time

primary fever fever which develops as the first signal of a pathology without any other apparent signs; essential fever

primary treatment the first and principal in a series of treatments

prime *n.* the best or most vigorous stage of life; a horse's prime is generally considered to be between the ages of 6 and 10

Primeval Pony a type of pony that has been discovered to have roamed all over Europe and Asia in the ancient past; it had a two-layered coat and short legs

primidone *n.* an anticonvulsant drug

primordial cyst a defect of the tooth bud (cellular foundation of the tooth) which may appear shortly after birth

pritchel *n.* a steel tool with a point used by a farrier to open and resize nail holes in a shoe

privet *n.* an evergreen shrub of the genus *Ligustrum* that has small white blossoms and, if ingested in significant amounts, is poisonous to the horse; most well fed horses are not interested in eating it but some may do so, particularly during winter when grass is either scarce or nonexistent

Prix des Nations an international jumping event held at an international horse show and involving competing teams; each team comprises four members who jump the course twice, and the three best scores of each team are counted in each round; in the event of a tie, a jump-off is held in which faults and time are totaled for a final result, counting only the three best scores and time of each team

prize money in rodeo, the money earned by winners of each event; it consists of the total of added money (that which is put up by the rodeo committee) and the competitors' entry fees

procaine *n.* a synthetic local anesthetic

procaine penicillin G a penicillin antibiotic agent used in intramuscular injections

process *n.* 1. a continuing action, as e.g. of training 2. a bony outgrowth

proctitis *n.* inflammation of the anus and rectum

proctoscope *n.* a tube used for insertion into the anus for examination purposes

Professional Rodeo Circuit System a system of rodeo circuits in 12 geographical regions across the United States that provide a means for skilled professional cowboys to compete and qualify for rewards close to home in their particular circuit. Each circuit, although part of the PRCA (Professional Rodeo Cowboys Association), functions independently, having its own board of directors; contestants must compete in their own circuit in order to earn circuit points. Champions are determined by their accumulated points at the end of the year; additionally, at the end of each 12-month season, top circuit cowboys are invited to Circuit Finals Rodeo and the winners from these finals are then eligible to enter the Dodge National Circuit Finals Rodeo.

progenitor *n.* a parent or ancestor

progeny *n.* offspring

progesterone *n.* a hormone, secreted by the corpus luteum of the female ovaries, which prepares the uterus for a fertilized ovum as well as the mammary glands for milk secretion

progestins *n.pl.* hormones secreted by the corpus luteum of the female ovaries, 95 percent of which comprise progesterone

prognosis *n.* an advance calculation of the course of a disease and individual's chances of recovery

progressive *adj.* 1. moving onward 2. continuing step by step 3. in disease, increasing in severity

progressive loading a conditioning system of methodically subjecting a horse to progressively increasing exercise periods with intervals allowing for physical response and adaptation

prolactin *n.* a pituitary hormone that stimulates milk production

prolan *n.* a hormone produced by the pituitary **gland**

prolapse *n.* the outward dislocation of an internal organ — *vi.*

proliferate *vi.* to reproduce or grow in profusion, as in similar cell production — *vt.* to produce (new parts) — **proliferation** *n.*

prolific *adj.* producing many offspring

promazine hydrochloride a tranquilizer

promethazine hydrochloride an antihistamine; trade name Phenergan

propagate *vi.* to reproduce or multiply — *vt.* 1. to breed (a horse); to reproduce or multiply (itself) 2. to transmit (hereditary characteristics) — **propagation** *n.*

prophase *n.* the first stage in mitosis (division of body cells)

prophet's thumb a muscle impression observed usually on the neck and caused by pressure on the developing muscle of the fetus; resembles the impression left by a human thumb when pressed on something soft, such as clay

prophylaxis *n.* preventive measure(s) taken against a disease, as a vaccine — **prophylactic** *adj.*

propionic acid preservation a technique for preserving hay which allows hay to be gathered and stored at a higher moisture content than when it is processed naturally

proprioception *n.* the instinctive sense that motivates horses to stay on their feet, always alert and ready to run from danger

propulsion *n.* a driving forward, as in describing the power of the horse's hind legs as they propel or push the horse forward — **propel** *vt.* — **propulsive, propulsory** *adj.*

proquamezine fumerate a mild tranquilizer; trade name Myspamol

prostaglandin *n.* a hormonelike fatty acid substance produced by body cells and affecting control of important body activities, such as reproduction, lowering blood pressure, inflammation, etc.

prostate gland a gland in the male behind the neck of the bladder; secretes a fluid with sperm

prosthesis *n.* an artificial substitute for a body part — **prosthetic** *adj.*

prostrate *adj.* totally exhausted and probably lying down — **prostration** *n.*

protease *n.* an enzyme that digests proteins

protective protein a protein that acts as a defense, such as an antibody or blood clotting

protein *n.* a constituent of animal and plant cells consisting of many elements; an essential component of a horse's diet

protein-losing enteropathy an intestinal disorder caused by loss of too much protein

proteinuria *n.* the presence of protein in the urine, symptomatic of kidney disease

proteoglycans *n.pl.* water-retaining molecules in cartilage

prothrombin *n.* a body protein that induces the production of thrombin, a substance essential to blood clotting; synthesized by the liver

protoplasm *n.* the essential material of animal and plant cells — **protoplasmic** *adj.*

prototype *n.* 1. the original being of a species 2. a model example of a particular type — **prototypical, prototypic** *adj.*

protozoal mylitis inflammation and degeneration of the spinal cord caused by protozoa

protozoan *n.*, *pl.* **-zoa** any of various single-celled microscopic animals of the phylum *Protozoa,* some of which can cause parasitic disease

protraction *n.* forward stride of the foreleg

protuberance *n.* something which bulges out, such as a swelling — **protuberant** *adj.*

proud flesh granulation tissue which becomes raised above the level of the skin around a wound; it is raw and delays healing, sometimes making healing impossible without medication or surgery

proximal *adj.* closest to the center of the body or closest to the point of attachment of a body part — **proximally** *adv.*

Przewalski *n.* the only surviving species of a true wild horse; found on the border of China; it is quite distinct from all other horses; named after Colonel Przewalski who discovered this type in 1881; very few remain in the wild but some are held in zoos; dun-colored with black points and black dorsal stripe; about 12 h.h.

psammoma *n.* a brain tumor

pseudoglanders *n. see* **epizootic lymphangitis**

pseudohermaphrodite *n.* a horse that has the rare abnormality of having internal reproductive organs of one sex and external ones resembling those of the opposite sex — **pseudohermaphroditism, pseudohermaphrodism** *n.* — **pseudohermaphroditic** *adj.*

pseudomonas *n.* a type of bacteria that prevail in open wounds and are resistant to treatment; characterized by a green color in the wound and an odor of rotten grapes

psoas major a back muscle that flexes the hip joint and revolves the thigh outward

psoas minor a back muscle that flexes the pelvis on the back

psoriasis carpi a dermatitis character-

ized by scabs; affecting the knee mallenders

psoriasis tarsi a dermatitis characterized by scabs affecting the front of the hock; sallenders

psoroptic mange mange caused by psoroptic parasites, occurring mainly on areas covered with long hair

PSS physiologic saline solution

psychogenic *adj.* of the mind —**psychogenically** *adv.*

Pteridium aquilinum see **bracken fern**

ptermalid *n.* stingless wasp that indirectly acts as a type of larvicide; it lays eggs on fly pupae that flies have laid on dung; as both mature, the ptermalids devour the flies, thus forming a type of fly control and ultimately an exterior type of larvicide for the horse

pterygoid *adj.* wing-shaped; used in relation to a part of the body, as a bone

pterygoideus lateralis a muscle that controls the jaw

pterygoideus medialis a muscle that controls the side to side movement and closing of the mouth

ptosis *n.* a falling or drooping of a body part, such as the upper eyelid

ptyalin *n.* an enzyme in saliva that converts starch to sugar

ptyalism *n.* excessive secretion of saliva; slobbering; causes are many and varied: effect of certain drugs, stomatitis, teeth abnormalities, presence of a foreign object or wound in the mouth, inability to swallow due to a paralysis, esophageal blockage

puberty *n.* the physical developmental stage at which sexual reproduction becomes possible —**pubescent** *adj.*

pubis *n.* one of the three pelvic bones (other two being the ischium and the ilium) —**pubic** *adj.* of or in the area of the pubis

puddle *vi.* to shuffle, dragging the feet, instead of lifting them and stepping properly; lazy or old horses are sometimes prone to this

puff disease *see* **anhidrosis**

puffer *n.* at an auction, a person who bids up the price of a horse for the seller but does not plan to buy

puff the glims (eyes) to puff up or inflate the hollows above the eyes to make an old horse look younger; a small hole is cut through the skin and air blown into the cavity through a quill

puissance *n.* strength or power; a jumping contest in which the strength of the contesting horse is judged by the height and distance that it can jump —**puissant** *adj.* —**puissantly** *adv.*

pull *vt.* 1. in racing, to restrain (a horse) 2. to stretch or strain (a ligament or muscle) 3. to draw in harness, as a carriage 4. to force out, as a tooth —*vi.* to strain on the reins, as when a horse ignores the rider's aids

pull corn blood in the white line of the hoof due to bleeding from strain on the laminae caused by too long a toe and low heels; push corn

pull leather in saddle bronc riding, to hold onto any part of the saddle during the 8-second ride, as a result of which the rider is disqualified; grab the apple

pulmonary *adj.* relating to the lungs

pulmonary alveolar emphysema *see* **heaves**

pulmonary artery the artery that carries oxygen-depleted blood to the lungs

pulmonary edema excessive fluid in lung tissues

pulp *n.* the soft, sensitive substance under the enamel and dentine of a tooth

pulse *n.* the intermittent beat of an artery caused by the contractions of the heart; the normal pulse of a horse at rest is 24–44 beats per minute but can rise to 70 beats when a horse is excited or sick

pumiced feet the rough, pumice-stone-like appearance of hoofs that have had corinitis or laminitis for an extended period and have thus lost their concavity

punter *n.* a person who regularly bets on race horses

pupa *n., pl.* -ae a developmental stage of an insect, as the fly, between the larval and adult forms, often enveloped in a cocoon — **pupal** *adj.*

pupil *n.* the black center of the iris of the eye through which light enters; in young horses the shape is roundish but by 5–6 years it is elliptical — **pulillary** *adj.*

pupillary dilator a drug that causes the pupil of the eye to widen

purebred *n.* a horse of a distinct breed whose sire and dam are registered in the same studbook; one of unmixed descent

purgative *n.* a strong laxative — **purge** *vt.* to empty (the bowels) by means of a laxative — *n.*

purpura *n.* a hemorrhage into the skin characterized by edema, swollen lips and nostrils and sometimes eyelids, sore muscles and inflammation of mucous membranes; several causes which may include inadequate platelets or an allergy to bacterial antigens in the bloodstream; also called anasarcous fever, putrid fever, petechial fever

purulent *adj.* containing, resembling, or discharging pus

pus *n.* the slightly thick, yellowish fluid containing bacteria, white blood cells, etc., and produced in certain infections

pushball *n.* a mounted game involving two teams, each of which tries to push a large soft ball over the opponent's goal; the horses do most of the pushing

push corn a pink or red spot on the sole of the foot resulting from bleeding in the angle of the sole or the white line adjacent to it; caused by a low heel receiving too much concussion; pull corn

pustular stomatitis a form of horse pox affecting the mouth and involving eruptions on the lips, gums, and tongue; like any pox, it is contagious

pustule *n.* a small, pimple-like abscess containing pus

put down to destroy — *see also* **euthanasia**

putrefaction *n.* rotting of tissue caused by bacteria or fungi, as in gangrene

putrefy *vt., vi.* to decay or become rotten — **putrefier** *n.* — **putrid** *adj.*

putrid fever *see* **purpura**

pyelitis *n.* inflammation of the pelvis of one or both kidneys

pyelo-nephritis the involvement of the pelvis of the kidney in nephritis

pyemia *n.* the presence of pus-producing bacteria in the blood — **pyemic** *adj.*

pyemic pneumonia a type of pneumonia involving pyemia that may attack young foals; characterized by numerous abscesses in the lungs; because it is usually well advanced before detection, it is usually fatal; external symptoms include cough, nasal discharge, and lethargy

pylons *n.pl.* a playday event in which competitors ride down the center of six pylons or cones and circle around a seventh pylon placed at the end between the last two then return down the center

pylorus *n.* the opening from the stomach into the duodenum or first

part of the small intestine — **pyloric** *adj.*

pyogenic *adj.* pus-forming — **pyogenesis** *n.*

pyometritis *n.* an uncommon condition of inflammation in the uterus characterized by vaginal discharge of pus; occasionally occurs in older mares and results from trauma to the uterus or infection of the endometrium

pyorrhea *n. see* **alveolar periostitis**

pyramidal disease *see* **pyramiditis**

pyramiditis *n.* an abnormal bone growth that pushes up the front of the coronary band; buttress foot; pyramidal disease

pyrantel *n.* a dewormer used to combat most intestinal parasites, excluding botfly larvae

pyretic *adj.* pertaining to, causing, or characterized by fever

pyrexia *n.* fever — **pyrexial, pyrexic** *adj.*

pyridoxine *n.* a component of vitamin B

pyrogen *n.* a substance that causes fever when injected, such as may be found in outdated medicines — **pyrogenic** *adj.* causing fever

pyrrolizidine alkaloid a toxin found in certain weeds, such as ragwort, groundsel, rattleweed (crotalaria), fiddleneck (amsinckia); if ingested, causes damage to the liver

— Q —

quadratus femoris a muscle that extends the hip joint and adducts the thigh

quadratus lumborum a muscle that flexes the pelvis on the back

quadriceps femoris a four-headed muscle of the femur

quadriga *n.* a two-wheeled chariot, drawn by four horses abreast, used in medieval times

quadrille 1. dressage movements in unison by four or more horses and riders 2. a horse "dance" involving 2, 4, or 8 riders; this kind of performance has a very long history, dating back to about 700 B.C., but declined for centuries until the late 19th century when it was revived; today quadrille competitions are held in England as well as other countries

quadruped *n.* a four-footed animal, like a horse

quality *n.* the fineness of a horse, as differing from substance — *see* **substance**

quantity intervals the intervals in a conditioning exercise between periods of strenuous work when the pulse is raised to 180–200 beats per minute for 1 to 2 minutes and relief periods of jogging when the pulse returns to 110–120 beats per minute

quarantine *n.* 1. a detention imposed for a period of time on horses imported from a foreign country for the purpose of preventing the spread of any disease that they may carry 2. the state of being quarantined 3. the place where the quarantined horses are kept 4. the isolation of a sick horse — *vt.* to place under quarantine; to isolate — **quarantinable** *adj.*

quarter *n.* the part of the hoof between the heel and toe

quarter boots *see* **bell boots**

quarter crack a vertical split or crack in the hoof wall between heel and toe; it may start at the coronet and work

quarter crack

down or start at the bottom of the hoof and work up —*see also* **crack**

Quarter Horse an American breed widely used in the West for working cattle; originally bred by English colonists by crossing imported English stallions with Mustangs; the breed's name derives from quarter-mile races for which it is famous; a very muscular horse with an intelligent, calm disposition that makes a good pleasure mount; average of 15.2 h.h.

Quarter Horse poles a timed playday event in which competitors ride up on one side to the last of six poles set in a straight line, weave back around each one, then up again in the same pattern to the last pole, and finally back on the other side in a straight line to the starting point

quartering *n.* the procedure of grooming a blanketed horse by first throwing the blanket back and grooming the front, then throwing the blanket forward to groom the quarters

quarter masks hair patterns made on a horse's quarters for appearance only, usually on racehorses or show horses; a design is made by brushing the hair in reverse to the hair growth with a wet brush

quarters *n.pl.* the hind legs and adjoining parts; specifically, the rear part of the horse between the flank and root of tail and down to the upper part of the gaskin

quarter sheet a rectangular sheet that covers a horse's back and sides from withers to root of tail; when a horse is

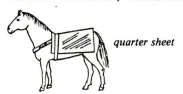

quarter sheet

being exercised, the front corners are folded back under the girth strap to form what is called a **galloping sheet**

Queensland itch an allergic reaction to certain flies, specifically the saliva of certain small flies such as culicoides, midges, etc.; so named because it is common in Australia; causes severe itching and exuding sores

quick *n. see* **laminar corium**

quidding *n.* a condition in which a horse rolls food about in its mouth after partially chewing it and then eventually rejects it; may be caused by some condition of the tongue or, as is most frequently the case, a problem involving the teeth —**quid** *vi.* —**quiddor** *n.* a horse who quids

quinella *n.* in racing, a type of betting in which to win, a bettor must pick the first- and second-place finishers in any order

quinidine sulfate a drug used to steady the heartbeat

quinine *n.* a crystalline alkaloid, a compound of which is used for medicinal purposes

quinsy *n.* an abscessed condition of the throat which can occur in various diseases, such as strangles —*see also* **strangles**

quintain *n.* in medieval sports, an object, such as a shield, on a pivoted crossbar, balanced on the other end of the bar by something like a bag of sand; a rider had to strike the quintain and try to escape the sandbag as it swung around from the impact of the strike; the sport itself was also called quintain

quinuronium sulfate a drug used to treat biliary fever; has almost immediate side effects that may include e.g., muscular spasms and salivation persisting for several hours, but can be counteracted with adrenaline or atropine

quirt *n.* a bullwhip

quittor *n.* a persistent suppuration from the coronet of the foot caused either directly by an injury, such as a

quirt

tread, or indirectly from suppuration inside the hoof from a puncture, corn, or crack; characterized by lameness and severe tenderness in the affected area

quiver *vi.* to tremble *—n.*

quotation *n.* in racing, the odds on a horse quoted by a bookmaker

— R —

rabicano *adj.* a color pattern that may be limited to a few white hairs on the flank and base of the tail or may involve more numerous white hairs on these same areas or may cover such an extensive area as to be confused with roan; squaw tail *—n.*

rabies *n.* a contagious disease transmitted chiefly in the saliva of rabid animals, such as skunks, racoons, dogs, etc., that might bite a horse on the nose or leg. This is not a common disease among horses but it does occur and once symptoms appear, recovery is considered hopeless. The infected horse usually goes through two phases; the first is the "dumb" phase, characterized by depression and listlessness with long, totally inactive periods; the second is the "furious" stage, which brings on restlessness and sometimes violence which can be dangerous; there may be grinding of teeth and foaming at the mouth and, as the disease progresses, retention of urine and feces; finally, paralysis ensues and death occurs within 5 to 8 days

race¹ *n.* a riding competition of speed *—vi., vt.*

race² *n.* a narrow, white facial marking usually starting from the forehead with a wide area which narrows down into an irregular line to the muzzle, sometimes veering off at the end to one nostril

race card a printed card that contains information pertaining to horses races, including type and time of each race, horses' names and their owners and trainers, and handicaps

racecourse *n.* a race track for various types of horse races as well as all the accompanying facilities, such as grandstand, paddock, stables, office buildings, etc.

racehorse *n.* a horse bred and trained for racing

race track a course for racing, especially an oval one

raceway *n.* a race track for harness racing

racing plate a thin, very lightweight horseshoe used on racehorses

racing saddle *n.* a saddle especially suited for use in racing; may range from a very light weight of less than two pounds, used for flat racing, to the heavier type used for hurdling and steeplechasing

racing seat the singular position a jockey maintains when racing as he leans forward and above the saddle on very short stirrups

rack *n.* a fast, even gait in which each foot strikes the ground separately in quick succession; it resembles the pace in that the forefoot and hind foot on the same side leave the ground at the same time, but, unlike the true pace, because of high forefoot action, the hind foot hits the ground before the forefoot; it is a gait of the American Saddlebred; also called single-foot; *—see also* **stepping pace**

radial nerve paralysis a degenerative condition of the elbow caused by damage to the radial nerve when it has been overstretched; loss of elbow function and severe lameness result;

the foot is unable to lift normally and, with complete paralysis, the horse stands with shoulder drooping and knee flexed with only the toe resting on the ground; the nerve is stretched when there is repeated slipping forward of the foreleg, as may be seen when playful youngsters race about and make sliding stops on slippery surfaces up to a fence, thereby overstretching the forelegs; also called dropped elbow

radiograph *n.* an image produced by X-rays on a special sensitized film and taken of internal parts of the body that cannot be seen externally; X-ray — **radiographic** *adj.* — **radiographically** *adv.*

radioimmunoassay *n.* technique used to analyze antibody protein by introducing radioactive tracers into body fluid and measuring the emission

radioisotope *n.* a radioactive atom whose measurable decay makes it an important diagnostic and therapeutic tool in medicine and research; radioactive isotope

radiology *n.* the science of X-raying internal body parts for diagnosis — **radiological** *adj.* — **radiologically** *adv.*

radiotherapy *n.* the use of radiation to treat diseases

radium *n.* a radioactive metal whose emissions can be used to destroy malignant cells

radius *n.* the long bone in the foreleg between the elbow and knee; forearm

radon *n.* a radioactive gas of radium

ragwort *n.* groundsel

rainrot *see* **rain scald**

rain scald a fungal skin condition that erupts in wet weather and affects mainly the mane and tail and sometimes the back; not to be confused with sweet itch; exudations at the roots of the hair form scabs that mat the hair and leave the coat, including lower limbs and heels, with bare patches; so called because it is caused by prolonged moisture on a dirty, neglected coat; also called rainrot, mud fever, dermatophilosis, mycotic dermatitis, greasy heel

rake *n.* in rodeo, the spurring action of a competitor — *see also* **reef a horse**

rales *n.pl.* abnormal bronchial sounds; referred to as **crepitant rales** (fine crackling sounds), **dry rales** (wheezing or whistling), **moist rales** (gurgling sounds)

ramp *n.* a sloping surface on which to ascend to or descend from an upper level, as that used for horses to enter or exit a trailer

ramus *n.* a branch in the body, as of a nerve

R.A.N.A. Registered Animal Nursing Auxiliary; a qualified animal nurse

ranahan *n.* (Western) a good rider

ranch *n.* an acreage, including buildings, etc., used for raising horses (and or other livestock) — *vi.* to work on or manage a ranch — *vt.* to raise (livestock) on a ranch

rancher *n.* a person who owns, manages, or works on a ranch; a cowboy

random *n.* three harness horses driven in single file

range *n.* an extensive open area of land on which livestock can graze or run

range horse a horse that has lived on the range without human contact

rapping pole a pole used to train jumpers to lift their hind legs properly when clearing a jump by rapping their belly right after the forelegs have gone over; sometimes used indiscriminately, which is cruel

rash *n.* a spotty skin eruption — *see also* **urticaria**

rasp *vt., vi.* 1. to file with a rasp, as in

rasping the teeth or hooves   2. to make a grating sound — *n.*   1. a rough file; rasper   2. a grating sound —**rasping** *adj.*

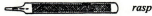 *rasp*

rasper *n.* in hunting, a large fence

rate *n.* in cutting, the ability to maintain the correct cutting position in relation to the cow being worked — *vt.* in hunting, to discipline (the hounds)

ration *n.* a determined portion, as of feed — *vt.* to supply with a ration

rattles *n.* pneumonia (because of the rattling sound when breathing)

rattleweed *see* crotalaria

rawhide *n.*   1. *see* **leather**   2. a whip made of rawhide — *vt.* to beat with rawhide

rear *vt.*   1. to breed (animals)   2. *vi.* (of horses) to rise up on the hind legs

reata *n.* *see* **riata**

recalcitrant *adj.* defiant and difficult to handle —**recalcitrance** *n.*

receptor *n.* an organ that senses or receives stimuli, as a nerve ending

recessive gene a gene whose trait will appear in offspring only when paired with an identical corresponding gene; many recessive traits remain hidden for generations before unexpectedly appearing in a foal

recessive trait a non-apparent genetic trait that is suppressed by a corresponding dominant trait and appears only when both of its corresponding alleles are identical so that it cannot be suppressed by the presence of a dominant counterpart allele (example: the recessive trait of blue eyes will appear in offspring only if both parents pass on the blue-eye genes; otherwise, a dominant brown-eye gene will subdue the blue-eye gene and the offspring will be browneyed)

reciprocal muscle action the responsive action of one muscle contracting while another corresponding muscle relaxes; this cooperation between muscles not only enables movement but also provides smooth rather than jerky movement

recombinant vaccine a vaccine derived from combining parts of a genome (heritable material) from two different viruses

recombination *n.* the appearance in offspring of new combinations of genes differing from those of the parents, resulting from cross-breeding —**recombinant** *n.* the offspring possessing these combinations

recto-vaginal fistula an abnormal opening between the rectum and vagina caused by a foal's hoof during delivery

rectum *n.* the last portion of the large intestine

rectus abdominis a muscle that compresses the abdomen to aid in birth, defecation, and expiration

rectus capitis dorsalis major and **minor** muscles that extend the head

rectus capitis ventralis major, minor, and **lateralis** muscles that flex the head

rectus thoracis a chest muscle that helps in respiration

recumbent *adj.* in or relating to a lying-down position —**recumbency** *n.*

recurrent uveitis periodic ophthalmia or moonblindness

red blood cell one of the components of blood; a tiny, circular disk with concave faces that contains hemoglobin that provides oxygen to body tissues; erythrocyte

red dun *see* **dun**

red flag a flag used in equestrian sports to mark the right-hand extremity of any obstacle; also used to mark a set track and must always be passed on the left-hand side

red ribbon one that is tied around the tail of a horse, especially when hunting, to indicate that he has the habit of kicking

red-tailed botfly nose botfly — *see also Gastrophilus hemorrhoidalis*

redtop grass a rhizome type, moisture-loving grass that grows in cool temperatures and usually has reddish floral clusters, used for hay or pasture

redworm *n. see* **strongyle**

reef (a horse) in rodeo, to slide one's legs back and forth along a bronco's sides to make him buck harder; rake; fan; scratch

reflex *n.* an automatic response to a stimulus

reflex arc the whole nerve path relating to a reflex action

refusal *n.* a horse's declining to jump an obstacle either by passing it or stopping in front of it

regeneration *n.* the natural replacement of an injured or lost part or tissue

regimen *n.* a set therapeutic plan or routine of diet, exercise, etc., to maintain or improve health or condition

regurgitate *vi.* to flow backward, as blood may due to faulty heart valves, or when stomach contents are vomited — *see also* **vomit** — **regurgitation** *n.*

rein *n.* one of a pair of straps attached to a bit and used for guiding and controlling a horse — *vt.* to control (a horse) by means of the reins

rein back to make a horse back while being ridden or driven — *see also* **back**

rein in to slow down a horse with the reins

reject *vt.* 1. to refuse to accept, as a mare may a stallion 2. to abandon, as a mare may her foal

relapse *n.* a recurrence of an illness after apparent recovery — *vi.*

relapsing fever *see* **intermittent fever**

relax *vt., vi.* to release tension; to become less tense — **relaxation** *n.* — **relaxed** *adj.*

relaxant *n.* a drug to reduce tension

relaxin *n.* a hormone which is released in the mare just prior to foaling to relax the pelvic muscles

relay race a race between teams involving competitors who run in turn only part of the way; each team member will run to a designated stop and be replaced by another member

remedy *n.* 1. a medicine or treatment that heals a disease or physical disorder 2. a corrective course of action directed towards something like bad behavior

remission *n.* in regard to illness, a relief of the symptoms — **remissive** *adj.*

remittent fever a fever whish rises and falls at short or daily intervals

remount *vt.* 1. to mount a horse again 2. — *n.* a fresh horse to replace another — *vt.* to supply with a fresh horse

remuda *n.* a group of riding horses standing as remounts

renal *adj.* relating to the kidneys

renin *n.* an enzyme

renvers *n.* a dressage movement on two tracks in which a horse, slightly bent, goes forward at an angle of not more than 30 degrees with hind legs on the outer track and forelegs on the inner track, looking straight ahead

reorganize *vi., vt.* to cue a horse back into the proper stride or way of going

rep *n.* a cowboy who rounds up cattle that have strayed from the employer's ranch

reproduce *vt., vi.* 1. to generate offspring 2. to regenerate lost tissue or organs — **reproduction** *n.*

re-ride *n.* in rodeo, another opportunity given to a competitor in a particular event when either the competitor or the animal has not had a fair chance, such as may happen when an animal in

the chute makes mounting impossible or falls

resilience, resiliency *n.* 1. the elastic quality of springing back to normal shape, as the skin after being swollen 2. the ability to recover normalcy — **resilient** *adj.* — **resile** *vi.* — **resiliently** *adv.*

resist *vt., vi.* 1. to oppose or try to avoid, as to resist being caught or trained or to refuse to obey, etc. 2. to engage in self-defense by kicking and biting — **resistance** *n.* — **resistant** *adj.*

resistance *n.* the body's ability to ward off infection through either immunity or the naturally defending white blood cells

resolution *n.* the reduction or disappearance of a swelling or disease symptoms

resonance *n.* the percussive sound produced within the body — **resonant** *adj.*

respiration *n.* breathing — **respirational, respiratory** *adj.*

respirator *n.* an apparatus used during surgery to facilitate breathing

respire *vi., vt.* to breathe

responsive *adj.* tending to react quickly and easily to a rider's aids

rest *n.* a period of ease and relaxation; sleep — *vi.*

restive *adj.* nervous and impatient, especially under restraint

restrain *vt.* 1. to hold back under control 2. to deprive of liberty, as in an enclosure — **restraint** *n.*

resuscitate *vt.* to revive

retention *n.* the holding in the body of a substance or fluid normally excreted

reticuloendothelial system a netlike structure of phagocytic cells in bone marrow and liver; can absorb bacteria

reticulum *n.* a weblike structure as found in various cells of the body

retina *n.* the light-sensitive membrane at the rear of the eye on which images are focused by the lens and are then in turn transmitted to the optic nerve and on to the brain — **retinal** *adj.*

retinal *n.* a product of digested vitamin A used by the body for bone growth and chemistry of vision

retinal cones bodies within the retina that generate electrical impulses when struck by light

retinal detachment a detachment or loosening of the retina from the eyeball; may be caused by retinitis or injury and may cause blindness

retinal rods cylindrical, retinal structures of the eye that give off electrical impulses under stimulation of light

retinitis *n.* inflammation of the retina

retinoblastoma *n.* a malignant retinal tumor

retinol *n.* a chemical produced by the retina that helps the eyes to focus in darkness

retinopathy *n.* retinal disease

retinosope *n.* an instrument for examining the retina of the eye

retract *vt.* to draw back, as in (a) surgery when the tissues are held back by an instrument (retractor) to allow penetration into deeper areas or (b) the action of a muscle when it withdraws an organ, etc.

retractor *n.* 1. an instrument used in surgery to hold back tissues or allow work in deeper areas 2. a muscle that withdraws an organ or other body part

retrobulbar *adj.* behind the eyeball

retrocecal *adj.* behind the cecum

retrocolic *adj.* behind the large intestine

retroflex, retroflexed *adj.* turned or bent backward, as an organ of the body — **retroflexion** *n.*

retrogress *vi.* to go backward or de-

cline in condition — **retrogressive** *adj.* — **retrogressively** *adv.* — **retrogression** *n.*

retrolental *adj.* behind the lens of the eye

retroverted *adj.* tilted backward, as an organ of the body — **retroversion** *n.*

retrovirus *n.* a virus imbedded in the body beyond the immune system

reversed hide *see* **leather**

revive *vt., vi.* to bring or come back to (a) consciousness or (b) a healthy condition after a decline — **revival** *n.*

reward *n.* something given in response to a desired behavior; it may be in the form of a treat to eat or a relaxation of restraint — *vt.*

rhabdomyoma *n.* a muscle tumor

rhabdomyosarcoma *n.* a malignant muscle tumor

Rhenish *n.* a heavy, powerful German cold-blood breed with short legs developed in the Rhineland early in the 20th century; commonly chestnut with flaxen tail and two-sided mane; nearly extinct now due to farm mechanization; 16–17 h.h.; Rhineland

rheum *n.* 1. a watery discharge as of the eyes, nose, or mouth 2. a cold — **rheumy** *adj.*

rheumatism *n.* an affliction of the joints, muscles, and tendons characterized by stiffness, inflammation, and pain, like arthritis

Rh factor a component of the blood so named because it was first discovered in the blood of rhesus monkeys (Rh is an abbreviation of rhesus); when present, the blood is termed Rh positive and when absent Rh negative; when an Rh negative mare bears an Rh positive foal, serious complications occur that can lead to death of the foal

Rhineland *see* **Rhenish**

rhinitis *n.* an inflammatory condition of the nasal mucous membranes

rhinopneumonitis *n.* a contagious viral disease characterized by fever, mild respiratory catarrh and, in mares, abortion; transmitted from the mucous membranes through direct or indirect contact; equine virus abortion; equine herpesvirus

rhinosporidiosis *n.* a nasal fungus infection characterized by growth on the mucous membranes

rhinovirus *n.* a virus that causes colds and other respiratory tract ailments

rhizoctonia leguminicola a toxic fungal growth on legumes; can adversely affect horses who graze on infected legumes or eat hay from them; characterized in these horses first by slobbering and oral irritation but may cause more serious symptoms or death; black patch disease

Rhodococcus equi an organism that causes pneumonia in foals; usually fatal; also called *Corynebacterium equi*

rhododendron *n.* a shrub that is poisonous to horses

rhodopsin *n.* a retinal pigment that enables the eye to adapt to darkness

rhomboideus muscle the neck muscle that lies along the crest

rhonchus *n.* a loud wheezing sound heard when the chest is auscultated; it is a symptom of mucus in the bronchial tubes

rhythm *n.* a flowing, regular movement as that of a rider who posts in rhythm with the horse's trot

riata, reata *n.* a rope; lasso; a **riata strap** is a strap used to tie the riata to the saddle

rib *n.* any of the row of bones encasing the chest and attached to the vertebral column, coming down on either side; the horse has 18 pairs (except the Arabian which has 17), of which 8 are true and 10 are false (*see* **false ribs**)

ribbon *n.* a strip of colored cloth

awarded as a prize; a rosette with strips hanging from it

riboflavin *n.* a B-complex vitamin essential to good health

ribonucleic acid (RNA) an acid in all living cells which, with DNA, is instrumental in the transmission of inherited traits

ricked back an abnormal, unsound condition of the hindquarters characterized by side to side swaying motion at the trot, lack of hind leg coordination, a jerky stop when pulled up out of a trot, and sometimes considerable wobbling of the quarters; may be caused by a variety of injuries, including traction incurred when cast for castration; also called jinked back

rickets *n.* a bone disease caused by vitamin D deficiency and characterized by failure of normal bone growth

rickettsia *n.* minute microorganisms that transmit Potomac horse fever through the bite of parasitic ticks, lice, etc.

ridable, rideable *adj.* 1. (of a horse) capable of being ridden 2. (of a track, path, or road) capable of being negotiated by a mounted horse

ride *vi., vt.* to be mounted on a horse in motion — *n.* 1. a trip made on horseback 2. a trail for riding

ride in a huntsman's pocket in hunting, to ride too closely behind the huntsman (the undesirable action of an inexperienced hunt participant)

ride off in polo, to interfere with an opponent's play of the ball by pushing that person's horse with one's own horse

rider *n.* a person who rides a horse — *see also* **horseman; horsewoman**

riderless *adj.* having no rider (usually applied to a saddled horse from which the rider has fallen)

ride straight to ride without detouring around obstacles

ridgeling, ridgling *n.* a stallion having one or both testes undescended into the scrotal sac; rig, cryptorchid

riding bat *see* **whip**

riding fracture an overlapping impacted fracture

riding master a person who teaches horseback riding

Riding Pony a British type developed principally from crosses of small Thoroughbred stallions with Welsh or Dartmoor ponies and some Arab blood; has much presence and good conformation; popular in the show ring; up to 14.2 h.h.

riding school a place where people are taught to ride; has horses for hire, or serves as a facility where horses may be taken for livery, or both

rig *n.* 1. *see* **cryptorchid; ridgeling** 2. a vehicle drawn by a horse or horses 3. a horse trailer

rigid *adj.* stiff, as in such diseases as tetanus, or in relation to a limb, or in relation to the body after death (rigor mortis) — **rigidity** *n.* — **rigidly** *adv.*

rigid saddle tree a saddle frame that is not of the spring type — *see also* **spring tree saddle**

rigor *n.* 1. a rigidity or stiffness of the body with immunity to stimuli 2. shivering, as in illness or antecedent to fever

rigor mortis rigidity of the body after death

rim firing in rodeo bronco-busting, the insertion of a burr under the saddle pad to make the bronco buck harder

ring *n.* 1. a circular enclosure used for shows or exhibitions, competitions, and the like 2. a ridge around the hoof horn

ring-a-pole a timed playday event in which a competitor rides up to a pole set between two others and throws a plastic ring around that pole while circling around it, then gallops back to the starting point

ring bit 1. called *la gineta* in Spanish from the name of a Moorish tribe; it is circular with small rings around part of it that act as a curb behind the chin 2. a Chifney bit

ringbone *n.* generally, abnormal new bone (osteophyte) formation between fetlock and hoof; specifically, there are two types: articular, which results from arthrosis of the pastern joint (high ringbone), caused by overdorsiflexion of that joint, and non-articular, which results from tearing of ligaments attached to bones; when the coffin joint is affected, the condition is called low ringbone

ringer *n.* 1. a horse illegally substituted for another in a race   2. an Australian cowboy

ring scar an obstruction consisting of scar tissue around the intestine

ring ulcer an ulcer on the shank caused by the horse getting a foot tangled in a rope

ringworm *n.* any of a variety of contagious fungal diseases which appear on the skin in the shape of a ring covered with small scales and which usually break out on the face and neck but spread anywhere on the body; incubation in the host is four days to one month

river bottom disease *see* **equine infectious anemia**

RNA ribonucleic acid

roach (a mane) to cut the mane off entirely

roach back a malformed, arched back; hogback

road founder founder caused by running on hard surfaces

roan *adj.* a color consisting of dark hairs thickly sprinkled with white hairs — *n.* a horse with this coloration

roaring *n.* an abnormal sound made while inhaling; caused by vibration of a paralyzed vocal cord, specifically a paralysis of muscles on the left side of the larynx; the nerve to the vocal cord may be damaged due to overstretching or injury but is seen usually in long-necked horses, and the condition can be caused by heredity or any of various diseases, such as strangles; also called laryngeal hemiplegia — *see also* **whistling**

rocker-toe shoe a horseshoe having an upward tilt to the toe for ease of breakover and reduction of stress to the coffin joint and hoof wall; the toe of the hoof is rasped to fit the shoe

rocker-toe shoe

Rocky Mountain Horse an American breed whose registry was formed in 1986 after the breed nearly became extinct. Possessing a smooth, ambling gait, these horses are said to have originated in the late 19th century from a Spanish-bred stallion in the Rocky Mountains; he was chocolate brown with flaxen mane and tail, strongly built with a broad chest, and gaited; evidently, he was bred to mares of a similar type descended from Spanish Barbs and other gaited horses imported during colonial times. In 1986 only 45 of these horses were known to exist, but by 1990 there were 1,000 names registered; they have an easy-going disposition, are surefooted, and are in popular demand; although various solid colors are accepted for registry, a chocolate-brown coat with flaxen mane and tail are preferred; 14.2–16 h.h.

rodeo *n.* (from the Spanish word for "round-up") a competition that originated in the United States in the 1870s involving riders exhibiting their skills in such events as bronco-busting, barrel-racing, and bull riding, among others

rodlet *n.* one of many minute reflective structures within the eyeball

rods *n.pl. see* **retinal rods**

rogue *n.* a vicious horse

roll *vi.* to lie down and rotate the body from side to side (or halfway and back) several times; a horse has a penchant for rolling when its body is wet, particularly in mud after a rain

rollback a Western maneuver in which the horse gallops in one direction, does a sliding stop and pivots 180 degrees, then gallops back on the opposite lead in the return direction; also called a set and turn

rolled heel an abnormal hoof condition wherein the wall bends under at the heel due to heels that are too low or shoes that are too small

roller-toe shoe a shoe in which the hoof surface is flat while the ground surface has a rounded toe to facilitate breakover

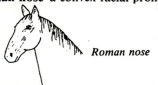
roller-toe shoe

rolling up turning a horse around several times when it refuses to move out

romal *n.* a whip used in Western riding which is attached to the end of a pair of closed reins that are wound together into a loop enabling the romal to "button" through the loop, thus forming a sort of completion to the reins

Roman nose a convex facial profile

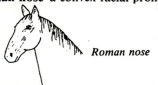
Roman nose

root *vi.* to extend the neck and muzzle to try and slacken or pull the reins — **rooter** *n.*

rope *n.* a cord made of intertwisted strands of various types of material; lasso — *vt.* to rope or lasso a horse or cattle

rope twitch *see* **twitch**

roping horse a horse trained to cooperate with the rider in roping cattle

Rosinante *n.* 1. Don Quixote's decrepit horse in the famous 17th century novel by Cervantes 2. an old nag

Rosinback *n.* the name given to a bareback circus horse used by acrobatic riders to perform their acts

Rosinback riding machine a safety device used by circus acrobatic riders who are in training; the rider wears a belt which is attached to a rope hanging from a moving crane above him which supports the rider in case of a fall

rostral teeth upper teeth (caudal teeth being the lower ones)

rotary gallop a disunited gallop involving a circular type of limb-placement pattern; for example: a right-lead rotary gallop begins with the right hind leg, then moves to the left hind and left fore and finally the leading right fore; round gallop

rotavirus *n.* a virus that causes diarrhea, lack of appetite, and sometimes colic in foals

Rottaler *n. see* **Oldenburg**

rough *n.* the area where horses favor leaving their droppings; they do not like to defecate where they graze so usually choose a particular spot or spots for this purpose

rough shoeing shoeing for slippery surfaces by usage of calks or frost nails

roundup *n.* 1. the act of driving free-ranging cattle or horses together into a collected herd for a particular purpose such as branding, inspection, etc. 2. the herd thus collected

roundworm *n.* a nematode parasitic worm that may inhabit the intestines

rowel *n.* a small wheel of projecting points forming the back end of a spur — *vt.* to prick a horse with a rowel

rowel

rowen *n.* the second yield of grass or hay in a season

ruano *adj.* a chestnut color, usually of a light shade, with flaxen mane and tail — *n.*

rub *vt.* 1. to move (the body) against an object, as when a horse rubs against a tree, post, etc. to relieve irritation 2. to massage (part of the horse's body) for a particular purpose 3. to wipe a cloth over (a horse's body) as to dry the horse or apply anti-fly solution 4. to make sore by rubbing, as by a girth or bridle

rubdown *n.* a massage-type rubbing of the horse's body with a cloth, as when the horse is sweated after a workout

rubefacient *n.* a substance that, when rubbed into the skin, increases blood supply and causes redness

rump *n.* the buttocks or hind part of the body

run *vi.* 1. to compete in a race 2. to finish a race in a particular position, e.g. to run third 3. to gallop rapidly 4. to flow, e.g. as relating to blood — *vt.* to discharge; e.g., a mare may run colostrum prematurely

runaway *n.* 1. a horse which is running away or has run away or has broken away from the control of his rider; a team of horses doing the same thing 2. the act of running away 3. a race won by a large margin — *adj.*

run-down *adj.* in poor physical condition — *n.* a condition of the fetlock wherein it has dropped due to injury of the suspensory ligament; suspensory sprain

run-down boots flexible padded leather boots worn on the fetlocks to protect them from contact with the ground

runner *n.* 1. a horse competing in a particular race 2. a loop to hold straps on tack in place; keeper

running martingale a strap that runs from the girth, between the forelegs, splits at the breast and attaches to the reins by two rings through which the reins run freely

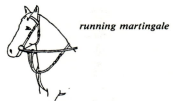

running martingale

running mute in hunting, the hounds' act of running without baying

running W a device used to throw a horse down by pulling its front legs out from under it

running walk a gait typical of the Tennessee (Plantation) Walking Horse; it can reach the speed of a medium trot and consists of a reach-slide motion of the hind legs and rhythmic bobbing of the head; the hind legs have an extended reach and step wide of the forefeet to avoid forging

run out in competition, (a) to avoid an obstacle to be jumped by running by it, or (b) to pass on the wrong side of a marker flag

Russian Heavy Draft a small cold-blood breed, active but good-natured and very strong; recognized as a breed in 1952; used extensively for draft work; 14.2–15.3 h.h.

Russian Trotter a fast trotter developed from crossing Orlov Trotters with American Standardbreds and officially recognized as a breed in 1949; 15.3–16 h.h.

rustle *vt.* to round up and or steal (cattle), which may be done on horseback

rye *n.* a cereal grass grown as forage; its grain is used as feed

— S —

sabino *adj.* of a color pattern that has variable white patches on a basic color but is distinct from paint; sometimes the patches vary from being sharply defined to consisting of small spots of white and usually both exist on one horse; usually the head is largely white with pigmented upper lip

Sable Island Pony a breed indigenous to Sable Island (about 200 miles off Nova Scotia) where only a few hundred live today; descended from French horses left there in the 18th century; 13–14 h.h.

sabulous *adj.* gritty; sabulous matter may sometimes be found in the bladder by rectal examination

sac *n.* a pouchlike covering of a body cavity, as the peritoneal sac which covers the abdominal organs

sack out to gently slap (a horse) with a sack or other soft material as part of gentling and training

sacro-coccygeus dorsalis and **-lateralis** muscles that raise the tail and turn it sideways

sacro-coccygeus ventralis a muscle that clamps the tail

sacrum *n.* a triangular bone situated at the end of the spinal column — **sacral** *adj.*

saddle *n.* 1. a seat made of leather or synthetic material used for riding a horse 2. a padded part of a harness worn over a horse's back to hold the shafts 3. the part of a horse's back where a saddle is placed — *vt.* to put a saddle on (a horse); saddle up — *see also* **Australian s.; English s.; McClellan s., Western s.**

saddle airer *see* **airer**

saddle-backed *adj.* having a low, concave back — *see also* **sway back**

saddle bag *n.* a bag, usually one of a connected pair, carried on a horse's back just behind the saddle — *see also* **saddle pouch; cantle bag**

saddle bag

saddle bars metal supports for stirrup leathers

saddle blanket *see* **saddle pad**

saddle bow the arch or front part of a saddle, the top of which is the pommel; saddle head

saddle bracket a saddle rack that attaches to a wall

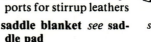

saddle bracket

Saddlebred *n.* an American breed whose registry was formed in 1891; an all-purpose horse originally called the Kentucky Saddler, as it was first developed by Kentucky pioneers, and bred from Thoroughbreds, Morgans, Trotters, and (now extinct) Narragansett Pacers; has animated action, an attractive advantage in the showring, and some have five gaits, two of which are 4-beat gaits, including the rack, which is very smooth for the rider; 15–16 h.h.; **Saddler; American Saddle Horse**

saddle-bronc riding a rodeo event in which a cowboy rides a bucking bronco on a specially designed saddle. When the horse first jumps out of the chute, the rider must have his spurs over and touching the bronco's shoulders and must then maintain a fore and after spurring motion from start to finish; one hand holds a rope attached to the halter while the other hand must remain free. The rider may not change hands and may not touch himself or the horse or tack with his free hand; nor must the rider lose a stirrup. The object is to stay mounted for 8 seconds.

saddle cloth *see* **saddle pad**

saddle head *see* **saddle bow**

saddle horse *n.* 1. a horse trained or suitable for riding 2. a wooden stand on which a saddle or saddles can be placed when not in use

saddle-horse seat *see* **seat**

saddle marks small patches of white hair caused by rubbing by an ill-fitting saddle

saddle pad a thick pad placed under a saddle to protect the horse's back; various shapes accommodate different saddles; also called saddle blanket, saddle cloth

Western saddle pad   English saddle pad

saddle panel the cushion under an English saddle; visible at the rear, sometimes in a contrasting shade of leather, as it projects from under the flap

saddle pouch a bag that attaches to the side of an English saddle

saddler *n.* a person whose work is making, repairing, or selling saddles, harnesses, etc.

Saddler *n.* *see* **Saddlebred**

saddle rack a stand on which a saddle can be stored; usually can be folded and sometimes has wheels —*see also* **saddle bracket**

saddlery *n.* 1. the craft of a saddler 2. the articles, as saddles, tack, etc., made by a saddler 3. a shop where saddles and tack are made

saddle rack

saddle-seat *n.* a style of riding in which the rider sits close to the cantle of the saddle, with very little bend of the knee; toes and knees are in line with feet parallel to the horse's sides

saddle soap a preparation for cleaning and softening leather

saddle sore 1. an irritation on a horse's back caused by friction of a saddle or rider 2. the discomfort that is sometimes felt by a rider after riding; usually caused by a badly made saddle or by improper riding

saddle tree the frame of a saddle, the three main parts of which are the fork, bars and cantle

saddle up to place a saddle on a horse

Sadecki *n.* *see* **Malapolski**

safe *n.* 1. a flap of leather on a saddle under a buckle that prevents the horse from being galled 2. either of the underflaps on an English saddle

safety catch a release device on the bar that holds a stirrup to a saddle

safety snap *see* **panic snap**

safety stirrups English stirrups that in an emergency will open, allowing the rider to fall free of the stirrups

safety stirrups

St. John's wort a weed that contains the toxin hypericin, which is a skin irritant

Salerno *n.* an Italian breed popularly used as a general purpose riding horse; 16. h.h.; also called Persano

salicylate *n.* any of a class of drugs used to relieve arthritic pain but which may cause intestinal irritation and diarrhea; aspirin is a salicylate

saline solution a solution of usually 0.9 percent salt in water which is used to clean wounds

saliva *n.* the watery fluid in the mouth, secreted by the salivary glands, which aids in swallowing and digestion; on average, a horse produces 10 gallons of saliva per day —**salivary** *adj.*

salivary glands three pairs of glands in the mouth that secrete saliva, the largest of which is the parotid gland near the ear

salivate *vi., vt.* to produce saliva excessively, as in the case of oral inflammation, defective teeth, taking certain drugs, etc.

saliva test a test performed to determine the possible presence of dope when there is suspicion regarding a horse in competition; blood and urine may also be tested

sallenders *n.* a skin disease affecting the front of the hock wherein the skin scabs and sometimes develops fissures, causing lameness; **psoriasis tarsi**

salmonellae *n.pl.* enteric bacteria that cause disease in humans and animals —*see also* **salmonellosis**

salmonellosis *n.* infection caused by salmonella bacteria ingested with food; characterized by gastrointestinal disorders, high fever, blood-stained diarrhea, and usually death

salpingitis *n.* inflammation of the fallopian tube

salpinx *n., pl.* **salpinges** a tube in the body (used chiefly in reference to the fallopian tube)

salt *n.* 1. sodium chloride which is (a) a natural element of the body and (b) a crystalline substance which may be added to feed or used in medicine

salt lick a brick or block of salt made available to horses to lick at will; it may be plain or mixed with other minerals

Sandalwood *n.* an Indonesian pony breed used for bareback racing; 12.1–13.1 h.h.

sand colic *see* **colic**

sandrack *n.* a fine, shallow crack in the hoof horn; may be complete, extending from the coronet to the ground surface of the wall, or partial, extending partway; there may be one crack or several; can admit foreign matter into sensitive tissues within, causing infection and inflammation resulting in lameness —*see also* **crack**

sandy bay a light tan coat color

San Fratellano a mountain breed from the Nebrodi Mountains of Sicily; used for riding, light draft and as a pack horse; gentle but spirited; always black, brown, or bay; 15–16 h.h.

sanguinary *adj.* flowing with blood or bloodstained

sanguineous *adj.* relating to blood

Sanho *n.* a subtype of the Mongolian breed

Sanpeitze *n.* a subtype of the Mongolian breed

sarcoceps *n.pl.* one-celled parasites

sarcoid *n.* a virus-caused tumor on the skin or in a wound; can have a thick, crusty surface or a raw, fleshy one that bleeds when touched; angleberry

sarcoma *n.* a type of malignant growth

Sarcoptes equi a parasite that causes sarcoptic mange

sarcoptic mange a crusty skin disease caused by the parasite *Sarcoptes equi*; these mites burrow into the skin and cause thickened areas and bald patches; resultant itching makes the horse rub the affected areas until they break open and are then subjected to other infectious organisms

Sardinian *n.* a pony breed indigenous to the island of Sardinia; sure-footed and tractable; up to about 13.2 h.h.

Sardo *n.* an Anglo-Arab breed developed in Italy for the Palio —*see also* **Palio**

sartorius muscle a thigh muscle that flexes the hip joint and adducts the leg

sausage boot a stuffed leather ring worn around the pastern to prevent capped elbow incurred by a shoe when the horse lies down

sausage boot

savage *vt.* to attack (another animal or a person) —*adj.* vicious

scab *n.* 1. a crust that covers a sore or wound as it heals 2. scabies —*vt.* to become covered with a scab —**scabby** *adj.*

scabies *n.* any itchy skin disease caused

by tiny mites that burrow into the skin; lesions result and the condition spreads to other parts of the body and to other horses, especially by contaminated equipment; also called scab or mange

scald *n.* a burn — *vt.*

scalder *n.* a type of horse boot fitted as a protection against scalping

scalenus *n.* a neck muscle

scalping *n.* a faulty action in which the hairline at the coronet of the hind foot hits the toe of the forefoot as it breaks over

scapula *n.* the shoulder blade

scar *n.* a mark that is left after the healing of a wound, burn, ulcer, etc.

schistosome *n.* any of a genus, *Schistosoma*, of parasitic blood

Schleswig-Holstein *n.* a German medium-sized draft breed from the province of Schleswig; strong and energetic but very manageable; usually chestnut with flaxen mane and tail, but occasionally some are gray or bay; 15.2–16 h.h.

school *n.* an enclosed area, either open or covered, where a horse is trained — **school** *vt.* — **schooled** *adj.*

schooling *n.* a training regime that begins at birth, in which a horse is taught to lead, tie, and respond to voice commands and riding aids for all gaits; dressage horses and jumpers are usually referred to as **schooled** horses

Schweiken *n.* an old German breed used for centuries on East Prussian farms. Crossed in the 18th century with Arab, Thoroughbred, and some Turkoman blood it formed the foundation of the Trakehner

scintigraphy *n.* a diagnostic procedure in which a **scintiscanner** is used to evaluate radioactive tracer substances injected into the body that have concentrated in injured areas

scirrhus *n.* a hardened swelling of connective tissue — **scirrhous** *adj.*

sclera *n.* the white part of the eye or white fibrous membrane covering all of the eyeball except the area covered by the cornea; sclerotic layer — **scleral** *adj.*

scleritis *n.* inflammation of the sclera

scleroderma *n.* a hardening of the skin due to rubbing by a harness

sclerostome *n.* an intestinal parasite; large strongyle

sclerotic layer *see* **sclera**

scoliosis *n.* a congenital curvature of the spinal column, caused by underdevelopment of the articulations on one side of the column, with a consequent pulling to that side; when this underdevelopment occurs on both sides, the spine is pulled downward so that the foal is born with severe lordosis

scope *n.* a horse's range of perception, particularly applied to jumping, in which a horse's scope determines its ability to gauge the height and breadth of an obstacle and clear it

score *n.* 1. the marks given to competitors in an event 2. in rodeo, the distance between the chute opening and the scoreline; the headstart given to timed-event cattle in roping and steer wrestling

scoreline *n.* in rodeo, a strip of material, like leather, rubber, or elastic, about 6 feet long, which is secured on the ground at a determined distance in front of the chute from which time-event cattle are released; once an animal crosses the scoreline, a contestant starts to run; contestants who start too soon are said to "break the barrier" and have 10 seconds added to their time made in the arena

Scotch Bottoms the 7 lb. shoes worn by Clydesdales

Scotch hobble a restraining device by which one hind leg is restrained off the ground by a rope passed around the horse's neck into a bowline, thereby forming a kind of loose collar; the free

end of the rope is then passed around the hind pastern, preferably several times, and back up through the loop, pulling the leg off the ground, and then tied into the collar; used when a mare is being serviced

scours *n.* watery diarrhea

scratch¹ *vt.* 1. to withdraw (a horse) from a sports event, particularly a race 2. to spur, especially in a certain motion as a cowboy does in rodeo when riding a bucking bronco (*see* **reef [a horse]**) — *vi.* to rub on something to relieve itching

scratch² *n.* 1. a horse withdrawn from a sports event 2. a superficial tear or wound on the skin 3. the act of scratching — *adj.* in reference to a team, as in polo, for example, organized hurriedly without careful selection

scratches *n.* a scabby and or oozing skin inflammation on the back of the pastern above the heels which occurs after the area has been cut or scratched and subsequently exposed to unclean stalls or paddocks or excessive moisture; grease; greasy heel

screw *n.* a nag

screwdriver fracture a fracture that slants to one side, often seen in fractures of the pastern long bone; caused by slippery surfaces and sharp turns made in barrel racing, cutting, etc., especially when the feet have been shod with caulks

screw-worm *n.* a larva of any of several American flies, which hatches from an egg that is laid in a wound or scratch where there is blood; it eats into the flesh and degrades a horse's condition seriously

scrotum *n.* the sac on a male horse that holds the testicles — **scrotal** *adj.*

scurry *n.* a jumping contest scored on speed; each fault incurs a penalty of one second

sea horse 1. in mythology, a creature of the sea depicted as half fish and half horse 2. a small marine fish of the genus *Hippocampus* whose head vaguely resembles that of a horse

season *n. see* **estrus; heat**

seat *n.* 1. when used with "proper" or "good," the way a rider sits the horse 2. the part of the saddle where the rider sits; **balanced seat:** middle of saddle on pelvic bones, knees moderately bent, feet in stirrups on ball of foot but no further, toes pointed approximately straight forward with very slight outward direction, inside of bent knees against saddle; **classical seat:** fairly long stirrups, toes parallel to horse's body; **saddle-horse seat:** straight legs forward with leathers at forward angle, seat back near cantle (often used on gaited horses); **English hunt seat:** legs slightly farther back than in the balanced seat; **jockey** or **racing seat:** flat saddle, stirrups extremely short with feet all the way in, rider hunched over and off the saddle; **cowboy seat:** a deep seat with long stirrups and very little knee bend, so that a gallop may be taken standing in stirrups off the saddle

seat of corn in the foot, the part of the sole that is located in the angle of the wall and bar at the heel and forms a "seat" for the development of a corn in unfavorable conditions, such as an improperly fitted shoe or one that has been left on too long

seatworm *n. see* **pinworm**

seaweed *n. see* **kelp**

sebaceous *adj.* relating to fat or sebum, as in a sebaceous cyst

seborrhea *n. see* **chorioptic mange**

sebum *n.* the greasy secretion of sebaceous glands; a slightly waxy lubricant of each hair follicle just below the surface of the skin which keeps the skin pliable, impermeable, and partially protected from bacteria, and which waterproofs the hair shafts — **sebaceous** *adj.*

second horseman in hunting, a groom who takes a fresh hunter to the master to relieve a tired one that the master has been riding

secrete *vt.* to form and release (a substance) as e.g. the salivary glands secrete saliva —**secretion** *n.* the substance thus released

sedate *vt.* to calm by giving a sedative

sedative *n.* a drug which has a calming effect —*adj.*

seed *n.* 1. sperm or semen 2. the part of a plant that develops into a new plant when sown. Horses enjoy eating the seeds of certain grasses and the grain fed to horses comes from seeds of food plants such as corn, oats, etc.

see daylight to observe that a rider is failing to keep his or her seat when cantering or galloping (a spectator can *see daylight* between horse and rider)

seedy toe a separation between the outer and inner layers of the hoof wall at the toe (when this occurs in areas other than the toe, it is merely called separation); caused by laminitis, poor hoof trimming and shoeing, or a foreign body, as a stone, wedged between sole and wall

segment *n.* any of the sections or parts into which a substance, as a part of the body, is divided —**segmentary, segmental** *adj.* —**segmentally** *adv.* —**segmentation** *n.* the process of being divided or dividing into segments

segmental myelitis a nervous disease caused by inflamed segments of the spinal cord and characterized by hind leg incoordination; usually serious deterioration occurs

Seine Inferieure *n.* a French breed used under saddle as well as for draft purposes; 16 h.h.

selenium *n.* a chemical element, one isotope of which is a trace mineral essential to muscle formation

seleniuim poisoning caused by inges

tion of certain plants, such as vetch; in an acute case a horse dies within hours after symptoms of difficult breathing, bloat, and colic; in sub-acute cases, progression of poisoning is more gradual, with symptoms of weight loss, lethargy, staggering, reduced vision, colic, inability to swallow, paralysis, and finally death; in chronic cases (alkali disease), there is weight loss, loss of hair from mane and tail, anemia, and depraved appetite; rings may also appear on the hooves and there may even be separation and shedding of the hooves

Selle Français a French hunter established as a breed in 1965; 15.2–16.3 h.h.; also called French Saddle Horse

sellers posits a special network of vessels in the body that reallocates blood from a damaged artery through alternate routes

selling race a race immediately after which the winning horse is obliged to be auctioned

semen *n.* the fluid secreted by the male reproductive organs and containing spermatozoa —**seminal** *adj.*

semimembranosus muscle a thigh muscle that extends the hip joint and adducts the leg

semitendinosus muscle a large, thick muscle of the buttock

sensation *n.* the response of nerves to such stimuli as pain, light, sound, etc.

sense 1. normal reasoning power, reflected in behavior —**sensible** *adj.* 2. sensation

sensitive laminae see **laminar corium**

sensitivity *n.* a natural aversion of body tissue to a particular substance, such as insect saliva; intensity of reaction is related to genetic factors as well as to the amount of the irritant, as e.g. the number of insect bites

sensory nerves nerves that transmit

feelings or sensations, as touch, heat, cold, pain, etc.

separation *see* **seedy toe**

sepsis *n.* decay; bacterial infection and the body's reaction to it —**septic** *adj.*

septic arthritis bacterial infection in a joint

septicemia *n.* a bacterial infection of the blood which sometimes affects newborn foals; signs vary according to site of bacterial colonization, as in the brain (convulsions), joints (swelling and lameness), etc.; often fatal despite treatment —**septicemic** *adj.*

septum *n.* a partition between two cavities or tissue masses, as in the nose

sequestrum *n.* a piece of bone, cartilage, or any hard tissue which has separated from the main mass and consequently undergone necrosis

serology *n.* the study of antibodies in the blood or other body fluid

serotonin *n.* a hormone secreted by the pancreas, which causes an increase in blood pressure by constricting the smallest arteries

serous arthritis *see* **closed arthritis**

serpent tail a concave dock

serratus *n.* a large, fanlike muscle which forms the chief attachment of the foreleg to the body; comprises two parts: the **serratus cervicis** (neck part) and the **serratus thoracis** (chest part); the **serratus dorsalis ansterior** aids in breathing in (inspiration); the **serratus dorsalis posterior** aids in breathing out (expiration)

serum *n.* 1. thin, watery tissue fluid; the fluid from blisters and wounds; the yellowish liquid portion of clotted blood 2. such fluid taken from the blood of an animal immunized against a specific disease; used for diagnosis and antitoxin 3. such fluid containing antibodies against a specific disease

and injected into a patient for immunization against that disease —**serous** *adj.*

serum gonadotrophin a sterile preparation of follicle stimulating hormones taken from the serum of a pregnant mare; trade name: Gestyl — *see also* **pregnant mare serum gonadotrophin**

serum lactate *see* **blood lactate**

serum protein protein substances in blood serum

serve *vt.* (of a stallion) to mate with or inseminate; service; cover —*see also* **settle**

service *vt.* serve —*n.* the act of copulating or the act of bringing a stallion to mate with a mare

service collar a collar that protects a mare from a stallion's bite during copulation

service hobbles *see* **breeding hobbles**

sesamoid bones two small, pyramid-shaped bones at the back of the fetlock joint; they act as a pulley for the flexor tendons that pass over them and provide attachment for the suspensory ligament

sesamoiditis *n.* a severe lesion of the sesamoid bones characterized by swelling, lameness, and pain when pressure is applied or on bending the fetlock joint; caused by excessive pulling or overflexion of the fetlock joint, causing the partial tearing away of the attached ligaments; new bone mass (osteophyte) finally forms; may be brought on by long-toe, low-heel trimming, or long, sloping pasterns, especially under stressful conditions such as making repeated sharp turns under excessive weight (of both rider and horse)

set and turn rollback

set fast *see* **atypical myoglobinuria**

seton *n.* a strip of threads drawn through tissues to create a drainage tract

set tail a tail in which the tendons of the

dock are cut for a high tail carriage; widely viewed as a cruel practice

settle *vt.* 1. to serve or impregnate (a mare) 2. *vi.* to calm down

shadbelly *n.* a dressy type of hunting coat, usually worn with a top hat; swallowtail; cutaway

shaft *n.* 1. the main part of a long bone 2. either of the two bars between which a horse is harnessed when pulling a vehicle

Shagya *n.* a Hungarian breed named after its foundation Arab sire, a gray Syrian horse, Shagya, imported in 1836; Arab mares and local mares, only some of which were purebred, were used to start this breed which is similar to the Arab; a harness and all-purpose riding horse; color is mostly gray; 14.2–15 h.h.

shaker-foal syndrome a progressive, often fatal weakness of a newborn foal which is attributed to botulism infection of the intestines

Shan *n. see* **Burmese**

shank *n.* 1. a lead line of half leather or rope and half chain 2. the lower extension of certain bits, either straight or curved, to which the reins are attached 3. the bone between the hock and fetlock

shear *n.* a force that develops in a bone at about a 45 degree angle to the compression force, resulting in what is called a shear fracture when excessive load or pressure is applied

sheared heel hoof damage resulting when one side of the heel receives more downward pressure than the other side

shear mouth a faulty condition of the cheek teeth wherein, due to malocclusion, there is uneven wear of the teeth surfaces, causing spear-like points on one side and perhaps wear as far as the gumline on the other

sheath *n.* 1. a covering, as the membrane around a tendon (tendon sheath) 2. the organ which encases the unextended penis

shed[1] *vt., vi.* to cast off the coat; horses shed twice a year, in spring and autumn, with the heaviest shedding in spring when their natural cold-weather protection is no longer needed

shed[2] *n.* a building, sometimes quite rustic, used for storage or shelter; often has the front end open — *see also* **lean-to**

shedding blade a device with curry-comb teeth pulled over a horse's coat to pull away loose hair when the horse is shedding

shedding blade

sheet *n.* a light covering used to cool a sweated horse or to protect a horse from flies — *see also* **cooler**

shelly hooves hooves that are brittle and split easily

Shelt *n.* a Highland pony used in England by deer hunters to carry carcasses

Shetland *n.* a pony breed that originated in the Shetland Isles off the north coast of Scotland; now bred in many countries around the world and popular as a child's mount; 9.2–10.2 h.h. — *see also* **American Shetland**

shigella infection *see Bacterium viscosum equi*

shin *n.* the front of the cannon bone

shin boots boots fitted to a horse to protect the shins when jumping

shine *vi.* to gleam; to be bright (as a horse's coat when it is clean, reflecting good health) — *n.* — **shiny** *adj.*

shipping fever a horseman's term for strangles or other respiratory infection sometimes caused by prolonged physical stress, a term now seldom used as the ailments that come under its heading are more specifically categorized

shippon *n.* a stable

Shirazi *n. see* **Darashouri**

Shire *n.* a very large English breed of ancient heritage with thickly feathered legs; originated in the Shires of England; the tallest and heaviest of coldbloods; very strong but gentle; makes an excellent farm worker and draft horse; very popular in shows where the breed's enormous size delights spectators; up to 18 h.h.

shivering *n.* 1. trembling, as from cold 2. a disease of the nervous system involving muscle tremors, usually of the hind limbs; when the hind leg is flexed and lowered to the ground, it trembles; not to be confused with trembling from cold or a foal's normal shivering immediately after birth — **shiver** *vi.*

shock *n.* a condition of mild or severe collapse that may be categorized into two forms: (a) primary shock, involving a sudden onset after an accident, due to nervous collapse, and (b) secondary shock, involving a delayed onset, 30 minutes to 12 hours after an accident such as a severe burn, and due to diminished circulation

shod too close a farrier's term for having a nail driven too close to the sensitive part of the hoof, a condition also called nail bind

shoe *n.* a U-shaped bar made to fit the bottom edge of the hoof for its protection; horseshoe; technically comprises three unseparated sections: the heel (ends), the branches (sides), and the toe; among the large variety of shoes used for various purposes, the commonly used shoe for general purpose riding has a groove (fullering *or* swaging) on the ground surface of each branch, having several holes for nailing on; the most widely used shoes are made of iron or steel; others can be of aluminum, plastic, natural or synthetic

shoe

rubber and various composite materials; some models are constructed with springs to absorb concussion and render a kind of shove on breakover — **shoe** *vt.*

shoe boil *see* **capped elbow**

shoe boil boots protective boots used in the presence of shoe boil

shoe boil ring *see* **doughnut**

shoeing *n.* the fitting of a shoe to a horse's hoof; farriery

shoeing block a tripod on which a horse's foot is placed to facilitate certain shoeing procedures

shoeing forge *see* **forge**

short *see* **go short**

short-coupled *adj.* having a back that is not too long, with well sprung ribs

short of rib having an exaggerated space between the last rib and point of hip — *see also* **slack loins**

shoulder blade the flat bone on the side of the chest to which the muscles of the shoulder and forearm are attached; scapula

shoulder-in *n.* a suppling, training exercise in which a horse in forward motion is asked to turn its head and laterally bend the body away from the direction in which it is going; the terms "inside" and "outside" in this exercise refer to the shoulder, the inside shoulder being the one in the direction of which the neck bends; the inside foreleg crosses in front of the outside foreleg, and the inside hind leg steps in front of the outside hind

shoulder sweeney paralysis of the shoulder muscles, caused by a fall or other injury

show *n.* an exhibition of horses — *see also* **horse show** — *vt.* to exhibit (a horse) — *vi.* in racing to finish in third place; a bettor who bets on a horse "to show" wins if the horse comes in first, second or third

show-jumping a sport wherein horses and riders compete in clearing a number of obstacles, trying to incur the least number of faults within a time limit set according to the course

shuttle bone *see* **navicular bone**

shy *vi.* to swerve to one side or suddenly stop or take off in fear of some startling object or sound

Sicilian *n.* a breed indigenous to Sicily and developed from Arabian stock; used for riding and light draft work; 15.1–15.3 h.h.

sickle-hock *n.* a conformation fault wherein the angle of the hock joint is too great — **sickle-hocked** *adj.*

sidebone *n.* a swelling or abnormal bone formation (ossification) on one or both lateral cartilages of the foot starting at the coffin bone. When the flexible, springy, lateral cartilages turn to bone, they are referred to as sidebones; they may or may not cause lameness. Age, especially in big, heavy horses, may be a cause; large, painful sidebones may, however, result from such injuries as concussion, barbed wire cuts, etc.

side clip *see* **clip**[1]

sideline *vt.* to tie (a rear foot) by a rope to a loop around the neck — *n.*

sidepass *vi.* see **sidestep**

side reins headsetting reins running from the bit to the girth, surcingle, or saddle

siderocyte *n.* red blood cell having non-hemoglobin iron, large numbers of which indicate a pathology; sidero-iron; cyte-cell

sidesaddle *n.* a variant of an English saddle designed for women in skirts; a large, hook-like pommel supports the rider's right leg, which hangs over the left side of the horse, while the left leg is held in a conventional stirrup — *adv.* on or as if on a sidesaddle

sidestep *vi.* (of a horse) to move sideways, passing one foot over the other, front over front, rear over rear; side-pass *n.*

side-stick *n.* a short stick, with snaps at each end which fasten to a halter and to the surcingle, used to prevent a horse from biting while being groomed or from biting a wound

sidestrap *n.* see **gaiting strap**

side-wheeler *n.* a pacer that rolls its body sidewise as it paces

Siglavy *n.* an Arabian subtype bred in Russia

silage *n.* green crops (cut at an earlier stage than hay) preserved in a silo for use as fodder; can be fed in equal parts with hay

silks *n.pl.* the racing colors or jacket and cap worn by jockeys

silo *n.* an airtight storage structure for green fodder

silver dapple a color pattern in which light dapples occur on a basic coat color of various shades of brown with flaxen or almost white points

silver dun *see* **dun**

silver nitrate a compound used in a weak solution as an astringent or antiseptic; **silver nitrate poisoning** can occur in an overdose

silver weed a poisonous plant, *Potentilla anserina,* fatal if eaten in large quantities

simple fracture a bone fracture in which there is a clean break in the bone at one place

simulcasting *n.* the live telecasting at one racetrack of a race held at another track to enable betting and viewing by television at a track other than the one where the race is actually held — **simulcast** *vt.*

sinew *n.* a muscle tendon

single bank a jump consisting of a bank with a ditch on one side

single-foot *n. see* **rack** — *vi.* to move in a rack

singletree *n.* the pivoted or swinging bar to which harness traces are fixed; in a team, a singletree is fixed at each end of the doubletree; also called whippletree; whiffletree; badikins

sinus *n.* a body cavity or a channel leading from a cavity; sinuses of the skull connect with the nasal cavities (4 pairs: maxillary, frontal, sphenopalatine, and ethmoidal)

sinusitis *n.* a bacterial infection of a sinus or sinuses, especially of the head; characterized by a thick discharge from one or both nostrils (usually one), lymph node swelling in the lower jaw, and pain

sire *n.* 1. the father of a horse 2. the "top line" in a pedigree — *vt.* (of a stallion) to beget (a foal)

sitfast *n.* a partial necrosis of the skin caused by pressure of a saddle or harness; it may extend in depth to subcutaneous tissues; the affected area is usually circular and raised, with a narrow groove around it, separating it from healthy tissue

Siwalik Pony an unattractive but hardy Indian breed originating in the Himalayan foothills of Siwalik; 13.2 h.h.

skeletal muscles the muscles that react only when stimulated; they bend limbs and move bones and bone-based structures at their joints by contracting

skeleton *n.* the framework of bones of the body

skewbald *n.* a two-colored horse whose coat is white with any color except black; paint

skill drills neuromuscular training exercises required for participation in a particular sport

skin *n.* the covering of the body that comprises two layers — the outer layer, or epidermis, which is covered with hair, and the inner layer, or dermis, with hair roots, sweat and oil glands, nerves, blood vessels, and tissue

skin itch *n.* an allergy to the bites of certain flies, occuring during hot, humid weather; rubbing and biting cause hair loss and abrasions of the skin, mainly in the areas of the ears, mane, tail, and withers

skinner *n.* a horse considered by a horse dealer to be worthless except for horse meat

skirt *n.* on an English saddle, the flap that protects the rider from the stirrup bar and buckle; on a Western saddle, either of two flaps (the upper flank skirt and the lower skirt) which extend behind the cantle

Skogsruss *n. see* **Gotland**

skull *n.* the head's framework of bones, including the cranium and facial bones: 3 auditory ossicles in each ear; 10 cranial: occipital, sphenoid, ethmoid, intraparietal (single bones) and parietals, frontals, temporals (paired); 21 facial: vomer, hyoid, mandible (single bones) and maxilla, incisive, palatine, pterygoid, nasal, lacrimal, zygomatic upper and lower turbinates (paired); lower jaw: mandible — 2 branches called rami

skunk tail *see* **frosty**

Skyros *n.* a Greek pony breed used as a pack pony or child's riding pony; 11 h.h.

slab fracture a fracture of the knee joint in which a slab of the broken bone is detached from the joint

slab-sided *adj.* having a conformation fault wherein the ribs are not curved (well sprung) but inclined to be flat; flat-sided

slackening *n.* the relaxation of pelvic ligaments of a mare shortly before foaling; it is seen in the appearance of a groove on either side of the root of the tail

slack loins too long a back, showing an exaggerated space between the last rib and point of hip; a horse with this fault is also called short of rib

slack time in rodeo, the period before or after the show; if there are too many contestants to compete in the allotted show time, they compete in slack periods

slake *vt.* to satisfy, as thirst

sleep *n.* a state of rest during which the eyes are usually closed; adult horses sleep intermittently, either standing or recumbent, 4–7 hours per day, of which time usually only about 45 minutes are spent lying down — *vi.* — **sleepy** *adj.*

sleep epilepsy *see* **narcolepsy**

sleeper *n.* a horse that surprisingly wins a race after formerly being a loser

sleeping sickness *see* **encephalomyelitis**

sleepy foal disease *see Bacterium vicosum equi*

sleepy staggers *see* **stomach staggers**

sleigh *n.* a vehicle, often horse-drawn, that has runners instead of wheels for traveling over snow or ice

slicker *n.* an oilskin coat used by a cowboy on the range, large enough to protect himself as well as his saddle

sliding stop a sudden stop made when a horse tucks in its rear and slides its hind feet on the ground

sling *n.* a device to support a horse in a standing position for a period of

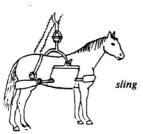

sling

time while it is undergoing medical treatment; it is made up of a wide belly band, a breast collar (to prevent slipping back), a singletree (to keep the straps separated over the back), and a chain hoist attached to a ceiling; the horse must support its own weight partially, otherwise the pressure on the belly can be fatal

slip *vi.* to abort

slip fillets small wood strips put on top of a hurdle; if dislodged, they prove that a jumper has touched the hurdle

slippers *n.pl.* lightweight horseshoes put on temporarily

slipping point in jumping, the point at which a rider begins to get the horse into the proper stride to make the jump

slobber *vi.* to salivate excessively — *n.*

slough *n.* a castoff layer, as of skin or dead tissue — *vt.*

slow gait the slower of two artificial gaits performed by the five-gaited American Saddle Horse; it is a slow stepping pace in which each foot in turn is raised and held up momentarily before coming down

slow-twitch muscle fibers (ST) muscle fibers that consume oxygen and contract during prolonged exercise and do not produce explosive bursts of activity but are steady and sustained in their action

Slypner *n.* in Norse mythology, a gray horse that belonged to the chief god, Odin; he had eight legs and danced on water, in the air and over ground

Slypner shoe a horseshoe that consists of two parts: a base, shaped and nailed to the hoof, and an interchangeable, shock-absorbing, urethane sole which varies to suit conditions and wear

small colon the section of the large intestine where digestive fluid is absorbed and solid food residue is formed into balls of dung; lies between the large intestine and the rectum and measures

3–4 inches in diameter and 10–12 inches in length

small intestine that portion of the intestines between the stomach and the cecum and large intestine; approximately 60 feet long with a 50-liter capacity

small strongyle a parasite whose larval migrations are limited to the intestinal walls; roundworm

smegma *n.* the cheesy secretion within the sheath of the male

smith *n.* blacksmith

smithing *n.* shoeing

smithy *n.* a blacksmith

smokey *adj.* having a coat color with a blue tinge

smooth mouth a defective dental condition in which the grinding surfaces of the cheek teeth are worn smooth; very old horses are susceptible but it may happen in youngsters too; not to be confused with a type of smooth mouth in 12-year-old horses that have lost the cups in their incisors; it may affect only two opposing teeth but otherwise the condition renders proper chewing impossible and the horse suffers from malnutrition

smooth muscles involuntary muscles which are capable of independent activity

snaffle *n.* a type of bit which may be either straight or broken; considered to be very mild; the thicker the mouthpiece, the milder it is; a smooth one is milder than a twisted one

snakebite *n.* a snake's bite or condition caused by it; can be fatal if from a rattlesnake; usually happens on the legs or the head (when a horse lowers its head to eat or investigate). Swelling at the site results, and if the bite occurs near the nostrils, they can swell shut, requiring the insertion of tubes in the nostrils to ensure breathing. Movement spreads the venom, so the horse

should be kept quiet until or while remedial measures are taken.

sneeze *vi.* an involuntary, explosive and noisy expiration through the nose

snide *n.* a horse with a fault or faults

snip *n.* a white or pink mark between or in the region of the nostrils

snore *vi.* to breathe noisily as the result of an abscess, tumor, or other swelling in the pharynx or nasal passages

snort *n.* a sound similar to a human snore which some horses make when they feel nervous about something they see or curiously investigate and nose it — *vi.*

snotty nose a viral disease of the respiratory tract causing a secretion of nasal mucus; rhinopneumonitis; cold; catarrh; coryza

snowflake *n.* a type of coat marking that features white spots on a background of any color; these spots can increase with age until they finally stabilize but sometimes they keep increasing until the horse appears white with contrasting spots, at which point the marking can be called speckled; snowflake marking is typical of the Appaloosa

snub *vt.* to secure (a horse) to a post by means of a rope turned around the post

sociable *n.* a low, closed, four-wheeled carriage, drawn by two horses, which seats four passengers in two rows facing each other

sock *n.* a marking of white hair completely surrounding the leg below the fetlock joint; sometimes called white fetlock, or white pastern if lower

sodium *n.* an alkaline metallic element found in body fluids and cells; **sodium acid citrate:** an anticoagulant added to transfusion blood; **sodium acid phosphate:** used to treat low phosphate conditions; **sodium bicarbonate:** used

to treat excess staling or diarrhea; **sodium calcium edetate:** used to treat lead poisoning; **sodium chloride:** salt; **sodium cromoglycate:** used in cases of broken wind; **sodium fusidate:** used in ointment form to treat infections with staphylococcus bacteria; **sodium glycarsamate:** used to treat infestation of redworm; **sodium morrhuate** and **sodium oleate:** used to treat fractured bones (hardens tissues); **sodium salicylate:** aspirin; **sodium sulfate:** a laxative; **sodium thiosulfate:** reduces flatulence and fermentation in stomach and intestines

soft eyes eyes that show an absence of tension, with the upper lid and brow being relaxed into wrinkles

soft palate the fleshy part at the rear of the mouth, separating the mouth from the nasal passages; in the horse its average medial length is 6 inches

Sokolsky *n.* a Polish light draft breed, also bred in Russia; calm and hardworking; 15–16 h.h.

sole *n.* the bottom of the hoof, formed of a horny substance that protects the inner tissue of the foot; slightly concave and soft enough to maintain a flexible wall that will give when the horse puts weight on the foot; flakes off naturally as it thickens and should not be trimmed

Solupen *n.* trade name for benzylpenicillin

somatotrophin *n. see* **growth hormone**

soogan *n.* (Western) a bed roll

sore¹ *vt.* to tenderize (the coronet area of the foot) with chemical irritants in order to produce high-stepping action; the horse snatches the sored forefeet up in reaction to the pain — **sored** *adj.*

sore² *adj.* tender; painful — *n.* a painful spot on the body

sore shin inflammation of the cannon bone — *see also* **bucked shin**

sorghum *n.* a genus of cereal grass used as animal feed, of which there are four distinct types, one of which is milo; molasses is made from sweet sorghum

Sorraia *n.* a Spanish pony breed of a primitive type with an eel stripe and zebra markings on the legs; native to western Spain and Portugal near the Sorraia River where it runs wild; 12.2–13 h.h.

sorrel *n. see* **chestnut¹**

sound *adj.* 1. free from disease and ailments and from any structural imperfections that may interfere with usefulness — **soundness** *n.*

soup plates round hooves, larger than normal for a given horse's size and usually having low heels

sour cattle in cutting, cattle that have become inactive and unresponsive to the cutting horse due to being continually worked

sour horse a horse that is no longer desirable due to bad handling

South German Cold-Blood a lighter version of the Noriker (Austrian); has an old history and was once extensively used for army artillery and pack transport in the mountains; still sometimes used today for that purpose, as well as by farmers; 16–16.2 h.h.

sow mouth *see* **undershot jaw**

soya-bean meal a high protein feed (as high as 45 percent), having 6 percent oil, sometimes fed in small quantities to young and breeding horses and those who are worked very hard

spade bit a severe Spanish bit with a high, solid port

Spanish American hip disease a disease found in Central and South America in wet areas and contracted from flies; characterized by extreme weight loss, anemia, swinging of the hindquarters, local edema, paralysis, and sometimes patches of dried exudate on the skin; also called mal de caderas

Spanish Horse *see* **American Indian Horse**

Spanish Riding School of Vienna the oldest riding school in the world, founded in the 16th century; so named because the horses used there are of Spanish origin

Spanish walk a dressage movement wherein each of the horse's feet in turn is raised high, then out and held for an instant before stepping down lightly and continuing

spasm *n.* a sudden, forceful muscle contraction that is painful

spasmodic colic an irritability caused by overactivity of the gut wall, resulting in painful spasms

Spasmodin *n.* trade name for benzyl benzoate

spavin *n.* a disease of the hock of which there are several kinds, most of which are characterized by a swelling; **blood spavin** is an enlargement or varicosity of the saphenous vein, which angles across the front of the hock joint, and is considered a blemish rather than an unsoundness; **bog spavin** is a large, fluid-filled swelling of the tibiotarsal joint, bulging out on the front-inside area and back of the joint; **bone spavin (jack spavin)** is the worst type, and is an incurable arthrosis causing lameness; **occult spavin (blind spavin)** involves the joint surfaces of the hock and, while it shows no bony enlargement, is a permanent and ugly blemish but rarely, if ever, causes lameness

spay *vt.* to remove (a female horse's) ovaries for the purpose of sterilization

species *n.* a biological classification, making up a subdivision of a genus, of animals (or plants) similar to each other in type (e.g., *Equus caballus,* the horse, is a species of the genus *Equus*)

specimen *n.* a sample, as of urine, blood, etc., collected for analysis

speculum *n.* a device used to (a) dilate a body opening for examination purposes or (b) hold the mouth open for dental work

speculum

speed *n.* 1. the ability to move rapidly 2. the rate of motion; the maximum speed of horses is about 40 m.p.h. over a short distance; the average speed for the Grand National is about 28 m.p.h. and for the Kentucky Derby about 35–36 m.p.h.

speedy cut a cut anywhere on the inner surface of a leg between the knee or hock and coronary band inflicted by the opposite foot

spell *vt.* to give (a horse) a period of rest — *n.* a period of rest

sperm *n.* spermatozoon

spermatic cord a cord to which each testicle is attached

spermatozoon *n., pl.* **-zoa** the male reproductive cell found in semen

Sphaerophorus necrophorus an anaerobic bacterium that can cause thrush

sphagnum *n. see* **peat moss**

sphenoid bone a bone at the base of the skull

sphincter *n.* a ring of muscle fibers which controls the opening and closing of a natural opening — **sphincteral** *adj.*

spicules *n.pl.* the porous, lattice-like interior of a bone

spider *n.* a very light type of phaeton carriage

spider

spin *n.* a maneuver in which a horse is asked to stop, plant hind feet on the ground and turn in a circle — *vi.*

spinal cord the part of the central nervous system within the spinal column

spinal nerve a nerve that originates in the spinal cord

spine *n.* 1. the backbone or spinal column 2. a slender bone projection —**spinal**

spiraling *n.* lunging or riding a horse in a spiral fashion, in either a constantly increasing or decreasing circle —**spiral** *vt.* —*adj.*

spirilla *n.pl.* various aerobic bacteria of the genus *Spirillum,* shaped like a spiral thread; can be found in the discharge present in seborrhea (grease)

spirited *adj.* full of energy —**spirit** *n.*

spirochete *n.* any of several spiral-shaped, disease-producing bacteria of the order **Spirochaetales** —**spirochetal** *adj.*

Spiti *n.* an Indian pony breed, named for the area of the Himalayas to which it is indigenous; hardy and very sure-footed; has a short strong back, short thick neck, short legs and hard round hooves; typically gray; 12 h.h.

splanchnic nerve a nerve that supplies the chest and abdomen

splayfoot *n.* a horse that stands with toes pointing outward —**splay-footed** *adj.*

spleen *n.* a lymphatic organ in the upper left area of the abdominal cavity —**splenic** *adj.*

splint *n.* an exostosis (bony growth) involved in a condition referred to as *splints* which affects the inside of the foreleg and very occasionally the outside of the rear leg; tearing of the ligament between the cannon bone and splint bone causes a periostitis appearing as a hot, painful swelling, which is followed by the formation of a splint; usually caused by excessive concussion in young horses, poor conformation, and sometimes improper calcium-phosphorous ratio

splint bones the two slender bones in the leg lying on either side of the cannon bone and closely attached to it; now non-functional, they are the second and fourth metacarpal bones in the forelegs and metatarsal bones in the hind legs

splint boots padded boots fitted to protect the splint bones; secured with straps and various types of fasteners: velcro slide-through-buckle closures, loop-n-lock fasteners, or ordinary buckles

splint boots

splinter bar a crossboard attached to the front of a carriage to which the traces of the wheelers are connected

split hoof *see* **crack**

split pastern a fracture of the first phalanx; a crack starts in the bone but rarely runs the entire length of it or the fracture may be comminuted; causes extreme lameness and distress to the horse; complete recovery is attained with the right treatment, unless arthritis develops

spondylitis *n.* inflammation of the vertebrae or spinal column, usually in the lumbar area; causes include positioning the saddle too far back, especially when a horse is ridden by a heavy rider, and bucking

spondylosis deformans a tearing of the lower part of an intervertebral disk, usually in the center of the back, due to a downward bending of the vertebral column and causing pain which leads to a horse being cold backed; new bone then forms on the bottom of the vertebrae, making that section rigid, thereby preventing further bending —*see also* **cold back**

sponge *n.* a porous, soft, absorbent mass that forms the skeleton of certain salt-water invertebrates of the phylum *Porifera*; useful for parts of grooming a horse, especially washing sensitive areas like the eyes, nose, and ears

sponsor *n.* in regard to equine activities, a person, group, or agency that endorses and assumes various responsibilities relating to competition riders or horses in such sports events as show-jumping, eventing, racing, etc. — *vt.* — **sponsorship** *n.*

spontaneous fracture a bone fracture that occurs without seemingly significant cause, such as may happen when a horse suddenly shies

spook *vi., vt.* to shy or bolt or cause to shy or bolt — *n.* a horse given to shying or bolting

spoon bit a type of curb bit similar to a spade bit but with a moderately high port

sporadic lymphangitis *see* **Monday morning leg**

sporotrichosis *n.* a contagious fungal disease characterized by nodules and ulcers, chiefly on the limbs

sport of kings horse racing

spot *n.* a white facial hair marking which is a small version of the star; flake

spots *n.pl.* *see* **coital exanthema**

spotted horse *see* **Appaloosa**

sprain *vt.* to tear or wrench (a muscle, ligament or joint) — *n.* — **sprained** *adj.*

spread *vi.* to stretch or pose

spread fence in show-jumping and cross-country events, an obstacle that is not only high but wide, such as parallel bars, triple bar, water jump, or hog's back; a **spread jump** is usually a wide water jump

spread plate a loose shoe

spring a leak *see* **leak**

spring bar a stirrup bar that has a spring-mounted safety catch

springer *n.* in racing, a horse on which bets suddenly increase

spring mouth a jointed, sometimes serrated snaffle bit with no rings which, for more severity, can be attached with spring clips to another snaffle

spring tree saddle a modern popularly used saddle that has springs, actually metal strips, in the tree which make it flexible, allowing the rider good contact with the horse; it is comfortable, helps the rider to sit correctly, and is conducive to using the seat as an aid

sprinter *n.* a horse that can move at high speed over a short distance

spur *n.* a device with a rowel, either blunt or sharp, that straps or clips onto a rider's heel and is used as an aid to impel a horse — *vt.* to prick with a spur or spurs

spur

spurious cyst *see* **false cyst**

squamous cell carcinoma lumpy cancer of skin cells near body openings

squared toe shoe a shoe squared at the toe for ease of breakover and set back from the toe of the hoof, which may be rasped or left to wear off naturally

squared toe shoe

squatter's rights *see* **take a squatter's rights**

squaw tail *see* **rabicano**

ST *see* **slow-twitch muscle fibers**

stable *n.* 1. an enclosure to house a horse or horses 2. a number of horses owned by one person or two or more co-owners, or kept in one place — *vt.* to house (a house or horses) in a stable

stable fly a blood-sucking fly that breeds on decaying vegetation, especially urine-soaked hay and soggy, fermenting grain; active on warm, sunny days and is particularly noticeable just prior to rain; highly irritating to confined horses; transmits habronema stomach worms

stable pneumonia *see* **arteritis**

stadium jumping a term relating to show-jumping, especially the show-jumping phase of a three-day event

stagecoach a four-wheeled coach that was once a primary means of transport; it had seats inside as well as on top, was pulled by two to eight horses and maintained a scheduled route carrying passengers and mail

stagger *vi.* to walk in an uncoordinated way, as if about to fall down

staggers *n. see* **wobbles** or **megrims**

stagnation edema *see* **stocking up**

stained line in hunting, a quarry's line that has been camouflaged by other animals crossing it; foil

stake class a class at a horse show that offers money prizes

stake money in racing, the total money taken in, out of which the winner and placed horses are paid

stake race a playday event which involves riding around six barrels in a pattern somewhat resembling an X

staking injury a wound caused by the penetration by a piece of wood or other material into a part of the body

stale *vi.* to urinate

stalking-horse *n.* a blind in the shape of a horse, or a real horse behind which a hunter may hide when stalking game

stall *n.* an enclosed area for a horse

stallion *n.* an uncastrated male horse, four or more years of age

stampede *n.* a sudden, uncontrolled running away of a herd of horses — *vi.* to run in such a manner — *vt.* to cause (a herd of horses) to run in an uncontrolled rush

stampeder *n.* one of a group of stampeding horses

stance *n.* a way of standing

Standardbred *n.* an American trotter breed, the fastest in the world for harness racing; developed chiefly from Thoroughbreds; has been exported to many countries to improve other harness racers; 14–16 h.h.

standard event any of five rodeo events recognized by the Professional Rodeo Cowboys Association, which are bareback riding, calf roping, bull riding, saddle-bronc riding, and steer wrestling

standing martingale a strap that runs from the girth between the forelegs, through a neck strap, to the noseband; controls the height of the head but has no effect on the bit

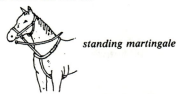

standing martingale

stand off in jumping, to take off far in advance of the fence

stand up in shows, to cause (a horse), in hand, to stand evenly on all four legs so that the judge can assess its conformation

Stanhope gig a light, topless, two-wheeled carriage for two people; named after the first owner (1787–1864) of such a carriage

stapes *n.* a small bone, shaped like a stirrup, in the middle ear

star *n.* a white facial marking that somewhat resembles a star

star gazer a horse that holds its head too high with its face more horizontal than the proper vertical position

starting gate in racing, a mechanical gate behind which all the horses in a race line up to get an even start when an official (starter) operates a control to release and raise it

starting stall in racing, any of the individual stalls in which the horses and their jockeys stand behind the gate in readiness to take off

stasis *n.* a slowing or stoppage as of the intestines or blood circulation

stay apparatus a linkage structure in each of the legs that locks them to enable a horse to sleep while standing

staying power stamina

steed *n.* a spirited horse for riding

steeldust *n., adj. see* **iron gray**

steeplechase *n.* a cross-country horse race over a specially prepared obstacle course. There are two kinds — the hurdle race, in which the fences are built to give way when knocked, and the steeplechase proper, which features some very difficult and dangerous obstacles to be jumped. The length of the course may be over four miles long. The name apparently originated in the mid–18th century with races between two riders to a goal, such as a church steeple, jumping any existing obstacles en route in an effort to maintain the most direct way.

steeplechaser *n.* a type of horse used for steeplechasing; specially bred for speed, strength and endurance coupled with a calm character; most are Thoroughbreds and others are halfbreds; also chaser

step mouth a condition in which one or more of the cheek teeth is much longer than the others, giving a step-like appearance

Steppe Horse a type of primitive horse that has been discovered to have roamed in the past over a huge area from the Atlas mountains and Spanish Sierras in the west to what is now Russia in the east; these horses had long, large heads with large ears and some were as tall as 18 h.h.

stepping action high lifting of the legs when in motion, either naturally or because of training; a horse with this action is called a high stepper

stepping pace a gait that is spectacular in its restraint; the horse is collected and held back by the rider, and there is an instant's hesitation with every step; the action is high, with exaggerated motion of knees and hocks, yet very slow and controlled; it is a gait of the Saddlebred and is similar to but slower than the rack

stereotype *n.* a compulsive, abnormal behavior (in horses) regularly repeated, such as cribbing, self-biting, etc. — **stereotypic, stereotypical** *adj.*

sterility *n.* 1. infertility; inability to produce offspring 2. purity; absence of microorganisms — **sterile** *adj.* — **sterilize** *vt.*

sternal recumbancy lying down on the breastbone with legs partly tucked underneath the body

sternocephalicus *n.* a muscle that moves the head and neck; lameness can be caused by a sprain of this muscle

sterno-thyro-hyoideus *n.* a muscle that aids in swallowing and sucking

sternum *n.* the breastbone — **sternal** *adj.*

steroid *n.* any of a group of organic compounds based on a system of four interlocking rings of carbon atoms. Included are the sex hormones, sterols, corticosteroids, Vitamin D, etc.; a drug containing compounds including natural hormones, such as estrogen and testosterone, and the synthetic corticosteroids used to control allergy and inflammation — **steroidal** *adj.*

sterol *n.* any of a group of solid, cyclic, unsaturated alcohols, as cholesterol, found in the body; a subdivision of the steroids

stertor *n.* the sound produced in sleep or coma by the soft palate

stethoscope *n.* an instrument used to amplify and listen to sounds from the body, as those of the heart or lungs

steward *n.* an official at a horse race who sees that all rules are carried out properly

sticker *n.* a thin metal wedge on the ground surface of the heel of a horseshoe used on racehorses to give better traction

sticky *adj.* hesitant to jump; describes a horse that almost refuses the fence and jumps from a standstill or trot

stiff line a headsetting harness device consisting of a one-foot piece of straight steel attached to the reins; it presses against the horse's neck if the horse turns its head

stifle *n.* the joint at the end of the thigh, corresponding to the human knee; formed by the lower end of the femur and upper end of the tibia with the patella

stiffle lameness a condition made apparent when a horse lifts its quarters on the lame side and bends the stifle and hock as little as possible; can be caused by arthritic pain

stilbestrol *n.* a synthetic estrogen used to induce estrus, treat uterine infections, dilate the cervix at parturition and expel afterbirth; diethylstilbestrol

stile *n.* in show-jumping and cross-country, an obstacle to be jumped

stilette *n.* 1. a fine instrument used to probe a body cavity 2. a wire used to insert into and clear a catheter or cannula

stillbirth *n.* the birth of a dead foal that is over 300 days old (if the fetus is younger, the term used is abortion) — **stillborn** *adj.*

stimulant *n.* 1. anything that excites or incites to action, as perhaps high wind or cold weather 2. any agent that invigorates, as a drug; stimulus — **stimulate** *vt., vi.*

sting *n.* an insect bite. Can raise significant welts on a horse's body and may cause a horse to gallop about, sometimes dangerously. If a horse lies down on an ant nest, thereby getting ants crawling over and stinging its body, the horse will most likely race around bucking in an effort to rid itself of the attackers; hosing the horse down with a strong spray of water will wash off the ants, relieve the pain and usually calm the horse.

stirrup *n.* 1. a device, of leather (Western) or metal (English), hung by a strap from a saddle to support a rider's foot in mounting and riding 2. a bone shaped like a stirrup — *see also* **stapes**

English stirrup   *Western stirrup*

stirrup cup in hunting, drinks offered by the host of the hunt before starting off

stirrup iron *see* **irons**

stirrup webs light tubular webbed supports for stirrups used for racing

stitch *vt.* to suture or join together (the edges of a wound or laceration) using a needle and any of various types of material such as catgut, nylon, or wire — *n.* (a) the act of stitching (b) the material used (c) a single loop made when stitching

stock *n.* 1. (a) the first in a line of descent of a particular breed; (b) individuals with the same ancestry 2. livestock 3. a supply, as of feed — *adj.* (a) for breeding, as a stock mare (b) used on a ranch, as for driving cattle

stock class a show class for stock horses

stock contractor in rodeo, a person or organization that provides all the livestock used in the rodeo; sometimes, especially in small rodeos, the contractor also promotes, rents the arena, manages ticket sales and concessions, and collects gate receipts

stocked *adj.* 1. (of a mare) serviced 2. (of a field) occupied by livestock

stocking *n.* a white coloration or marking surrounding the leg and extending from hoof to above the knee or hock (full stocking), or to the knee or hock (half stocking), or halfway up the cannon (quarter stocking)

stocking up a swelling of the legs or filling of the tendons, usually as a result of poor circulation which can be caused by conformation faults; many horses left standing for long periods after hard work will stock up; also called stagnation edema

stock saddle a Western saddle

stock seat the correct Western seat; a rider sits on seat bones with a slight bend at the knee, toes under knee, and feet parallel to the horse's sides

stock whip *see* **whip**

stomach *n.* the digestive organ between the esophagus and small intestine having a capacity of about two to four gallons

stomach staggers a condition which in chronic cases may be attributed to cirrhosis of the liver or to hydrocephalus; more commonly affects carthorses; characterized by a staggering gait, sleepiness and lack of interest in anything, including finishing food in the mouth; grass staggers; sleepy staggers

stomach tube a flexible tube used for the administration of oral drugs directly into the stomach

stomatitis *n.* inflammation in the mouth which can be caused by any of various irritants, such as chemicals, foreign agents such as thorns, certain feeds, tooth irregularities, fungi, bits, etc.; contagious in its pustular form; characterized by appetite loss, particularly for dry food, copious salivation, and an offensive mouth odor

stone *n. see* **calculus**

stone bruise a bruising or inflammation that occurs in the sole of the foot due to stepping on a sharp object, as a pointed stone

stone-cold *adj.* in racing, not making a vigorous effort, as if having given up

stone horse a stallion

straightaway barrels in playday com-petition, a timed event wherein a rider must weave through three barrels set in a straight line and return in the same way

straight behind a conformation fault wherein there is too little angle in the stifle

straight fence in show-jumping and cross country courses, any obstacle whose parts are all in a straight line, such as a gate, post and rails, etc.

straightness *n.* the quality of having no curve throughout the length of the body; many horses are not totally straight in their movement and some tend to curve quite significantly while galloping; when the hindlegs follow exactly the same track as the forelegs, the horse is traveling straight

straight pastern a pastern that is too upright instead of angled

straight stall an enclosure, usually 8 × 5 ft., in which a horse is tied, with manger and bucket at its head; tie stall

strangle *vt.* 1. to kill by squeezing the throat, as might be done with a rope 2. to suffocate or choke, as might be done by smoke — *vi.* to be strangled

strangles *n.* a highly contagious bacterial infection of the lymph nodes, chiefly in young horses, usually of the head; caused by *Streptococcus equi*; abscesses form and may become large enough to obstruct the airway (hence the name); these may break internally, draining a creamy nasal discharge; the condition can be spread to other parts of the body and localize in areas such as the lungs, this being called **bastard strangles**; although this disease is also known as **distemper**, it is unrelated to the viral distemper in dogs and cats; a vaccine is available — *see also* **coryza**

strangulate *vt.* 1. to strangle 2. to constrict a body channel — *vi.* to become constricted — **strangulation** *n.*

strangulated hernia a tightly constricted protrusion of an organ or

tissue through an abnormal body opening; this is a serious condition wherein there is a narrowing of the hernial ring, or mouth of the sac; the resulting compression affects circulation and causes hemorrhage, peritonitis, and necrosis, if not relieved; symptoms are pain, restlessness, patchy sweating, pawing the ground, and crouching as if to stale; the horse may lie down on its back; as the condition advances, the horse groans frequently, pulse quickens, and temperature rises to 104–105 degrees F.; finally, pain symptoms disappear, skin becomes cold and hiccuping and neighing may ensue; then the horse sways, falls, and dies

strangury *n.* a urinary disorder in which there are frequent attempts to stale with only small results

strap[1] *n.* a narrow strip of leather or other material used for fastening one thing to another, as, for example, to hold a blanket on a horse

strap[2] *vt.* 1. to groom 2. to lash with a strap 3. to fasten with a strap

strappings *n.pl.* same as trappings

straw *n.* 1. the stalk of grain 2. plurally, stalks when cut and threshed; certain types of straw can be fed to horses but have little or no nutritional value; sometimes used for bedding

strawyard *n.* a yard covered with straw for horses at rest or recuperating from illness

stray *n.* a horse that joins a herd from outside — *vi.* to wander off from one's usual habitat or herd

streak *n.* *see* **stripe**

Strelets Arab a grouping of three Arabian subtypes bred in the Kirghiz region of Russia: the Kuhailan, Munighi, and Siglavy; used as racehorses and in harness

streptococcus *n.* any of various spherical or oval-shaped bacteria of the genus *Streptococcus*; some species occur normally in the upper respiratory tract, while others produce diseases such as strangles —**streptococcal, streptococcic** *adj.*

stress fracture a fracture caused by repeated concussion or force

stretched *adj.* *see* **camped**

striation *n.* a fine groove or ridge, as e.g. a bit may make on a horse's teeth by contact with them; also stria —**striated** *adj.*

strike *n.* an act of aggression or defense by a horse — *vt.*

string *n.* 1. (Western) a cowboy's group of horses 2. two or more racehorses exercising together

stringhalt *n.* spastic overflexion of a hind leg, observed when a horse is in motion and raises one or both hind legs with a high-stepping, jerky, spastic action; mild cases ease out with exercise but severe cases render the horse useless to ride

strings *n.pl.* the leather strips that hang from a Western saddle; can be very useful for tying things to the saddle

stripe *n.* a narrow white facial marking extending from forehead to muzzle —*see also* **race; streak**

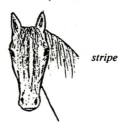

stripe

stroke volume the amount of blood being pumped through the heart with each beat

Strongid-C *n.* a parasiticide pelleted with alfalfa that is given on a daily

basis to keep the recipient worm-free; as such it is a preventative rather than a curative agent; its active ingredient is pyrantel tartrate, and it is given at the rate of 4 ounces per 1,000 lbs. of body weight

strongyle *n.* a roundworm parasite whose larvae can permanently damage the intestinal blood vessels and walls and cause death by intestinal failure; eggs are passed in excrement; redworm, *Strongylus vulgaris, Strongylus equinus*

strongylidosis *n.* infestation of strongyles

strychnine *n.* a poisonous stimulant obtained from the seed of the nux vomica plant

stub *n.* a stone bruise

stud[1] *n.* a removable steel cleat screwed into a horseshoe to increase traction

stud[2] *n.* 1. a stallion used for breeding 3. a place where stallions and mares are kept for breeding purposes

studbook *n.* a registry in which all the purebred ancestors of a breed are recorded

stud groom a senior groom

stud ring a ring, made of plastic or metal, that may be placed around the horse's penis to discourage erection

stumble *vi.* to trip or fall when walking or running; usually a horse will recover after tripping over something, but occasonally a horse will either fall forward onto its knees and then recover or come down altogether; some horses are prone to stumbling because of laziness, bad conformation, or a pathology such as arthritis, but fatigue or bad horsemanship can also be a cause with any horse — *n.* — **stumbler** *n.* a horse prone to stumbling

sty, stye *n.* a small swelling of a sebaceous gland on the rim of the eyelid

stylo-hyoideus muscle the muscle that pulls back the tongue and raises the larynx when swallowing

styptic *adj.* having astringent qualities and able to contract blood vessels and halt superficial bleeding — *n.* a styptic substance — **stypticity** *n.*

subacute *adj.* less than acute or between acute and chronic, as a disease — **subacutely** *adv.*

subchondral bone cyst a cyst in bone beneath joint cartilage

subclinical *adj.* without apparent disease symptoms

subconjunctival *adj.* beneath the conjunctiva

subcutaneous *adj.* beneath the skin

subscapularis *n.* a muscle between the scapula (shoulder blade) and the chest wall

substance *n.* the strength and endurance of a horse, as differing from quality

substrate *n.* a substance, as blood or tissue, acted upon by a chemical, such as an enzyme, and made usable for muscles of any other body tissues

suck *vt.* to draw in (liquid), as milk from an udder — *vi.* to draw from the udder

suckle *vt.* to nurse or cause to suck at the udder — *vi.* to suck at the udder

sudaderos *n.pl.* the fenders of a Western saddle

Suffolk *n.* the purest of British cold-blood breeds, with a lineage that can be traced back to 1760; first registered in 1877; always some shade of chestnut in color; strong and very wide, with short legs; very good temperament; up to 17 h.h.; also called Suffolk Punch

sugar beet poisoning *see* **beet poisoning**

sulcus *n., pl.* -ci a groove such as one of those on either side and the center of the frog

sulfa *adj.* chemically related to sulf-anilamide

sulfamethazine *n.* generic name for an antibacterial sulfa drug

sulfanilamide *n.* a compound used to inhibit bacterial infection

sulfate *n.* a salt of sulfuric acid

sulfur *n.* an element used to inhibit bacterial infection

sulky *n.* a light, two-wheeled, one-horse carriage having a seat for only one person, especially today one used in harness races; bike

Sumba *n.* an Indonesian pony breed; intelligent and agile; dun-colored with a black eel stripe and upright mane; used in the local sport of lance-throwing and in dancing competitions in which the horse dances in time to the beat of tom-toms; about 12.2 h.h.

summer sores *n.* sores found usually on the legs, flanks, back, neck, and penis, which begin as inflamed lesions which refuse to heal; soon ulcerations and rawness appear and the sores grow, sometimes reaching huge proportions; caused by migrating larvae of common stomach worms deposited by flies on wounds; these sores resemble proud flesh, benign tumors and cancer, so diagnosis to determine treatment requires care; habronemiasis

sunburn *n.* inflammation of the skin due to prolonged exposure to the sun in fiercely hot conditions; areas around the head and back are susceptible to sunburn, although non-pigmented and hairless skin, as on the muzzle, is more easily burned; these areas become swollen and ooze serum

sunfish *vi.* to twist the body in the air when bucking — **sunfisher** *n.* a bucking horse that twists its body

sunstroke *n.* a condition brought on by exposure to intense heat and glare of the sun, chiefly caused by fatigue from working under that exposure, especially when the horse is deprived of sufficient fluid intake; an ill-ventilated hot stable, perhaps with direct exposure to the sun, may also bring on the condition; characterized by the horse suddenly collapsing into an insensible state, with hindquarters paralyzed, then in a convulsive manner struggling to rise but in so doing often inflicting serious injury to itself; staring eyes; rapid respiration; weak pulse; in mild cases the horse recovers, but severe cases are fatal

superficial digital flexor muscle a muscle which flexes the toe and extends the hock

superficial flexor tendon an outer tendon that connects the superficial muscles of the upper leg to the back of the pastern bones

superficial line firing a type of firing in which the iron is used to draw lines through only the superficial layers of the skin

superficial pectoral muscle a muscle which advances and adducts the leg

superior check ligament a muscle that supports the superficial flexor tendon above the knee

superior maxilla the upper jaw

suppurate *vi.* ooze — **suppuration** *n.*

supraorbital fossae the hollows above the eyes, which provide a safety area of retreat for the eyes in case of a blow; the eye lies in an orbit which has a layer of fat behind the eye; when the eye receives a blow, it is pushed into the safety of the orbit where, in turn, the protecting fat layer makes room by being pushed into the supraorbital fossa

suprarenal *adj.* above the kidney

suprascapular nerve the motor nerve that innervates the scapula (shoulder blade) muscles

suprascapular paralysis a type of

paralysis which causes a wasting of the shoulder muscles

supraspinatus *n.* a muscle that extends the shoulder joint — **supraspinous** *adj.*

suramin *n.* a substance used in worm medicines

surcingle *n.* a girth or strap that passes around a horse's girth to hold on a saddle, blanket, or pack

sure-footed *adj.* not prone to stumbling

surfactant *n.* 1. a chemical substance that reduces the surface tension of a liquid to promote absorption; sometimes added to injectable medications 2. a chemical substance in the lung that reduces the surface tension of the air sac lining, which enables the sac to retain its expansion; its absence causes the air sac to deflate, as in certain respiratory diseases

surfeit *n.* *see* **urticaria**

surgeon *n.* *see* **veterinarian**

surgery *n.* 1. the operative procedure for the treatment of disease or injury that should only be performed by a qualified veterinarian 2. an operating room

surra *n.* a usually fatal blood disease transmitted by flies and characterized by pernicious anemia

surrey *n.* a light, four-wheeled horse carriage with two seats facing forward

surrogate *n.* a mare that replaces a foal's dam

suspension *n.* a liquid (not solution) in which tiny particles float

suspensory *adj.* supporting or sustaining, as a muscle or bandage

suspensory ligament a thick strip of fibrous tissue extending from the back of the carpus (knee) and tarsus (hock) to the fetlock, just above which it splits into two major branches that connect with the sesamoid bones; two smaller branches extend across the fetlock and join the extensor tendon on the front of the pastern; supports the fetlock joint, preventing it from sinking to the ground

suspensory sprain *see* **run-down** — *n.*

suture *n.* 1. a surgical stitch 2. a uniting together or line of junction of certain bones, as of the skull

swab *n.* a small piece of cotton or sponge at the end of a stick used to apply medicine to, or clean, a wound or part of the body; also used to collect material, as from an infected site, for laboratory examination

swage shoe (*pron.* swej) a shoe that has a longitudinal groove or grooves in the bottom surface (usually including the nail holes) which increase traction

swaging *n.* a groove in a shoe to provide traction; also called **fullering**

swallowtail *n.* *see* **shadbelly**

swallow the head (of a bucking bronco) to lower the head all the way down between the forelegs while bucking furiously

swamp fever *see* **equine infectious anemia**

swan neck a neck that is too long and thin and becomes ewe-necked at its base

sway back a back that is concave, a mark of bad conformation or old age; an exaggerated dip behind the withers can be due to having sustained a sprain below the short ribs; lordosis; saddlebacked — *adj.*

sweat *vi.* to ooze a salty moisture from the pores of the skin; to perspire; hot sweating, with the skin being warm, occurs as a natural coolant for the body when it is subjected to heat from external conditions or exercise; cold sweating, the skin being cold, occurs under nervous stress or with certain diseases — *n.*

sweat scraper a device with a handle and curved attachment edged with rubber stripping, used to scrape sweat

off a horse or to scrape excess water off after bathing

Swedish Ardennes a heavy Swedish draft horse which originated in the 19th century with crosses of imported Belgian Ardennes with North Swedish horses; 15.2–16 h.h.

sweat scraper

Swedish Warm-Blood an attractive Swedish horse of good temperament used in dressage and competitions; registry dates back to 1874; 15.2–16.3 h.h.

sweeny *n.* a degenerative condition of the shoulder joint wherein the supra-scapular nerve is stretched and damaged, thereby causing eventual atrophy of the two adjoining muscles; characterized by a snap or popping outward of the shoulder as weight is put on the leg; caused by slipping back of the shoulder in a forward stride, which might occur on slippery ground when pulling a heavy load or climbing a steep incline

sweepstake *n.* in regard to horse racing: 1. a lottery in which the winners are determined by the results of the race   2. the winnings of such a lottery

sweetfeed *n.* a feed mixture of ingredients such as corn, oats, minerals, vitamins, etc., with molasses

sweet itch a dermatitis or skin allergy to the saliva of some insects or possibly to ingestion of certain plants; characterized by an inflammatory, itchy thickening and scabbing of the skin, causing exudation when the horse scratches; often affects the mane and tail

Sweet PDZ *see* **clinoptilolite**

swell *vi.* to bulge out or increase abnormally in size — *vt.* to cause to bulge or become abnormally large — **swollen** *adj.* — **swelling** *n.*

swells *n.pl.* the front projections of Western saddle below and on either side of the horn, 9–15 inches wide; the narrower width facilitates a quick dismount; the wider one offers more security

swim *vi.* to propel the body through water by movements of the legs; horses swim naturally even under the weight of a rider; swimming is a good method of exercise without putting strain on the legs, and is especially useful if the legs are undergoing physiotherapy — *vt.*, — *n.*

swing horse the center horse in a random or, if plural, the center pair of a six-horse team

swinging-leg lameness lameness caused by pain from moving the affected leg

swish *vt.* to whip (the tail) from side to side; a horse does so (a) as a sign of displeasure, (b) sometimes after defecation or staling, or (c) to brush off flies

Swiss Warm-Blood a new breed of sports horse developed in Switzerland for general riding, competition, and driving; 15.3–16.2 h.h.

switch *n.* 1. a hairpiece that ties into a horse's tail, matching its color and texture, to add length or fullness   2. a thin stick used as a whip   3. a lashing action by a rider with a switch — *vt.* to lash with a switch

switch-tail *n.* a tail that has the end hairs pulled to form a point

symbiosis *n.* an intimate and beneficial association of two different organisms — **symbiotic** *adj.*

symmetrical *adj.* in relation to a disease or infection, affecting corresponding parts of the body in the same way and at the same time — **symmetrically** *adv.*

symmetric focal cervical myelopathy a noninflammatory spinal pathology which affects both sides of the cord symmetrically

sympathetic nerve a nerve, one of the

functions of which is to cause constriction of blood vessels and increase of blood pressure; it is part of the nervous system which automatically stimulates involuntary action of various body organs

symptom *n.* a sign of a disease which may be used in diagnosis —**symptomatic** *adj.*

synapse *n.* an area of contact between two nerves where an impulse passes from the end of one nerve to the beginning of another

synarthrodial joint *see* **joint**

syncope *n.* unconsciousness caused by insufficient blood supply to the brain —**syncopal** *adj.*

syndicate *n.* a group of people with shares in a horse

syndrome *n.* a collection of symptoms which, when occurring together, form a pattern of a particular disease or abnormality

synergism *n.* 1. the combined action of different chemicals which, when administered together (as in certain drugs called **synergists**), have a greater result than the total of the results of each when administered separately 2. the joint action of different parts of the body, such as muscles —**synergistic** *adj.* —**synergistically** *adv.*

synovia *n.* the clear, sticky lubricating fluid in joint cavities, tendon sheaths, etc. —**synovial** *adj.*

synovial membrane the thin tissue that lines a joint

synovial sac the sac within a joint that secretes synovia

synovitis *n.* inflammation of the synovial membrane

syphilis *n.* an equine venereal disease —*see also* **dourine**

syringe *n.* 1. a device having a narrow tube at one end and a rubber bulb at the other, used to suck in fluid and then eject it; used to extract fluid from a body cavity or to cleanse a wound 2. a hypodermic syringe is a glass or plastic container with a hollow metal needle, used to inject fluid or extract it

system *n.* a set of body parts that are united to perform the same function, as e.g. the nervous system or respiratory system

systemic *adj.* acting system-wide in the body

systole *n.* the period of heartbeat when the heart contracts and expels the blood contained therein —**systolic** *adj.*

systolic blood pressure the pressure of blood exerted when pumped by contraction of the heart muscle

Sztum *n.* the largest of the Polish draft horses; originated from crosses of local horses with Belgian, Rhenish, Jutland, Ardennes and Dole stock; 16–17 h.h.

— T —

table *n.* the part of an incisor tooth that comes into contact with the corresponding tooth of the opposite jaw

tables *n.pl.* in show-jumping, the score boards showing penalties incurred for faults or for taking more time than that allowed in speed classes

tack *n.* saddle, bridle, and other equipment used in riding, handling a horse, and in harness; a shortening of **tackle**

tacked up saddled and bridled or harnessed

tacking race a gymkhana event in which contestants line up their haltered but unsaddled horses at one end

of the ring and at a signal lead them to be tacked up at the other end where saddles and bridles are put on; the winner is the first to finish and pass inspection

tack room a room next to a stable in which tack is kept

Tagamet *n.* trade name for cimetidine

tail *n.* the appendage formed by the prolongation of the backbone; it includes the dock with all the hair

tail blocking the cosmetic injection of small amounts of alcohol into the tail muscles to prevent a horse from swishing its tail

tail carriage the way a horse holds its tail when going; an elevated carriage is a mark of good breeding; the Arabian is known for its singular and gracefully elevated tail carriage

tail guard *see* **tail wrap**

tail hounds in hunting, the hounds that run some distance behind the main pack

tail-male line the top line of a pedigree

tail mark on New Forest ponies in England, a mark made by cutting the hair of the tail in a certain way to show that the fee (marking fee) required for the ponies pastured in the New Forest has been paid

tail pulling manicuring the tail by pulling out untidy or unshapely hairs

tail swishing *see* **swish**

tail wrap either bandaging or a one-piece wrap with self-gripping closure used on the tail to protect it when traveling, in preparation for showing, for veterinary examination, or when breeding; sometimes called a **tail guard**

take a squatter's rights to be thrown from a horse

take off in jumping, to lift the forehand to take a jump; also the place from which a horse jumps

taking your own line 1. in showjumping, selecting one's own route on the course 2. in hunting, departing from the field

tally-ho 1. in hunting, the announcement that a fox is seen 2. a four-in-hand coach

tamed iodine *see* **povidone iodine**

tandem *n.* a pair of horses harnessed one behind the other —*adj.* refers to horses so positioned

T'ang horses horses made of pottery during the Chinese T'ang Dynasty, AD 618–906, used as substitutes for living animals to be buried with their dead masters in their tombs

tantivy *adv.* at full gallop (term imitates the sound made by a horse's feet)

tapaderno *n.* (from Spanish, meaning "cover") the front covering of some Western stirrups that protect the feet when riding through thorny brush or in winter to keep the feet warm and dry; taps; hooded stirrup

tape suture a stitch made of linen

tapetum *n.* a layer within the eye between the choroid layer and retina, through which it reflects light to provide vision in dim light

tapeworm *n.* a long parasitic flatworm that infests the intestines

tap root in reference to horses, the main root of a female pedigree traced directly to its origin

taps *n.pl.* *see* **tapadero**

tarantula a large spider whose bite is painful but not fatal

tarantula

Tarbenian *n.* an Anglo-Arab breed from the plains around the town of Tarbes below the Pyrenees mountains; descended from the Iberian Horse; early in the 19th

century was improved with crosses of Arab stallions imported by Napoléon Bonaparte; subsequently, Thoroughbred stallions were introduced; a light-boned, handsome horse with attractive action and excellent all-a-round qualities; 15 h.h.

tarp *n.* a cover, usually of canvas, thrown over a loaded pack saddle

Tarpan *n.* originally a primitive wild Russian breed (*tarpan* being the Russian word for "wild horse") that no longer exists; however, today there is a forest pony breed that resembles the old Tarpan which is bred in Poland (*see* **Konik**); these ponies have a black eel stripe, zebra markings on the legs and sometimes on the body, which is either brown or dun-colored; about 13 h.h.

tarsal check ligament *see* **inferior check ligament**

tarsus *n.* 1. a group of six short bones in the area of the hock   2. a small plate of connective tissues that stiffen the eyelid — **tarsal** *adj.*

tartar *n.* brown dental calculus

taste *vt.* to sample by licking or taking a bit into the mouth — *n.*

Tat *n.* a native breed of India

tattoo *vt.* to mark (the skin) with coded numbers, as a means of identification, by searing or puncturing and filling the punctures with indelible ink or dye; this is sometimes done inside the upper lip of a valuable horse, especially race-horses — *n.*

taxus *n.* yew

TB 1. tuberculosis   2. Thoroughbred

T-cell *n.* a lymphocyte (white blood cell)

Tchenarani *n.* a breed that originated in Persia; used under saddle; 15 h.h.

TDN total digestible nutrients in any feed; the amount of nutrients actually used by the horse's system; oats, for example, have the highest TDN of all feeds, 80 percent

t.d.s. three times per day (ter die sumendum) (of medical prescriptions)

team *n.* technically, two or more horses harnessed together; generally, four or more horses harnessed together; a four-in-hand; also, the harnessed horses together with the vehicle (or plow) they are pulling — *vi.* to harness horses together

team chasing a sport that was first introduced in England in 1974; teams of four cross-country riders start together on a cross-country course and the team that gets three of its members back to the starting point first wins

team penning a sport in which a team of three riders tries to cut three numbered calves out of a herd of 30 and pen them at the designated end of the arena in less than two minutes; winners usually make a time of less than one minute

team roping a timed rodeo event involving two teamed competitors, a header and a heeler; a steer is given a head start out of a chute, then the first roper (header) chases after it and ropes it around the horns, taking two turns (dallies) of the other end of the rope around his saddle horn and slowing the steer; the second roper (heeler) then ropes the steer's hind feet; timing is complete when both ropes are tight and the horses face the steer; a five-second penalty is given for roping only one hind foot

team whip *see* **whip**

tear *vt.* to wound by pulling apart, as the skin or a muscle — *n.*

tear *n.* a drop of slightly saline fluid secreted by the lacrimal gland which normally lubricates the eyeball — *vi.* to shed tears, as in cases of infection or some foreign matter in the eye

tease *vt.* to flirt with or show a desire for mating with

teaser *n.* when breeding horses, a stallion, referred to as a teaser (not necessarily the one to be used for breeding), that is brought to a mare, with a partition between them, so that her reaction may be observed and her readiness to be settled judged

teat *n.* either of two protuberances on the female's udder; nipple

technical delegate at an international horse show and three-day event, someone who enforces pertinent international rules and ascertains that the course being used is as it should be

teeth clapping a foal's act of exposing its teeth and opening and closing its jaws, making a clapping noise as the teeth make contact; this is a submissive action performed toward an approaching strange horse; sometimes an adult horse under saddle may clap its teeth for no apparent reason

telemeter *n.* an instrument that uses radio signals to transmit electrical measurements of body functions; e.g. a telemeter can be strapped onto a horse to enable the recording of an electrocardiogram to be made at a distance while being ridden — *vt., vi.* to transmit by telemeter — **telemetric** *adj.* — **telemetrically** *adv.*

telemetry *n.* the usage of a telemeter to measure body functions

temperament *n.* character or disposition

temperature *n.* the degree of body heat; the average normal temperature of a male horse is about 100.5 degrees F., but very young or old horses have a temperature one degree lower, as do mares, except when they are in heat; temperature is measured by insertion of a thermometer into the rectum — *see also* **hyperthermia** and **hypothermia**

temple *n.* the flat surface on either side of the forehead — **temporal** *adj.*

temporalis *n.* a muscle that closes the mouth

tendinitis *n.* inflammation of a tendon

tendon *n.* the tough fibrous sinew connecting muscle to bone — **tendinous** *adj.*

tendon boots boots fitted to protect the tendons of the leg, especially in cases of bowed or sprained tendons

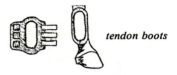

tendon boots

tendon graft the graft of a piece of normal tendon from one part of the body (of the same or another horse) to an injured tendon in another part

tendon sheath the covering of a tendon that lubricates it to reduce friction at certain points

tenectomy *n.* the surgical removal of a section of injured tendon

Tennessee Walker, -Walking Horse an American breed known for its comfortable running walk; the foundation sire was a Standardbred named Black Allan, foaled in 1886, which possessed this gait; the breed was developed for use on Southern plantations using Arab, Narragansett Pacer, Thoroughbred, and Morgan blood; its slow gaits are the flat-foot walk and running walk and its third gait is what is called a rocking chair canter wherein the forelegs move in a rotating motion while the hindquarters remain almost level; originally called Plantation Walker; 15–16 h.h.

tenorrhaphy *n.* surgical repair of torn tendons

tenosynovitis *n.* inflammation of a tendon and its sheath; tenovaginitis; can arise from over-reaching, a thorn, a kick, etc.

tenotomy *n.* the surgical cutting of a tendon, as to relieve a deformity

tension-band plate an implant for repairing and preventing separation of a broken bone

tension fracture a fracture caused by forces pulling a bone apart

tensor fasciae antibrachii a muscle that extends the elbow joint

teratoma *n.* a tumor consisting of misplaced tissue

teres major muscle a muscle which flexes the shoulder joint and adducts the leg

teres minor muscle a muscle which flexes the shoulder joint and abducts the leg

Terramycin *n.* trade name for tetracycline

Tersk, Tersky *n.* a Russian Arab-type breed officially recognized as a breed in 1948; used for general purpose riding; usually gray; 14.3–15.1 h.h.

test *n.* 1. an examination, as of blood or for pregnancy 2. a trial to ascertain ability to aptitude, as in a test ride — *vt.*

testicle, testis *n., pl.* -cles, tes either of a pair of male sex glands contained within the scrotum; they secrete spermatozoa and testosterone

testosterone *n.* male sex hormone produced by the testes

tetanic convulsion *see* **convulsion**

tetanus *n.* an acute, infectious disease produced by the bacterial agent *Clostridium tetani,* which lives in the soil and in manure and which enters the body via a wound; it may lie dormant for some time until conditions are suitable for spores to produce toxin; symptoms include muscle spasm, resulting in stiffness and rigidity (including rigidity of the jaw), drooling, and partial covering of the eyes by the third eyelid; death can occur in two or three days; also called lockjaw

tetany *n.* twitching or spasms of voluntary muscles, as in tetanus

tether *vt.* to tie with a rope — *n.* a rope used to hold a horse within a limited area

tetracycline *n.* an antibiotic; trade name Achromycin, Terramycin, and others

tetrahedral *adj.* shaped like a pyramid as is one type of enterolith — **tetrahedron** *n.*

thalamus *n., pl.* a part of the brain which relays sensory impulses in the cerebral cortex; also serves as a perceiver of some types of sensation — **thalamic** *adj.*

thallium poisoning a condition caused by ingestion of rat poison

thatching *n.* a means of drying a wet horse in cold weather by placing a layer of straw on its back under a blanket

theadore *see* **fiador**

therapeutic *adj.* able to cure or heal — **therapeutical** *adj.* — **therapeutically** *adv.*

therapeutics *n.pl.* the branch of medicine that deals with treatment and cure of diseases; therapy

therapy *n.* the treatment of diseases

theriogenology *n.* a branch of veterinary medicine that deals with reproduction

thermograph *n.* an instrument that automatically records variations in temperature in different parts of the body

thermography *n.* a diagnostic evaluation of body temperature variations using a thermograph

thermometer *n.* an instrument for detecting body temperature, inserted into a horse's rectum for this purpose

thermoregulation *n.* the body's system of maintaining a constant temperature

thiabendazole *n.* generic name for an oral dewormer used primarily against strongyles

thiamine, -min *n.* vitamin B; found in grains and cereals; deficiency of this vitamin is characterized by an abnormal walk and sometimes an arched appearance to the back while standing with rear legs set wide apart, muscle tremors, weakness and an abnormal heart rate

thick head horse sickness *see* **dikkop horse sickness**

thick wind a thickening of the respiratory mucous membrane, apparent both when inhaling and exhaling; characteristic of bronchitis

thief *n.* in racing, a horse that does not race up to the form it demonstrates when not competing

thigh *n.* the section of the hind leg between hip and stifle; the **second thigh** is the gaskin

thill *n.* either of the two shafts between which a harness horse is hitched

thiopentone sodium an anesthetic; trade name Pentothal

third eyelid *see* **nictitating membrane**

third phalanx *see* **coffin bone**

thirst *n.* the desire for water. A horse drinks 6–12 gallons a day, varying according to size, weather, and moisture content of food. Most drink less in very cold weather, and as a result food may become impacted in the intestines and cause colic. — *vi.* — **thirsty** *adj.*

thoracic percussion a test of a horse's chest for possible pain or tenderness by manually thumping on it; this is usually done by placing the palm of one hand on the area to be checked, then making a fist of the other hand and pounding once on the back of the first hand; the horse's reaction determines the diagnosis

thoracic wall the chest cavity, containing the pleura, ribs, muscles, skin, etc.; the chest cavity's enclosure

thorax *n.* the part of the body between the neck and abdomen; the chest — **thoracic** *adj.*

Thorazine *n.* trade name for chlorpromazine

thoroughbred *n.* purebred — *adj.*

Thoroughbred *n.* (from the literal translation of the Arabic *kehilan,* meaning "purebred all through") a British breed famous for speed, being the world's fastest horse and used worldwide for racing; originated by crossing native mares with three imported Eastern stallions: the Byerley Turk (1689), the Darley Arabian (1705), and the Godolphin Arabian (1728); sometimes referred to as TB; 14.2–17 h.h. Bulle Rock, in 1730, was the first Thoroughbred imported from England to America

thoroughpaced *adj.* thoroughly trained in all gaits or paces

thoroughpin *n.* a soft swelling of the lubricating tarsal sheath surrounding tendons on the sides and back of hock; caused by hard work, especially in immature horses; does not usually cause lameness except perhaps for the first day or two

threadworm *n.* an intestinal parasite, *Oxyuris equi,* that resembles a white thread and is about 1¼ inches long at maturity; the curved front end is thicker than the tail end which is thin and whip-like; an infestation is manifested by the horse rubbing its tail due to itching at the anus; also, a light yellow waxy substance (eggs) may be seen on the horse's skin just below the anus; the worms can also be seen in the dung; also called maw worm

three-day event a competition that continues over three consecutive days and tests the ability and versatility of both horse and rider; includes a dressage test, a cross-country event, and show-jumping

throat *n.* the area behind the tongue

which contains the soft palate, glottis, epiglottis, and openings to the larynx, eustachian tubes, and nasal cavities; pharynx

throat horse botfly *see Gastrophilus nasalis*

throatlatch *n.* 1. a bridle strap that goes under the throat 2. the underpart of the throat

thrombo-arteritic colic a thrombus-induced colic usually affecting the small intestine and cecum; the most frequent cause is the redworm parasite

thromboembolism *n.* a free-floating blood clot

thrombosis *n.* blood coagulation or clot formation in the heart or a blood vessel, causing an obstruction; can be caused by a wound; when the blood supply to muscles is obstructed, symptoms are apparent when the affected horse is exercised, such as a weakening of one or both hind legs and sinking of the croup; the limbs stiffen and finally the horse drops and struggles, sweats and then remains motionless later to rise and continue; in brachial thrombosis the forelegs are affected — **thrombotic** *adj.*

thromboxane *n.* a prostaglandin

thrombus *n., pl.* **thrombi** a blood clot

thrown *adj.* 1. (of a rider) dislodged from horseback 2. (of a horse) cast down for an operation

thrush *n.* a fungal disease of the hoof, characterized by black discharge from the grooves on either side of the frog and by a foul odor

thruster *n.* in hunting, a greenhorn who overrides hounds and jumps fences unnecessarily

thumps *n.* a quick, uncontrolled fluttering of the diaphragm sometimes due to mineral depletion

thymus *n.* an apparently functionless gland located in the upper thorax near the throat

thyroid *adj. see* **thyroid gland**

thyroid gland a large two-lobed endocrine gland in the neck on either side of the trachea which controls body growth and metabolism

thyroxine *n.* a hormone produced by the thyroid gland which regulates metabolic rate

tibben *n.* chaff of barley or wheat straw; bhoosa

Tibetan (Nanfan) a pony breed found in the Himalayan mountains of Tibet; sure-footed and strong and used as a pack pony on the steep mountain trails; adapts well to cold temperatures; 12.2 h.h.

tibia *n.* the thicker of the two bones of the hind leg extending between stifle joint and hock; forms the gaskin (second thigh)

tibialis anterior a muscle that flexes the hock joints

tibialis cranialis a muscle in the front of the gaskin

tibiotarsal bone a bone in the hock at the uppermost and largest joint with the lower end of the tibia

tick¹ *n.* a blood-sucking parasite which attaches itself to the skin and transmits diseases, such as Rocky Mountain spotted fever, equine encephalomyelitis, swamp fever, etc., by means of a secretion called attachment cement, produced by the salivary glands; its six rows of teeth also help it to grip onto its host; ear ticks live deep in the ear and cause a horse to shake its head, rub its ears, cock its head from side to side, and become ear-shy and hard to bridle

tick

tick² *vi., vt.* in jumping, to touch a jumping obstacle without knocking it down

tidal volume the amount of air inhaled in a single breath; the amount of change in the lung volume in one

breath; does not represent total lung capacity as there are residual gases left in the lungs with each breath

tied-in *adj.* very short of bone just below the knee

tie-down *n.* a Western martingale; a single strap runs from the noseband, between the forelegs, to the girth

tie-down

tied-up *adj.* having a muscle condition wherein lactic acid accumulates and is not expelled from the muscle tissue, thereby damaging the muscle fibers; if large areas are damaged or destroyed, it causes azoturia, a more severe form of tying-up; occurs most often in irregularly exercised horses; myostitis; Monday morning leg (or disease)

tie stall *see* **straight stall**

tiger trap a jump consisting of rails that angle over a deep ditch, either as one set of rails or two that form a cathedral ceiling–like shape

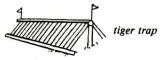

tiger trap

time allowed in show-jumping, the given period in which a competitor must complete a show-jumping course to avoid being eliminated or subjected to penalties

Timor *n.* an Indonesian pony breed native to the island of Timor; intelligent, agile, and strong, as well as sure-footed and gentle; used locally as a cow pony; 11–12 h.h.

timothy grass a tall perennial bunch (grows in clumps) grass with long, closely packed floral spikes; used for hay

tincture *n.* a solution of a drug in alcohol, as e.g. tincture of iodine

tip[1] *n.* 1. the pointed end of a body part, such as the tongue 2. a type of

corrective shoe or metal plate used on a foal 3. secret information given by a tipster

tip[2] *vi.* to tilt, as in relation to an inner part of the body —**tipped** *adj.*

tipster *n.* in racing, a person who provides information or tips about the horses

tissue *n.* a mass of cells of the same type; e.g., brain tissue, fat tissue, etc.

titer *n.* the measurement of the concentration of an antibody in blood serum or other substance

titration *n.* the measurement of a certain substance in a known volume of solution —**titrate** *vt., vi.* to conduct such a measurement

toad eye a bulging type of eye as typical of the Exmoor Pony

toad face pink pigmentation and spotted facial markings around the eyes and muzzle

toasted *adj.* having a coat coloration with dark patches, dull finish, or dark overcast

Tobiano *n.* a clearly marked color pattern with white as a base and another color, usually divided about half-and-half, throughout the coat; mane and tail are the color of the region from which they stem, legs are usually white, and the head is dark or combined with markings such as a star, stripe, snip, or blaze —*see also* **Pinto**

toe *n.* the front section of the hoof which meets the ground

toes out an undesirable position of a rider's feet with toes pointing outward in the stirrups

togavirus *n.* a mosquito- and tick-borne virus that can cause hemorrhagic fever; so named because it is contained in an envelope or "toga"

tolt *n.* a very rapid and smooth walking gait performed by Icelandic ponies

Tom Thumb bit a type of bit which has a mouthpiece with a port, straight bar, mullen mouth, or snaffle; may be made for single or double reins

Tom Thumb bit

tongue *n.* the muscular organ in the mouth used to taste, move food around, and swallow; when the horse is bitted, the tongue should lie under the bit

tongue grid a metal port hung in the mouth above the bit to prevent the tongue from getting over the bit

tongue lolling the unsightly habit of hanging the tongue out of the mouth when being driven or ridden

tongue strap a slotted strap to keep a horse's tongue down; sometimes used in racing; the tongue is put through the slot of the strap which is then fastened under the lower jaw; if fastened too tightly, it can cause enormous pain

tongue swallowing a condition sometimes seen during the latter part of a race when a horse makes a gurgling noise; said to be caused by neck muscles pulling at the larynx; gurgling; choking up

tonus *n.* the slight tension that muscles maintain when not contracting; this state prevents from extending or flexing too suddenly, maintains posture, and aids in venous circulation

tooth *n.* one of the bony structures set in the jaws and used for biting and chewing food as well as for attacking and self-defense; a mature male horse has 40 teeth: 12 incisors (6 in each jaw), 4 canines (tushes) except in females (which lack canines, except sometimes rudimentary ones), and 24 molars; sometimes there are also 4 wolf teeth, one in front of each first molar

top boots black or brown riding boots used for hunting

topical *adj.* local, as in the application of an ointment

top line 1. on a pedigree, the identification of a horse's sire 2. on a horse's body, the withers, length of back, croup, and tail set

top weight in racing, the maximum weight of jockey and lead carried by a horse in a handicap

Toric *n.* a Russian breed developed in the 19th century and popular for farm work; it is quite a heavy breed, but lighter types are used for sport and general riding; 15–15.2 h.h.

torsion *n.* 1. a twisting or being twisted, as of the intestines (volvulus) 2. a method of castration

tostado *adj.* a Spanish color term for a chestnut with brown points

total blood volume the amount of blood circulating in the body; a measure of the liquid capacity of the heart and blood vessels

totalizator, -sator *n.* an electro-mechanical apparatus used for a pare-mutuel form of betting which automatically records and totals all wagers made; also called a tote

tote *n.* *see* **totalizator**

touch and out a type of jumping contest in which a jumper who touches the hurdle is immediately eliminated

touched in the wind slightly unsound in respiration

tournament *n.* 1. a contest on horseback in the Middle Ages —*see also* **joust** 2. dressage, show-jumping, and three-day events

tourniquet *n.* a piece of rope or other material used to wrap around a part of the body to check blood flow in that area

toxemia, toxaemia *n.* blood poisoning —**toxemic, toxaemic** *adj.*

toxin *n.* 1. any of various poisonous compounds produced by some micro-

organisms and causing certain diseases 2. any of various similar poisons, related to proteins, formed in certain plants or secreted by certain animals, such as snake venom; toxins, when injected into horses, typically initiate the formation of antitoxins — **toxic** *adj.* poisonous

toxoid *n.* a toxin that has been treated, as with chemicals or heat, so as to eliminate the toxic qualities while retaining the antigenic properties

toxoplasma *n.pl.* intracellular protozoal parasites

trace clip the partial clipping of a horse, leaving the full coat on the top part of the body and lower part of the legs

traces *n.pl.* two straps, chains, etc., used to connect a horse's harness to the vehicle pulled; they extend from the collar to the singletree; when made of leather, they are called tugs

trachea *n.* the windpipe; a tube leading from the larynx to the lungs — **tracheal** *adj.*

tracheitis *n.* an infection of the trachea

tracheotomy *n.* an operation wherein a surgical opening of the windpipe, with insertion of a tube, is made to alleviate difficult breathing; may be temporary or permanent

trachoma *n.* granular conjunctivitis; inflammation of the eyelids

track *n.* 1. footprint 2. beaten path; trail 3. a course, as a racetrack — *vt.* 1. to trail or follow by means of footprints or marks 2. to wear into a path

tract *n.* a canal in the body, as e.g. the urinary tract

tractable *adj.* readily handled; manageable

tractive power a horse's pulling power, averaging approximately 2200 lbs.

tragacanth *n.* a gummy base used in medications

trail *n.* a track (def. 2) — *vt.* 1. to hunt or follow 2. to trample down into a path

trailer *n.* 1. a non-motorized vehicle for hauling horses, pulled by a truck or automobile 2. an extension of about ½-inch on the end of a horseshoe heel used for correction, usually on hind shoes

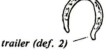

trailer (def. 2)

trailer tie a safety strap with a panic snap used to tie a horse in a trailer; usually made of one-inch nylon web

trailer tie

trail horse a horse used for cross-country rides

trail riding country rides along trails, which can be easy and relaxing, through forests or open country, but can also involve treacherous going along steep mountainsides or through rivers, etc.

train *n.* a line of horses in single file, with or without riders

train *vt.* 1. to tame and school (a horse) 2. to condition (a horse) for any of various athletic competitions 3. to teach (a horse) to perform tricks — **trainer** *n.* a person who trains horses and, in racing, supervises all preparations for the horse to race — **trainable** *adj.*

trait *n.* a characteristic

Trait du Nord a French draft horse established as a breed in 1919; very strong, hardy and gentle; 16 h.h.

Trakehner *n.* a very fine German breed whose origins can be traced to 1732; used to advantage in riding competitions, especially jumping; 16–16.2 h.h.

tramp *n.* any injury to the coronary band of one foot caused by the shoe of the opposite foot or by the foot of another horse, as when two draft horses are paired together or when horses are transported together without partitions between them; tread

trample *vt.* to tread down with the feet (also **trample on**)

trandem *n.* a harness team of three horses abreast —*see also* **triga**

tranquilize *vt.* to sedate or make calm by means of medication —**tranquilizer** *n.* —**tranquil** *adj.*

transfusion *n.* the transference of blood, blood plasma, or saline solution into a vein —**transfuse** *vt.*

transhumance *n.* seasonal herding or migration of livestock —**transhumant** *adj.*

transition *n.* a change of pace from one type of movement to another, as from a trot to a canter or a passage to a piaffe

transit tetany *see* **lactation tetany**

transplant *vt.* to take (tissue) from one part of the body and implant it in another part; graft —*n.* 1. the act of grafting 2. the tissue moved by this process —**transplantation** *n.* — **transplantable** *adj.*

transport protein a protein that transports various bound nutrients via the bloodstream to body tissues (*example:* hemoglobin)

transudation *n.* exudation from a blood vessel into surrounding tissues or onto body surface; serum —**transude** *vi.* —**transudate** *n.* the blood so exuded

transversus abdominis a muscle that compresses the abdomen to aid defecation, birth, and breathing

transversus nasi a muscle that dilates the nostrils

transversus thoracis a chest muscle that aids breathing

trap *vt.* to put trappings on (a horse) —*n.* 1. an ornamental horse cloth (*see* **trappings**) 2. any light two-wheeled carriage drawn by a horse

trapaderos *n.pl.* decorative pieces on a Western stirrup

trapezius *n.* a shoulder muscle

trapping *n.* a short, quick, choppy stride; a tendency of horses with short, straight pasterns and straight shoulders

trappings *n.pl.* decorative coverings for a horse, including tack

trauma *n.* a bodily injury or wound; traumatism —**traumatic** *adj.*

travers *n.* a dressage movement on two tracks in which a horse moves at an angle of not more than 30 degrees along the side of the arena with the forelegs on the outer track and the hind legs on the inner track and body bent in the direction of movement, with head facing forward

traversal *n.* *see* **half-pass**

travois *n.* a drag (something pulled along the ground) consisting of a platform supported by two long poles, the forward ends of which are fastened to a horse, the rear trailing on the ground; used by North American Indians to transport supplies

tread *vi.* *see* **tramp** —*n.* a coronet injury

treadmill *n.* a moving surface that is controlled mechanically and on which a horse walks, trots, etc., depending on the speed of the treadmill; used for observation as well as photographic study of a horse in action in confined quarters, and sometimes for training

treat *n.* a special, particularly enjoyable morsel to eat, such as cut-up carrots and apples, sugar lumps, etc.; care should be taken to avoid harmful treats, such as corn screenings (which

contain fumonisin, a substance toxic to horses)

treble *n.* 1. in show-jumping, an obstacle consisting of three separate jumps 2. in racing, a single bet on three horses in different races

tree *n.* the wooden, fiberglass, or plastic frame on the inside of a saddle

trekking *n.* long-distance pleasure riding

trematoda *n.* a fluke of the liver which causes anemia and diarrhea

tremor *n.* a trembling or quivering — **tremulous** *adj.*

trephine *n.* a small surgical instrument that may be used to bore a hole in a sinus for drainage in cases of sinusitis — *vt.* to use a trephine in surgery — **trephination** *n.*

trial *n.* a competition that tests a horse's endurance under controlled conditions and according to fixed standards

triamcinolone *n.* a synthetic cortisone

triathlon *n.* a relay competition involving teams of three: a runner, biker, and horse and rider; the course covers different types of terrain and takes an average of four hours to complete

triceps brachii a powerful three-headed muscle above the foreleg behind the shoulder

trichiasis *n.* a condition in which the eyelashes grow inward, thus irritating the eye

trichlorfon *n.* generic name for an organophosphate insecticide

trichoglyph *n.* a whorl

trifecta *n.* in racing, a bet in which a bettor wins only by picking the first, second, and third place finishers in exact order; a **twin trifecta** is won by picking two consecutive trifectas in the third and fourth races

triga *n.* in ancient times, a two-wheeled chariot drawn by three horses abreast — *see also* **trandem**

trim *vt.* to clip off, usually in reference to the lower edge of the hoof wall that has grown too long or extra long hair, as from the ears, coronet, or mane; the tail is also sometimes trimmed, especially when it is so long as to drag on the ground

trimethoprim *n.* an antibacterial drug

triple bar in show-jumping, a spread fence consisting of three sets of rails consecutively escalating in height with the highest last

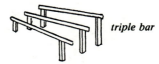

triple bar

trocar *n.* a sharply pointed instrument used with a cannula to extract body fluid, pus, etc.

trocha *n.* a type of the Paso breed; also, a gait comprising a four-beat single-foot diagonal with uneven intervals, shorter between the diagonals and longer between the laterals; the footfall is RF-RR-LF-LR; the leg action is high and the speed of the footfall very fast

trochanter *n.* any of several prominences of bone on the upper end of the femur or thigh bone — **trochanteric** *adj.*

trochanteric bursitis inflammation of the bursa between the greater trochanter and the middle gluteal-muscle tendon; usually secondary to other conditions; seen in show horses or racehorses that are turned frequently or forced to work in a cricle; characterized by lameness in the rear, a shortened stride and inward rotation of the leg as the horse tries to circumvent the pain; cause may be slipping on bad surfaces or trying to trot or pace too fast, as may happen in harness racing; may be confused with spavin; also called whorlbone or whirlbone lameness

trochlea *n.* a pulley-shaped anatomical structure, as the femoral trochlea — **trochlear** *adj.*

troika a Russian carriage drawn by three horses abreast; a team of three horses abreast —*see also* **trandem; triga**

Trojan horse in ancient Troy in Asia Minor, the large hollow wooden horse in which Greek soldiers were taken inside Troy's walls and from which they came out at night to open the city gates to attackers from outside

tropical horse tick *see* **dermacentor nitens**

trot *n.* a natural two-beat gait in which the forefoot and diagonally opposite hind foot strike the ground simultaneously: RF-LH-LF-RH —*vi.*

trotter *n.* a horse that trots at a fast speed

trotting races harness races in which light, two-wheeled carts or sulkies are pulled by horses either trotting or (more popularly) pacing, the trotters in separate races from the pacers; in the United States, Standardbreds are used for these races and, over short distances, are the fastest in the world

trotting vanner a tradesman's carthorse in England before motor vehicles were used; vanner

true arm the humerus bone of the foreleg

true osselet an abnormal bone growth in front of the fetlock

trumpet *vi.* to blow with force through the nose by the vibration of the false nostril; often done when the horse is first let out into an open field and prances about feeling exhilarated; blow —**trumpeting** *n.* —*see also* **high blowing**

trypanosome *n.* a parasitic protozoan organism that invades the blood, causing various diseases

trypsin *n.* an enzyme secreted by the pancreas

tryptophan *n.* an amino acid that converts to niacin in digestion

Tschiffely, Aime Felix (1895-1954) a famous Swiss-born naturalized Argentinian who rode two Argentine Criollo horses, Mancha, 16 years old, and Gato, 15 years, about 10,000 miles from Buenos Aires to Washington state. The journey started in 1925 and ended two and a half years later and was undertaken to prove the stamina of the Criollo. Mancha died at 40 years old and Gato at 36.

tsetse-fly disease *see* **nagana**

tube *n.* *see* **stomach tube; tracheotomy**

tuber calcis the bone which forms the point of the hock

tubercle *n.* a knoblike part, as on a bone; any abnormal hard swelling; the lesion typical of tuberculosis

tuberculosis (TB) *n.* a disease caused by *Myobacterium tuberculosis, Myobacterium bovis,* or *Myobacterium avium*; rare in horses but, when present, it is usually contracted from pasture used by cattle; symptoms are chiefly seen in advanced stages and include stiffness of the neck, excessive passing of urine, irregular defecation, and signs of colic; there are various forms, but the abdominal form is the most common; lungs are affected with consequent cough, nasal discharge, quickened respiration, and high temperature

tucked up having the skin drawn tightly over the stomach, hollow-looking loins, and a drawn appearance

tugs *n.pl.* leather traces

tumor *n.* an abnormal growth, either malignant or non-malignant

Tundra Horse the ancestor of the modern cold-blood; a wild horse that lived in the tundra (arctic regions), in marshlands, and Siberian swamps during the Ice Age; had a big head with a Roman nose and broad feet; 13.2-18 h.h.

turf *n.* 1. a race course   2. horse racing

turf ponies in the 19th century, before grandstands were used to attend horse racing, ponies that were ridden behind the rails by observers

turgid *adj.* swollen

Turkoman *n.* a horse of ancient heritage bred for centuries in Turkmenistan, a mainly desert area bordered by the Caspian Sea (west), Afghanistan (southeast), Uzbekistan (northeast), and Iran (south); has been used in founding a number of other breeds; one place where the Turkoman was originally bred was Persia, and today it is still bred on the Turkoman Steppes of Iran; has no registry; used for racing, espec. long distances; 14.3–15.1 h.h.

turnback help in cutting, two riders positioned in front of the cattle who are responsible for driving any strays back to the herd

turn on the forehand a movement in which a horse pivots on the forehand while forming circles with its hind legs

turn on the quarters a movement in which a horse pivots on its hind legs while forming circles with its forelegs

turnout *n.* a two- or four-wheeled vehicle with its harness horse or horses

turn out to put (a horse) out to pasture

tush *n.* any of four teeth, one each in the upper and lower jaws on each side between the incisors and molars; normally found only in males, but sometimes small ones occur in mares

twin *n.* either of a pair of foals born at the same birth

twist *n.* 1. *see* **volvulus** 2. *see* **waist**

twist colic *see* **volvulus**

twitch *n.* an implement used on a horse's muzzle for restraint; if the horse moves, the twitch causes pain and thus keeps the horse under control; used for such purposes as dentistry, drenching, etc. It does not cause injury if properly used but can do so and can be a cruel instrument of torture when in inexperienced or careless

hands. There are various kinds of twitches: the **lip twitch** (useful for short procedures) consists of a wooden handle attached to a loop of chain which is twisted around the horse's upper lip; the **nutcracker twitch**, a metal device that attaches to the halter, does not offer a safe method of restraint; a **rope twitch** is no longer often used; the

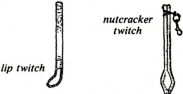

nutcracker twitch

lip twitch

chain twitch is a chain that runs through the lower left halter ring, over the horse's nose, around the noseband, and through the right halter ring (for more severity, the chain can be put under the horse's lip over the gums) — *vt.* to apply such a device

two-tracking the act of moving with the forelegs and hind legs on parallel but separate tracks without bending the body

two-year-old a colt, gelding, or filly that has reached two years but not three since its birth; a racehorse is described as a two-year-old from January 1 of its second year until December 31 of that same year

tying-up *n.* *see* **tied up**

tympan, tympanum *n.* a tightly stretched membrane; often refers to the thin membrane that divides the outer from the middle ear — *see also* **ear drum** — **tympanic** *adj.*

tympanic membrane eardrum

tympany *n.* a type of colic caused by temporary gaseous distension of the gut; caused by excessive fermentation of ingested food, taking large quantities of new food, working immediately after feeding, wind-sucking, and crib-biting

type *n.* a particular kind of horse, as a hunter or hack, as opposed to a breed

– U –

udder *n.* a mammary gland with two teats

uhlan, ulan *n.* a cavalryman who carried a lance; of Tatarian origin, especially prominent in Prussia during the 19th century

Ukrainian Riding horse a new breed of Russian sports horse whose breeding is centered in the Ukraine and derived from imports of various breeds and some Russian saddle horses; about 16 h.h.

ulcer *n.* a sore, either external or internal (rare in the horse) involving a necrosis of tissue and sometimes discharge of pus — **ulcerous** *adj.*

ulcerative enteritis *see* **enteritis**

ulcerative lymphangitis a contagious bacterial disease similar to epizootic lymphangitis but, unlike the latter, general inflammatory swelling is usually present in the area of the abscesses, which, after opening, convert into granulatory ulcers; also, the subcutaneous tissues are more involved; affects the legs and very rarely anywhere else; ulcerative cellulitis

ulna *n.* a small bone in the foreleg, the upper end of which forms the point of the elbow and the lower end of which is joined to the radius

ulnaris lateralis *n.* a forearm muscle that flexes the knee and extends the elbow joints

ultramicroscopic *adj.* beyond a microscope's power to be seen

ultrasonics *n.pl., sing. in constr.* the science of high frequency vibrations that are beyond human audible range; used to help in diagnosis and promote healing; ultrasonic waves (sound beams) are projected by an ultrasound machine through the body from an area of one density to one of a different density; when this occurs, some of the sound beam reflects back, like an echo, to a probe, or transducer, which sends a message to a computer; the intensity of the echo is transmitted as an image on a screen, which then may be analyzed

ultrasonogram *n.* a chart made from ultrasonic echo patterns

ultrasonography *n.* the use of an ultrasonogram in examining deep body structures for diagnosis; can detect pregnancy from 10 to 11 days after conception

ultrasound *n.* ultrasonic waves used to help in diagnosing physical disorders and to promote healing — **ultrasonic** *adj.* — **ultrasonically** *adv.*

ultraviolet *adj.* pertaining to light rays having a wavelength shorter than that of visible light but longer than that of X-rays and existing just beyond the violet end of the visible spectrum

ultravirus *n.* a virus so minute as to pass through the finest filter

umbilical *adj.* resembling or pertaining to a navel or umbilical cord

umbilical cord a thick, tough cord that extends from the navel of the embryo or fetus to the mare's placenta and serves to convey nourishment to the embryo or fetus and carry away waste from it

umbilical hernia a hernia that protrudes through the navel

umbilicus *n.* the navel

umbiliform *adj.* having the form or shape of an umbilicus

unbroken *adj.* not trained

unconditioned *adj.* inborn or natural, not acquired by conditioning

underbite *n. see* **undershot jaw**

under-horsed *adj.* (of a rider) too large or heavy for one's horse

under in the knees having a conformation fault wherein the knees bend toward each other; knock-kneed

under-reach *vi.* in trotting, the contacting of the hind toe by the front of the toe of the forehoof, scraping up the front of the hind hoof; may be counteracted by use of square-toed, well rounded up fore shoes

undershot jaw a malocclusion and unusual deformity wherein the lower jaw protrudes beyond the upper part of the mouth, hindering the horse's ability to graze in severe cases; underbite, sow mouth, bulldog mouth; monkey mouth

underweight *adj.* too lean — *adv.* (of a manner of riding) in a light, alert way and not slumping in the saddle; the opposite is known as riding overweight

undescended testicle a testicle which has not descended into the scrotum — *see also* **ridgeling**

unflappable *adj.* calm in exciting circumstances — **unflappability** *n.*

unfruitful *adj.* sterile

ungula *n.* a hoof — *Ungulata n.pl.* a former group comprising all hoofed mammals, including the horse

ungulate *adj.* 1. having hoofs 2. hoofshaped — *n.* a hoofed animal

unicorn *n.* 1. a mythical animal resembling a horse in its head and body but having a straight, spiral-twisted horn on its forehead, hind legs of an antelope, and a lion's tail; modern versions are often of a horse in every aspect except for the horn 2. a team of three horses, one leader and two wheelers

unilateral *adj.* relating to one side only

United States Trotting Association an association that registers all eligible Standardbred trotters and pacers

unsaddle *vt.* 1. to remove a saddle from (also *vi.*) 2. to throw (a rider) off — *vi.*

unsaddling enclosure in racing, an enclosure in the paddock next to the weighing room where there are separate places for the first three horses who reached the finish line at a race; other jockeys use the main part of the paddock

unsaturated *adj.* having an element capable of combining further with other elements as e.g. most vegetable fats

unseat *vt.* to dislodge from the saddle either totally or partially

unsettled *adj.* disturbed and nervous — **unsettle** *vt.*

unsound *adj.* not normal or healthy; physically unsuitable or not serviceable

unstable *adj.* easily upset and unreliable

unstrung *adj.* upset or in a nervous state

unthrifty *adj.* in an unhealthy physical condition

untried *adj.* having only maidens as offspring

unwind *vi.* to start to buck

upset *vt.* to disturb mentally or physically — *adj.* disturbed in such a manner — *n.* un unexpected defeat, as in racing

upsides in racing, evenly or in line with each other; said of horses exercising or in a race

upstanding *adj.* leggy

up to weight able to carry a particular rider's weight easily

urachus *n.* a tubal structure extending from the fetal bladder to the placenta

urea *n.* a compound, present in urine and blood, which is the waste product of protein metabolism

urea nitrogen a constituent of normal whole blood; urea is the chief nitrogenous component of urine in which it is excreted by the kidneys as a waste product; abnormal levels in the blood of urea nitrogen indicate kidney failure known as uremia — *see also* **BUN**

uremia *n.* a toxic condition caused by kidney failure and resultant excessive presence in the blood, instead of in the urine, of waste products from protein metabolism — **uremic** *adj.*

ureter *n.* either of two tubes that carry urine from the kidneys to the bladder

urethra *n.* a tube or canal that provides an outlet for urine from the bladder and in the male accommodates sperm ejection

urethritis *n.* inflammation of the urethra

urethroscope *n.* an instrument that can be inserted into the urethra to permit an illuminated view of it

uric acid a normal chemical substance excreted by healthy kidneys in urine

urinalysis *n.* an analysis or examination of urine

urinary calculus a calculus or stone in the urinary bladder; urolith

urinary eczema skin eruptions that occur in the presence of nephritis

urinary tubule any of the long, winding tubules of the kidney in which urine is formed

urinate *vi.* to excrete urine; to stale; a healthy horse normally excretes a light yellow urine about five to six times a day depending on fluid intake, diet, etc. — *vt.* to excrete with urine — **urination** *n.* — **urinary** *adv.*

urine *n.* the liquid waste product of the kidneys — **urinary** *adj.* — *for related disorders, see* **albuminuria, anuria, dysuria, hematuria, hemoglobinuria, ischuria, myoglobinuria, oliguria, polyuria, strangury**

urine pooler a mare with a condition wherein urine, air and or excrement are aspirated into the vagina and uterus; wind sucker; a surgical procedure called Caslick's operation can rectify the problem

uriniferous *adj.* carrying urine

urobilin *n.* bile pigment excreted in the urine

urogenital *adj.* pertaining to the urinary and genital organs — **genitourinary** *adj.*

urogenous *adj.* 1. producing urine 2. in or obtained from urine

urolith *n.* a urinary calculus — **urolithic** *adj.*

uroscopy *n.* the diagnostic examination of urine — **uroscopic** *adj.*

urticaria *n.* an allergic reaction, usually to something in the diet; in severe cases the face is swollen, especially the nose and eyelids; hives; nettlerash; surfeit

USCTA United States Combined Training Association; an association whose rule book governs eventing of one, two, or three days involving dressage, endurance (includes cross-country over obstacles) and stadium jumping

uterine *adj.* pertaining to the uterus

uterine atrophy the degeneration of the endometrium (uterine lining)

uterine culture a culture of uterine mucus for detection of bacteria

uterine horn either of a pair of upper projections in the mare's uterus that connect the oviducts with the uterine body

uterine inertia lack or slowness of uterine contractions during parturition

uterine milk a fluid produced in the mare's uterus that nourishes the fertilized ovum before it attaches itself to the uterine wall

uterine quiescence a reduction of uterine muscle action during or after parturition

uterus *n.* a mare's womb, which houses the fetus from conception to birth — **uterine** *adj.*

utility saddle a general purpose saddle

uvea *n.* the part of the eye that comprises the iris and blood vessels

uveitis *n.* inflammation of the uvea; iridocyclitis

— V —

vaccinate *vt.* to immunize by inoculation of a vaccine against a disease — **vaccination** *n.*

vaccine *n.* a preparation used in vaccination; produces immunity to a specific disease by causing the formation of antibodies

vagina *n.* a canal in the mare, leading from the vulva to the uterus, in which copulation takes place — **vaginal** *adj.*

vaginitis *n.* inflammation of the vagina characterized by a purulent discharge

vagus nerve *n.* a cranial nerve, the largest in the body, which extends from the brain to the heart, lungs, esophagus, larynx, and intestines

valine *n.* an essential amino acid

valinomycin *n.* an antibiotic that promotes movement of potassium ions in cells

Valkyrie, Valkyr, Valkyria *n.* in Norse mythology, one of Odin's handmaidens who, on horseback, monitored the soldiers in battle, selected those who would be killed and guided the souls of chosen heroes to Valhalla, Odin's palace

valve *n.* an anatomical membrane or structure that opens and closes an opening and permits organ contents to pass through in only one direction — **valvular** *adj.*

valvular endocarditis inflammation of the heart valves caused by bacterial infection from damage by redworm larvae; results in inefficiency of heart contraction with heart murmur, decrease in stamina, etc.

van *n.* a vehicle for transporting horses — *vt.* to transport (a horse or horses) in a van or trailer

vanner *n.* a cart-horse, so called by dealers, formerly used in England by tradesmen; typically was small, short-legged, strong and a good trotter

vapor-locked *adj.* a cowboy's term to describe a horse that refuses to move (from the same term applied to a car engine that shuts down or locks due to vapor in the fuel line)

vaquero *n.* a working Mexican or Spanish cowboy

varicose vein a dilated vein; rare in horses but can appear in various parts of the body or limbs

variola equina a viral disease characterized by pustular eruptions — **variolous** *adj.*

varmint *n.* in hunting, a fox

varnish roan a coat color that is basically white with contrasting splashes of a darker color called varnish marks

vascular *adj.* pertaining to blood vessels or the system of blood vessels — **vascularity** *n.*

vascularization *n.* the formation of new blood cells

vas deferens the canal in the stallion which carries sperm from each testicle to the penis

vasectomy *n.* surgical cutting of the vas deferens which causes sterility but not impotency; not a common procedure on horses but occasionally performed on a colt used as a teaser so that he may mount a mare without causing conception

vasoactive *adj.* temporarily altering the size of blood vessels

vasoconstriction *n.* the narrowing of a blood vessel — **vasoconstrictor** *n.* a nerve or drug that causes such narrowing — *adj.*

vasodepressor *n.* an agent that lowers blood pressure

vasodilation *n.* dilation or enlargement of blood vessels — **vasodilator** *n.* a nerve or drug which causes dilation of blood vessels — *adj.*

vasomotor *adj.* (of a nerve or drug) able to regulate the diameter of blood vessels

vasopressor a substance that causes a rise in blood pressure

vasospasm *n.* an abnormal contraction of a blood vessel

vasovagal *adj.* relating to the vagus nerve and its effect on the circulatory system, as in the case of losing consciousness

vault *vi.* to mount a horse by jumping onto its back, often while the horse is moving out; it is the fastest way to mount but requires a nimble rider — *n.*

vaulting surcingle a type of girth fitted with hand-grips for practicing vaults on and off or over a horse

vector *n.* a carrier, as an insect, that transmits a disease from one individual to another

VEE Venezuelan equine encephalomyelitis

vehicle *n.* in relation to medicines, a liquid or substance, often something sweet, with which the medicine is mixed

vein *n.* a blood vessel which conducts blood from a part of the body to the heart — **venous** *adj.* — **veined** *adj.* having veins

veld, veldt *n.* open grassland with no bushes and few trees

velum palati part of the soft palate

venation *n.* a system of veins in a part of the body

Vendeen Charollais a French crossbreed that since the 19th century has developed from crosses of native mares with Normans, Anglo-Normans, Thoroughbreds, Arabs, Anglo-Arabs, and Norfolk Trotters; about 15 h.h.

venereal disease any disease transmitted primarily by sexual intercourse — *see also* **dourine, equine syphilis**

venesection *n.* the cutting of a vein or the act of bleeding a horse for any purpose, as for diagnostic purposes or for blood transfusions

Venezuelan equine encephalomyelitis (VEE) *see* **encephalomyelitis**

venipuncture *n.* an injection of a vein with a hypodermic needle

venom *n.* the poison transmitted by the bite of a snake, insect, etc. — **venomous** *adj.*

venostasis *n.* the arrest of blood flow, as by applied pressure

venous hyperemia an increased blood collection in the body caused by partial obstruction of blood flow from the brain as from a tight throatlatch, tumors or enlarged thyroids, or indigestion; symptoms include cyonotic mucous membranes, difficult breathing, and low, frequent pulse; passive hyperemia

ventral *adj.* relating to the belly area of the body — **ventrally** *adv.*

ventral midline dermatitis a skin inflammation along the midline of the horse's ventral area

ventricle *n.* a cavity or hollow formation in the body, as the heart ventricles, which are the two lowermost chambers of the heart — **ventricular** *adj.*

ventricular septal defect a heart abnormality wherein there is a hole in the partition between the two lower chambers; this results in the oxygenated blood mixing with the stale blood that goes out to the lungs; the size of the hole determines the seriousness of the defect

venule *n.* a minute vein

vermicide *n.* a worm medicine given for intestinal parasites — **vermicidal** *adj.*

vermifuge *n.* a worm medicine given for intestinal parasites — *adj.* deadly to parasites

verminous aneurism an aneurism caused by the larvae of the redworm; when an artery supplying the intestine is partially blocked, recurring bouts of colic are a common symptom; when

totally blocked, the horse will eventually die

verminous arteritis blood vessel damage caused by parasites

vertebra *n., pl.* **-brae** any of the bones forming the spinal column — **vertebral** *adj.*

vertebrate *n.* a creature having a spinal column — *adj.*

vertigo *n.* dizziness

vesica *n.* bladder, e.g. the urinary bladder

vesicant *n.* an agent that causes blistering — *adj.*

vesicatory *n., adj.* vesicant

vesicle *n.* a small, fluid-filled sac; blister — **vesicular** *adj.*

vesicular gland an accessory sex gland in a stallion

vesicular stomatitis blisters or lesions affecting the soft tissues of the mouth

vesiculate *vt., vi.* to become or cause to become vesicular or like a blister — *adj.* — **vesiculation** *n.*

vessel *n.* a body tube that conducts fluids, as a blood vessel

vestibule *n.* a body cavity that leads into another cavity — **vestibular** *adj.*

vestige *n.* a part of the body that represents a structure that was once more developed or functional at an earlier stage of development; the chestnut on the horse's leg, for example, is considered a vestigial toe — **vestigial** *adj.*

vetch *n.* a vine-like leafy plant; the seeds of some species are toxic and can cause liver damage and photosensitization if ingested — *see also* **selenium poisoning**

veterinarian *n.* a person licensed to practice medicine and surgery on animals

veterinary *adj.* pertaining to the branch of medicine dealing with animals

veterinary boot a leather or plastic horse's boot that allows pressure on the frog while protecting the remaining part of the hoof

veterinary certificate a report made by a veterinarian on the physical condition of a horse, often requested by a prospective buyer

Vetidrex *n.* trade name for hydrochlorothiazide

viable *adj.* in relation to an embryo, able to live and develop

Viatka *n.* a Russian general purpose pony breed possessing an unusual trotting gait; usually dun and light brown with black mane and tail and often a dorsal stripe; 13–14 h.h.

vibrio *n.* a gram negative bacterium of the genus *Vibrio*. Various species include *Vibrio hepaticus* — *see also* **campylobacter**

vice *n.* a bad habit

vicious *adj.* mean; having dangerous habits

Victoria *n.* an open carriage partly protected by a top; dates back to the 1870s

villitis *n.* a condition of the coronet wherein the horn just below the coronet is whitish and somewhat powdery and may even extend farther down the hoof; caused by dietary deficiencies such as the absence of green fodder

villus *n., pl.* **villi** one of many hairlike projections from mucous membranes in various parts of the body, as of the small intestines where they function in the process of digestion

viral poliomyelitis inflammation within the nerve tracts of the spinal cord

virile *adj.* sexually potent — **virility** *n.*

virology *n.* the study of viruses

virulent *adj.* relates to a disease that is very serious or malignant, or to a microorganism that is very infectious — **virulently** *adv.* — **virulence** *n.* the quality of being virulent

virus *n.* 1. a microscopic organism

that causes various diseases 2. a disease caused by a virus — **viral** *adj.*

viscera *n.pl.* internal organs of the body, especially of the chest and abdomen — **visceral** *adj.*

viscid *adj.* 1. viscous; having a thick, sticky, fluid consistency resistant to flowing 2. covered with such a substance — **viscidity** *n.* — **viscidly** *adv.*

viscous *adj.* see **viscid** — **viscousness** *n.* — **viscosity** *n.* — **viscously** *adv.*

vitamin *n.* any of several organic compounds found in most foods and necessary for normal body function; can also be given as a supplement when necessary; the chief vitamins are: A (retinol), B (B1, B2, B12, panthotenic and folic acids, biotin, choline), C (ascorbic acid), D (calciferol), E (tocopherol), and K

vitiligo *n.* see **pinky syndrome**

vitreous humor the jelly-like, transparent substance between the retina and lens of the eye; also **vitreous body**

viviparous *adj.* bearing live offspring, as opposed to laying eggs

Vladimir Heavy Draft a Russian breed developed at the beginning of the 20th century in Vladimir province mainly from imported British stock; by 1946 it was recognized as a breed; used for draft work and in harness to troika sleighs; 15–16 h.h.

VMD (Veterinariae Medicinae Doctor) Doctor of Veterinary Medicine

vocal *adj.* uttered by the vocal chords

vocal cords the bands of tissue in the larynx which produce sound by regulating the flow of air from the lungs through the larynx

voice box see **larynx**

Volante *n.* a two-wheeled carriage having the body in front of the axle; once used in Latin American countries

volar *adj.* pertaining to the bottom of the hoof or back of the forearm, knee, fetlock, or pastern

volar annular ligament a band of fibrous tissue which holds the flexor tendons in place by crossing the back of the fetlock and bridging the sesamoids

volemia *n.* blood volume that circulates in the body — **volemic** *adj.*

volition *n.* 1. the use of the will 2. a deliberate decision to perform a certain act — **volitional** *adj.* — **volitionally** *adv.*

volte *n.* in dressage, a complete turn on the hind legs, which is the smallest circle a horse can make (about 20 ft. in diameter)

voluntary *adj.* by free will or choice — **voluntarily** *adv.*

volvulus *n.* a twisting of the intestines characterized by intense pain; parts of the intestines become entangled through tears in the mesentery, obstructing passage of contents and resulting in severe colic and, if not surgically corrected, death; torsion; twist; twist colic

vomit *vt., vi.* to regurgitate and eject (ingested food); extremely rare in horses and then usually only through the nose — *n.*

vomitus *n.* that which is vomited

Voronezh Harness Horse a Russian crossbreed that began to be developed in the 1930s from breeding local mares of the Voronezh Province with Orlov horses; 15.1–16.3 h.h.

vosal *n.* a variation of the basic hackamore bridle, similar to the bosal in shape, with leather side straps and metal-ring chinpiece

vulcan mouth a rubber-mouth bit

vulva *n.* the external genital organs of the mare

vulvitis *n.* inflammation of the vulva

vulvovaginitis *n.* inflammation of both the vulva and vagina

— W —

wagon *(also, especially British,* **waggon)** *n.* 1. a four-wheeled, horse-drawn vehicle, either covered or open, used for hauling   2. loosely, any horse-drawn vehicle

wain *n.* a farm wagon

waist *n.* the narrowest part of the saddle, just behind the pommel; twist

Waler *n.* an Australian breed used largely at one time as a cavalry mount; now it is known as the Australian Stock Horse breed and is used mainly on sheep and cattle ranches and rodeos; also used in eventing, polo, endurance competitions and some racing; 14.2–16 h.h.

walk *vi.* to move by alternately stepping in an even four-beat sequence: near hind, near fore, off hind, off fore; a horse can do so in various ways: (a) freely, with a free rein under saddle, (b) collected, with short, quick, elevated steps with no over-tracking, (c) medium, between collected and extended (d) extended, the longest stride, with over-tracking — *n.*

walkabout disease *see* **Kimberly horse disease**

walker *n.* a mechanized device that has revolving arms under which several horses may be tied, one to each arm, to be led in a circle for gentle exercise; *see also* **hot walker**

walkover *n.* in racing, an easily won victory

wall *n.* 1. in show-jumping, an upright obstacle made of hollow wooden blocks that are arranged in the form of a brick wall   2. in cross-country racing, an upright obstacle made of bricks, concrete blocks, sleepers, or stone

wall eye *n.* a blue eye circled with white; one or both eyes may be wall-eyed; **watch eye; glass eye; blue eye** — **wall-eyed** *adj.*

waltz *n.* a dressage movement in which a horse pivots the forehand and then the hind quarters in time to music — *vi.*

wander *vi.* to roam about or to stagger about aimlessly, as in the presence of an abnormality

wanderer-foal syndrome *see* **neonatal maladjustment syndrome**

warble *n.* 1. a lump or hard tumor on a horse's back caused by an ill-fitting saddle   2. a lump, usually on the back, caused by the presence of a maggot or larva of the warble fly or botfly — **warbled** *adj.*

warble fly a fly, the larvae of which burrow under the hide of horses and other animals causing warbles

war bonnet paint a color pattern that is like the medicine hat except with very pale body color

war bridle a rope bridle, somewhat similar to a halter, except that part of the rope passes through the mouth. War bridles are made as follows: a loop about five inches in diameter is made and placed over the lower jaw and tongue, then the rope is run up the right side of the face over the poll, from right to left, and through the loop on the left of the jaw. In a Pratt's Twitch, the free end of the rope is passed back over the head, left to right, under the lip and above the gums, through the loop on the left.

"'ware hounds!" in hunting, a warning by the huntsman to the followers that a hound is coming up from behind or side and to be wary of stepping on it

"'ware wire" in hunting, a warning from one hunter to another that there is wire in a fence

warfarin *n.* generic name of a crystalline powder that is used as a rat poison but when neutralized with sodium

hydroxide is used as an anticoagulant medicine

war horse a horse used in battle

warmblood *n.* a cross between a hot-blood and a cold-blood, as e.g. a Hanoverian

wart *n.* a contagious tumor-like skin growth caused by a virus, usually occuring on the muzzle, eyelids, or cheeks and sometimes present in young horses, especially any time up to three years old; they vary from a few to hundreds and usually regress within three months after they appear

washed red blood cells red blood cells that have been separated from other parts of the blood and cleansed for diagnostic purposes

wasp *n.* any of various stinging insects of the same order as the bee, but of a different family; its venomous sting can cause a swelling, which may exude pus

wasp

waste away to lose physical condition, as by disease or starvation; to become emaciated

watch-eye *n. see* **wall-eye**

water bag the fluid that surrounds a fetus in the uterus

water brush a grooming brush with longer bristles than a body brush; used damp on mane and tail and wet for quartering

water hole a pond or pool from which horses may drink water

water jump in show-jumping, a strip of water over which competing horses and riders must jump; sometimes has a fence of some sort on the take-off side

water soluble vitamin a vitamin which is dissolved in body fluids

wave mouth a condition in which the

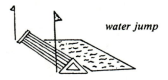

water jump

biting surface of the teeth, instead of being level, undulates to form one or more "waves"; mild cases are common and need regular floating; severe cases are difficult to help

wax *n. see* **earwax**

waxing *n.* a wax-like coagulation of leaking colostrum on a mare's teats about 2 to 4 days prior to foaling; waying up

waying up *see* **waxing**

wean *vt.* to cause (a foal) to discontinue suckling and substitute other food for the mother's milk; a mare weans her foal gradually, discouraging it from nursing by kicking, biting, etc. until at about 10 to 11 months old weaning is completed; when a human controls the weaning process, it is usually done at about 6 months by separating the foal from its dam — **weaning** *n.*

weanling *n.* a foal that has been weaned and is not yet a yearling

weave *vi.* to sway back and forth in a compulsive, repetitive behavior, usually in a stable where the horse may develop the habit out of boredom — **weaver** *n.*

web *n.* 1. the measured width of the branch of a horseshoe 2. a tissue or membrane in the body

web martingale a running martingale in which the split is filled in with baghide; bib martingale

web martingale

wedge shoe a shoe shaped like a wedge, with a high heel, sloping down to a regular low toe

WEE Western equine encephalomyelitis —*see* **encephalomyelitis**

weed *n.* 1. an undesirable plant that grows wild, often crowding out other desirable plants, such as grass; many weeds are poisonous to horses, affecting various parts of the body such as the intestines, nerves, blood, reproductive organs, and skin; these include locoweed, groundsel (ragwort), crotalaria (rattleweed), fiddleneck, yew, St. Johns wort, castor bean plant, nightshade, horseradish 2. a horse considered unsuitable for racing or breeding

weep *vt., vi.* to exude (fluid), as from the eyes or a wound —**weeping, weepy** *adj.*

weigh-in the process of weighing a rider immediately after completion of a competition that requires that a specific weight be carried by the horse; it ensures that the correct weight was carried during the event

weigh-out the process of weighing a rider before a competition that requires that a specified weight be carried by the horse; everything is included except the jockey's cap, whip, bridle and anything worn on the horse's legs and feet

weight *n.* a measure of heaviness; in show-jumping, FEI rules stipulate that competing horses carry a minimum of 165 lbs., including saddle and pad —**weigh** *vt., vi.*

weight calculation a determination of weight, found exactly be using a scale or estimated by using either a weight tape or the following formula: (girth^2 × length) ÷ 300 = weight (in pounds). The length is taken from elbow up to point of buttock; three-fifths of a horse's weight is distributed on the forelegs and two-fifths on the hind.

weight cloth in racing, a saddle cloth that has pockets in which lead weights may be inserted so that the required weight may be carried

weight for age in racing, a handicap in which older horses carry more weight than younger ones

weights *n.pl.* in racing, lead blocks placed in a saddle cloth to add weight when the jockey does not meet the required weight to be carried by the horse —*see also* **foot weights**

well sprung ribs ribs that are curved like barrel staves

Welsh Cob an old British breed of exceptional versatility, used by farmers for centuries; strong enough for logging work, tractable for riding, and showy for driving; allegedly developed from crosses of Welsh Mountain Ponies and Andalusians; 14–15 h.h.

Welsh Mountain Pony a pony breed indigenous to Wales and having an ancient heritage; intelligent and gentle; up to 12.2 h.h.

Welsh Pony a riding pony indigenous to Wales and developed by crossing the Welsh Mountain Pony with Welsh Cob and Thoroughbred blood; up to 13.2 h.h.

Western boot a rider's boot that forms part of a Western outfit; may have a flat heel or a raised one and have a design or be plain

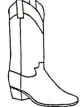

Western equine encephalomyelitis *see* encephalomyelitis

Western boot

Western hat a rather broad-rimmed hat, creased at the crown

Western saddle a saddle designed primarily for stock work; it has a high cantle and pommel with a horn for roping, one or two skirts at the rear, wide fenders, and wooden stirrups,

usually leather covered, and often two cinches

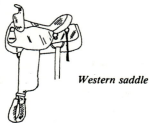

Western saddle

Westphalian *n.* a German warm-blood breed of mixed blood originating in Westphalia; strong and athletic and very successful in competition; 15.2–16.2 h.h.

Weymouth *n. see* **double bridle**

whanghee *n.* a riding cane made from the stems of bamboo

wheat *n.* a cereal grass that contains grains, the husks of which (bran) may be fed to horses; high in vitamin E

wheat germ part of the wheat kernel that is milled out and used in feed and vitamin preparations

wheel *vi.* to turn about in a circular movement —*n.* the act of doing so

wheeler *n. see* **wheel horse**

wheel horse of several horses harnessed to a vehicle, the horse, or either of two horses, nearest the vehicle wheels

wheeze *vi.* to breathe with a whistling, breathy sound —*n.*

whicker *n.* a gentle, barely audible blowing sound made in greeting —*vi.*

whiffletree *n. see* **singletree**

whinny *n.* a gentle neigh —*vi.*

whip *n.* a rod, usually leather-covered, that is either stiff or flexible and has a lash at one end; used on a horse either for discipline or to urge the horse to greater speed; a crop. A **riding whip**, or crop, has a looped lash and a short stock (handle), sometimes with a wrist

strap enabling it to hang from the rider's wrist when not in use; a riding bat has a leather slapper instead of the looped lash; a **coaching whip** (or **team whip**) is longer than a normal driving whip, the rod being shorter but the lash longer, enabling it to reach the leaders; a **hunting whip** has a lash at the top end and a handle for opening gates at the lower end; a **stock whip** has a short stock but very long lash and is used for driving cattle; it can be snapped to produce a very loud cracking sound —*see also* **lunge whip** —*vt.* to use a whip on.

whipper-in *n.* a huntsman's assistant who keeps the hounds together

whippletree *n. see* **singletree**

whip reel a round wooden wall knob on which driving whips may be hung

whipworm *n.* a type of roundworm, about two inches long, that has a whip-like front and is an intestinal parasite

whirlbone lameness *see* **whorlbone (whirlbone) lameness**

whirlicote *n.* an English horse-drawn vehicle of bygone days comprising four boards put together to transport a person

whirlpool *n.* water that movers in a rapid, circular manner; a **whirlpool bath** is a bath in which a device agitates warm water in a swirling motion; it is used in hydrotherapy

whiskey, whisky *n.* an old type of gig having a chair body

whisperer, horse a trainer who can handle dangerous, high-spirited horses

whistle *n.* the warning signal given by a stallion to his band; it is neither a nicker, neigh, nor snort

whistling *n.* a milder form of roaring in which the sound is high-pitched

white *adj.* in relation to a horse's coat, having the color of clear snow; an

albino is white; a gray horse may turn white with age

white blood cell one of the colorless cells that act to defend the body against infection; there are 5 types: neutrophils, lymphocytes, eosinophils, monocytes, and basophils; also called leukocytes; white blood corpuscles

white death *see* **lethal white foal syndrome**

white face *see* **bald**

white fetlock *see* **sock**

white flag a marker used in equestrian sports to mark the left-hand extremity of an obstacle; it is also used to mark a set track and must always be passed on the right; in racing, the lowering of a white flag is one method of signaling the start of the race

white heel a partial coronet mark at the back of the foot

white line the narrow boundary line between the wall and sole of the hoof extending around its periphery where the insensitive and sensitive laminae meet and grow out to the sole; formed of unpigmented, somewhat soft horn

white muscle disease a disease which damages the muscles and is caused by dietary selenium deficiency

white of the eye *see* **sclera**

white pastern *see* **sock**

white scour infectious diarrhea in a two- or three-day-old foal, caused by a microbe in the digestive tract; it is a yellowish gray or dirty white liquid with a fetid odor emitted with strong force; not to be confused with simple diarrhea

whole colored having one solid coloration all over the body

whoo-hoop *n.* the announcement in hunting that the fox is dead

whorl *n.* the circular pattern in which a horse's coat hair meets in certain areas; trichoglyph

whorlbone (whirlbone) lameness lameness caused by an inflamed bursa under the gluteus muscle tendon where it extends over the femur; pressure on the hip area causes pain; trochanteric bursitis

wide behind the conformation fault wherein the hocks are not parallel, making the horse look bow-legged

wide-web shoe a shoe having extra-wide web for increased strength

Wielkopolski *n.* a Polish warm-blood used for competition, draft, and general riding, for which its gentle nature is well suited; 15.1–16.1 h.h.

wild *adj.* 1. living in a natural, undomesticated environment 2. having an uncontrollable character

wild-eyed *adj.* staring in an excited way, usually with the whites of the eyes showing

Wild Goose Chase a 17th century horse race in which the competitors covered 219 miles and then had to follow the leader, and one another, no matter where he went and at specified distances of so many lengths, somewhat like wild geese in flight

wild horse *see* **Przewalski**

willful *adj.* stubbornly persistent

wind[1] *vt.* (of a hound) in hunting, to smell (a fox)

wind[2] *n.* 1. gas in the intestines; flatulence 2. breathing; used in terms describing respiratory infections (e.g., broken wind, gone in the wind)

winded *adj.* out of breath

windgall *n.* a soft swelling on the fetlock joint caused by pockets of fluid secreted from the bursa; may be caused by hard work that causes overextension or overflexion; wind puff —**windgalled** *adj.*

windpipe *n.* the trachea

wind puff *see* **windgall**

wind-sucking *n.* aerophagia 1. a stable

vice in which a horse swallows air, chiefly because of boredom, by tucking in the chin; can develop into an unsoundness because it can lead to indigestion 2. wind-sucking through the vagina is another phase and can cause infertility in the mare —**windsucker** *n.*

wind swept having a conformation fault wherein both knees are bent in the same direction, either to right or left

wing *n.* either of a pair of uprights that support poles used for showjumping

winging *vi.* a faulty way of going, often in horses who toe out, wherein the feet break over the inside of the toe and swing in an inward arc to the outside, as opposed to paddling

win in a canter in speed events, to pass the winning post first at an easy pace, leaving the rest of the competitors far behind

wink *vi.* 1. to close and open the eyelids quickly 2. to close and open the vaginal lips, as the mare may when she is in estrus

winkers *n.pl. see* **blinkers**

winners' enclosure the reserved area in a race course to which the first three winning horses and their mounted riders have to return immediately after the end of the race

winter horse a horse kept at a ranch for use during the winter

winter out to remain out in the field during the winter rather than in a stable

winter tick *see* **Dermacentor albipictus**

wire *n. see* **barbed wire**

wire cutter a cutting device with sharp blades used to cut wire in scissor-like fashion; useful for cutting baling wire or fencing

wire muzzle a round muzzle cover of woven wire which serves the same function as a box muzzle

wire stirrups stirrups made of stainless steel wire with leather foot pads

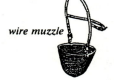
wire muzzle

wire stirrups

wisp *n.* a grooming device used to improve circulation; made of rope, hay, or straw formed into a kind of pad; it is dampened and used on the muscular parts of the body (quarters, shoulders, and neck)

with a stain well bred but having some common blood

wither pads two joined soft pads temporarily placed over the withers and under the forward part of an ill-fitting saddle or to protect subcutaneously bruised withers

withers *n.* the prominent ridge where the neck and back join, which is the highest part of the horse's back; at this ridge powerful muscles of the neck and shoulder attach to elongated spines of the second to sixth thoracic vertebrae; the height of a horse is measured vertically from the withers to the ground

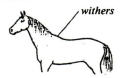
withers

wobbler *adj.* a horse that has the wobbles

wobbles *n.* a disease symptom which varies in severity from poor coordination and weakness, particularly in the hindquarters, to drunken, wobbling movements, even crashing into objects and falling down when galloping; onset

may be slow, over a period of months, or may appear within 24 hours; symptomatic of at least three diseases: cervical vertebral malformation, equine protozoal encephalomyelitis, equine degenerative myelopathy; also called staggers

wolf teeth one of two or occasionally four small, superfluous teeth which sometimes grow in just in front of the premolars

womb *n.* the uterus of the mare

wood chewer a horse that habitually chews or bites off chunks of wood, some of which it may swallow; a very bad and destructive habit; not to be confused with a cribber

wooden *adj.* lacking agility, collection, and attentive response to a rider's aids

wooden tongue *see* **actinomycosis**

work *vt.* to train or exercise and condition (a horse) — *n.* the act of so doing

working hunter a show class for hunters involving a course of "natural" type fences; performance and conformation are judged

World Arabian Organization (1970–) a group which acquires and promotes information on the Arabian breed worldwide and seeks to maintain the purity of the breed

worm *n.* any of various parasites that may infest a horse's intestines, such as roundworms, whipworms, strongyles, etc. — *vt.* to rid of intestinal worms with medication, as should be done on a regular basis

wormer *n.* a medication used to purge a horse of worms; vermicide; vermifuge

Woronesh *n. see* **Voronezh Harness Horse**

wound *n.* an injury to a part of the body; wounds vary in type and include open wound (a cut), lacerated wound (tear), and puncture wound (hole, as inflicted by a nail) — *vt.*

wrangle *vt.* to round up and care for (horses)

wrangler *n.* a cowboy who rounds up horses, especially saddle horses

wrinkle *n.* a crease in the skin, as that formed on the side of the mouth by a bit — *vt.* to form a wrinkle or wrinkles — *vi.* to become wrinkled

wry foot *see* **flare foot**

wry neck an abnormal birth in which the head or neck of the fetus is bent backward — *see also* **dystocia**

Wuchumutsin *n. see* **Mongolian**

Württemberg *n.* a German breed with very old ancestry; used under saddle and in harness; up to 16 h.h.

— X —

xanthos *adj.* a yellow coloration said to have been typical of Greek chariot horses

Xanthus *n.* in Greek mythology, an immortal chariot horse which, with Balios, was used by Achilles; able to speak, he foretold his master's death

X chromosome a sex chromosome in the male sperm which, when present,

causes a female embryo to result from fertilization of the mare's ovum

Xenophon *n.* a Greek historian born in the 5th century B.C. and famous for his writings on horsemanship, which are still read today

xerosis *n.* dryness of the skin or of the conjunctiva of the eyeball

X-ray *n.* an electromagnetic ray that

can penetrate body tissues and affect a photographic plate in such a way as to render an image of the internal parts of the body, thereby aiding in medical diagnosis —*adj.* relating to X-rays

—*vt.* to photograph by means of an X-ray

xylazine *n.* a local anesthetic

xylocaine *n.* a local anesthetic

— Y —

Yakut *n.* a Russian breed that lives around the Arctic Circle; because of the extremely cold winter conditions, these horses have to dig through ice and snow in winter for food; their pale gray coats are up to four inches long; they are named after the Yakut tribesmen of that area, who use them for riding, harness, and pack work

yard *n.* 1. an open area into which a horse or horses may be let out 2. a place of business dealing with horses (e.g., livery yard, dealer's yard, racing yard)

yaud *n.* an old mare or worn-out old horse

yaw *vi.* to toss the head and try to reach out and down when under saddle; certain kinds of nosebands are used to counteract this

yawn *vi.* to open the mouth wide and inhale while totally relaxed; yawning in horses, just as in humans, inspires the same behavior in others — *n.*

Y chromosome a sex chromosome in sperm which when present causes a male embryo to result from fertilization of the mare's ovum

yearling *n.* 1. a horse which is at least one but not yet two years old 2. in racing, a foal born on any date of the preceding calendar year —*adj.*

yeld mare a mare that did not produce a foal during the current season

yellow body *see* **corpus luteum**

yellow dun *see* **dun**

yellow star thistle a thistle-type weed, *Centaurea soostitialis*, that is poisonous to horses; has small yellow, star-shaped flowers; affects chewing function causing horses to starve to death

yew *n.* an evergreen shrub or tree that has red, waxy cones and broad flattened, needlelike leaves containing alkaloid taxine, which is fatally poisonous to horses; also called taxus

yolk sac a primitive embryonic placenta in which early blood cells form, and which nourishes the embryo for about the first 30 days and is then replaced by a permanent placenta

Yomud *n.* *see* **Iomud**

— Z —

zebra *n.* an African member of the genus *Equus* that resembles the horse and ass but has dark stripes all over a white or tan body

zebra dun *see* **dun**; **zebra stripes**

zebra stripes dark stripes on the legs, seen, for example, on the dun-colored horse (also **zebra markings**)

zebroid *n.* a cross between a zebra and a horse

Zemaituka *n.* a Lithuanian pony breed descended from primitive wild horses of the Asiatic steppes; extremely tough, surviving in very harsh climatic

conditions with little food, despite which it can cover 40 miles in one day; has a dark dorsal stripe and is usually dun in color; about 13.2 h.h.; also called Pechora Zhmud

zig-zag *n.* a wooden jump made of posts and rails at angles to each other; it may be jumped over the V-shaped points or over the slanting sides

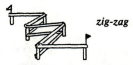

zig-zag

Zimecterin *n.* trade name for ivermectin

zinc *n.* an essential element in the body and a constituent of many enzymes

zinc oxide a white powder used in the form of an ointment to soothe and dry up skin irritations

Zmudzin *n.* a Polish pony

zoonosis *n.* a disease of an animal that can be contracted by human beings

zygoma *n.* the cheekbone — **zygomatic** *adj.*

zygomatic ridge the cheekbone

zygomaticus *n.* a muscle that retracts the angle of the mouth

zygote *n.* a fertilized ovum before it starts to divide and multiply